FOURTH EDITION

NURSING RESEARCH

READING, USING, AND CREATING EVIDENCE

The Pedagogy

Nursing Research: Reading, Using, and Creating Evidence, Fourth Edition demonstrates how to use research as evidence for successful nursing practice. Fully updated and revised, this reader-friendly new edition provides students with a fundamental understanding of how to appraise and utilize research, translating it into actionable guidelines for practice. Organized around the different types of research that can be used in evidence-based practice, it addresses contemporary methods, including the use of technology in data collection, advice for culturally competent research, and suggestions for accessing hard-to-reach subjects. Additionally, it explores both quantitative and qualitative traditions and encourages students to read, use, and participate in the research process. The pedagogical aids that appear in most chapters include the following:

Chapter 3

Ethical and Legal Considerations in Research

CHAPTER OBJECTIVES

The study of this chapter will help the learner to

- Describe fundamental ethical concepts applicable to human subjects research.
- Discuss the historical development of ethical issues in research.
- Describe the components of valid informed consent.
- Identify the features of populations that make them vulnerable in a research context.
- Discuss statutes and regulations related to conducting clinical research.
- Describe the history, functions, and processes related to the institutional review board.
- Identify the three levels of review conducted by institutional review boards.
- Relate protections for human subjects to guidelines for animal welfare in research.
- Discuss the major provisions of the privacy rule (HIPAA) that affect data collection for research.

KEY TERMS

A priori	Full review	Nontherapeutic research
Beneficence	Health Insurance Portability and	Respect for persons
Ethics	Accountability Act (HIPAA)	Right of privacy
Exempt review	Informed consent	Therapeutic research
Expedited review	Institutional review board (IRB)	Vulnerable populations
Full disclosure	Justice	

Introduction

Ethics is the study of right and wrong. It explores what one might do when confronted with a situation where values, rights, personal beliefs, or societal norms may be in conflict. In everyday life, we are often faced with ethical situations when we must ask a key question: What is the right thing to do in this particular situation?

49

Chapter Objectives
Objectives provide instructors and students with a snapshot of key information in each chapter. They can serve as a checklist to help guide and focus study.

Key Terms Found at the beginning of each chapter and in bold throughout, these terms create an expanded vocabulary in evidence-based practice.

VOICES FROM THE FIELD

I was on the Evidence-Based Practice (EBP) Council for my hospital, and one of the questions we wanted to study was whether hourly rounding—a nurse checking every patient, every hour, and documenting it—was worth the amount of time it required of the nurse. The policy had come down from administration, and the rank and file who were expected to carry it out were not sure it would achieve the expected outcomes of decreasing the number of adverse events and enhancing patient satisfaction.

We talked about designing our own little study, but concluded we would see if there was already enough literature to show its effectiveness. We started with the question, "What are the outcomes associated with hourly rounding?" and identified search terms. We found quite a bit of literature through our initial search, but much of it focused on physicians' rounds, not nurses'. We asked the health sciences librarian for help, and she combined our terms in novel ways that brought us more focused literature. She also helped us search dissertations and conference proceedings. This turned up a few dozen applicable abstracts. After applying our criteria to the list, we ended up with six articles that measured some aspect of hourly rounding. One of them was a review of other articles, so that was like hitting the evidence jackpot.

We started the study expecting to prove that hourly rounding did not really improve things. What we found—when we used objective criteria for including studies—was that evidence supported the effectiveness of this policy. Adverse events were decreased in two of the studies; patient satisfaction improved in almost all of them. So we were both surprised and a bit dismayed by the findings: We found something we did not expect that supported continuing a time-consuming policy.

When we looked closer, however, it became clear that it was the nurse contact that made the difference. That did not surprise us when we thought about it. There really was no evidence that we needed in-depth documentation of the rounding for it to be effective. So we suggested to our nurse administrator, "We recognize the evidence for hourly rounds, but can we find a faster way to show it was done?" We brainstormed for some time and decided the rounds could just be marked off on a small whiteboard in the room. Check the patient, check the whiteboard.

This was a case when the literature showed us something we did not expect but helped us pose alternative solutions. I think it convinced most of the team of the value of going to the literature first—you do not have to reinvent the wheel—and doing so in an objective, deliberate way.

Eunice Nolan, RN, DNP

SCENES FROM THE FIELD

Treatments that are planned but not delivered are a serious source of adverse events for patients in an acute care unit. Missed nursing care may be even more serious in the neonatal intensive care unit (NICU), where even small departures from the plan of care can lead to serious complications. Tubbs-Cooley and colleagues (2015) conducted a descriptive study to determine the frequency and type of missed care as reported by NICU nurses and the factors that may have contributed to these omissions.

These researchers surveyed a random sample of certified NICU nurses in seven states who provided direct care. They used an existing survey—the MISSCARE Survey—that consists of three sections: questions related to the characteristics of the nurses, questions about the frequency and type of missed nursing care activities, and questions about the possible reasons for the missed care. The data, which were collected via a web-based survey, comprised both ordinal and nominal (classification) data.

Tubbs-Cooley et al. (2015) reported the findings in tables with sufficient information to determine both the typical values and the ranges of responses. The ordinal data were represented in tables that allowed the reader to see the actual counts and percentages for responses by item. This helped support the credibility of the analytics and the interpretation of the results.

A range of care activities was found to be missed. Most frequently missed were routine rounds, oral care for ventilated infants, parent education, and parental involvement in care and oral feedings. The activities missed least often were reassuring—these NICU nurses were particularly attentive to hand washing, safety, physical assessment, and medication administration. The nurses reported the most common reasons for missed care were the frequent interruptions and urgent patient situations that arise in an intensive care environment. As would be expected, unexpected upturns in patient volume and care intensity were also reported as issues leading to missed treatments.

This evidence was presented well and the variables were measured and analyzed appropriately. NICU nurses can use this information as evidence in developing care plans and practice guidelines that enable nurses to ensure that every patient gets every treatment needed, at the time it is needed.

Voices from the Field and Scenes from the Field Found at the beginning of each chapter, these features share stories from practicing nurses, and analyze new research for practice.

Purpose, Importance, and Scope of the Literature Review

Literature reviews add credence to the researcher's assertions of the importance of the topic proposed for investigation. It is the researcher's responsibility to determine what others have discovered on the same topic. A thorough literature review may turn up studies that can be replicated, instruments that have been standardized and tested for use, or procedures that can be adapted to the proposed study. In addition, the literature often reveals an appropriate theoretical framework.

The literature review may enhance the body of knowledge on a particular issue, or it may establish that there is a paucity of knowledge on the subject in question. Although many researchers are discouraged by a lack of published findings on a specific topic, this may actually be a benefit. A gap in the knowledge of a healthcare issue creates an area that is ripe for exploratory or interventional study and signals that the researcher is pioneering a new issue for investigation. It also increases the likelihood of publication and can serve as the basis for advanced academic study. Either way, the literature review is the first step in evaluating the importance of a research question and potential methods for its study.

Although the researcher needs to provide substantial literature support that directly relates to the problem, it is important to resist the temptation to include everything. A researcher must decide when to stop searching—perhaps an obvious point in theory, but one that is sometimes difficult to put into practice. A researcher may want to consciously note that nothing new is being revealed or that literature resources are exhausted. The scope of a scholarly literature review will obviously go into greater depth than a literature review for a small bedside science project. Likewise, a study directed toward a journal focused on practice may have fewer references than one intended for publication in a research journal. The type of study, the expectations of the readers, and the level of scholarly sophistication required will drive the scope of the literature review.

Scholarly: Concerned with or relating to academic study or research.

Theoretical literature: Published conceptual models, frameworks, and theories that provide a basis for the researcher's belief system and for ways of thinking about the problem studied.

New Term Found in the margins, these notes provide definitions of key terms when they first appear in the chapter.

GRAY MATTER

A literature review will
- Add credence to the importance of the topic proposed for investigation
- Identify studies that can be replicated, instruments that have been standardized and tested, or procedures that can be adapted
- Reveal appropriate theoretical frameworks
- Contribute to the body of knowledge or establish the lack of published research on a subject

Gray Matter These notes cover information about key concepts for quick review.

Case in Point Case studies expand upon concepts in the chapter and test your knowledge in real-life settings.

CASE IN POINT Experimental Design

Preterm infants manifest pain and stress during traumatic procedures such as the heel stick for blood samples. A number of individual nonpharmacologic methods have been found to be effective in reducing pain in this population, including non-nutritive sucking, administration of oral sucrose, and facilitated tucking. While evidence shows a modest effect for each of these interventions, researchers wanted to test combinations of them as means to reduce pain in preterm infants. In the study carried out for this purpose (Yin et al., 2015), controlling for interactions between treatments was complex, requiring five randomly selected comparison groups, each of which was provided with a different combination of interventions. This in turn required a large sample—110 infants—to adequately test each group of interventions. All were compared to a control group that received routine nursing care during the procedure.

All of the procedures were effective alone and in some combination with other interventions, but the magnitude of effect of all three combined was the largest. Observable signs of pain decreased by more than 32% in this group. The results clearly support the use of all three interventions simultaneously to achieve the greatest benefit for the infant. The authors were also able to determine that heel stick procedures can, indeed, be atraumatic when conducted while infants are stable, quiet, appropriately positioned, and soothed with nonpharmacologic methods before gently sticking the heel and squeezing blood.

This randomized trial was a complex and well-executed example of isolating the effects of both individual interventions and groups of them. Randomization minimized a host of threats to the study's validity and made the results stronger as evidence for practice in the neonatal unit.

More Common: Quasi-Experimental Designs

Experimental designs provide clear evidence of the effectiveness of interventions, yet they are uncommon in nursing and health care in general. This rarity reflects the difficulty in achieving the high levels of control that are characteristic of experiments in

Where to Look This feature provides guidance on where to look for key elements of a research paper, the wording that might be used to describe them, and specific things to look for during the evaluation process.

WHERE TO LOOK

A review of literature can appear throughout a published research article, but typically will be concentrated in a special section that follows the introduction, purpose statement, and research question. Citations to literature that support and discuss the scope of the research problem generally first appear in the literature review section, which may be labeled straightforwardly as "Literature Review"; alternatively, it may be called "Background" or "Context of the Problem." On occasion, this information might not be presented in a separate section, but rather will be embedded into the introductory paragraphs.

Literature may also be cited to support the measurements that were used, the intervention protocol, or the data analysis procedures. The literature is often referred to during discussion and conclusions; it is there that the authors compare their findings to the findings of previous studies. In discussing the findings of their

own study, the researcher should identify results that confirm previous studies, clear up contradictions, or highlight inconsistencies with the findings of other studies. Each citation in the text should be linked to an entry in the references list.

The use and placement of the literature review is standardized in most quantitative studies. Qualitative studies, however, may refer to and cite the literature in various ways. Some qualitative researchers believe the researcher should not have preconceived notions about a study and so should complete the literature search only after completing the study. Others use a fairly traditional approach. The literature review for qualitative studies often appears sprinkled throughout the sections noted earlier but may also appear in the results section, supporting the themes recorded and the words of informants.

Checklist These lists support the "Where to Look" feature and provide students with an evaluation of specific research activities and issues.

CHECKLIST FOR EVALUATING AN EVIDENCE-BASED LITERATURE REVIEW

☐ The literature review relies primarily on studies conducted in the last 5 years.
☐ The relationship of the research problem to the previous research is made clear.
☐ All or most of the major studies related to the topic of interest are included.
☐ The review can be linked both directly and indirectly to the research question.
☐ The theoretical or conceptual framework is described.
☐ The review provides support for the importance of the study.

☐ The authors have used primary, rather than secondary, sources.
☐ Studies are critically examined and reported objectively.
☐ The review is unbiased and includes findings that are conclusive and those that have inconsistencies.
☐ The author's opinion is largely undetectable.
☐ The review is logically organized to support the need for the research.
☐ The review ends with a summary of the most important knowledge on the topic.

For More Depth and Detail Reference lists are provided for a more in-depth look at the key concepts covered in select chapters.

For More Depth and Detail

For a more in-depth look at the concepts in this chapter, try these references:

Brouwers, M., Thabane, L., Moher, D., & Straus, S. (2012). Comparative effectiveness research paradigm: Implications for systematic reviews and clinical practice guidelines. *Journal of Clinical Oncology, 30*(34), 4202–4207.

Cantrell, M. (2011). Demystifying the research process: Understanding a descriptive comparative research design. *Pediatric Nursing, 37*(4), 188–189.

Higgins, J., Altman, D., Gøtzsche, P., Jüni, P., Oxman, D., Savovic, A., . . . Sterne, J. (2011). The Cochrane Collaboration's tool for assessing risk of bias in randomized trials. *British Medical Journal, 343*(7829), 1–9.

Levin, G., Emerson, S., & Emerson, S. (2013). Adaptive clinical trial designs with pre-specified rules for modifying the sample size: Understanding efficient types of adaptation. *Statistics in Medicine, 32*(11), 1259–1275.

Lioddden, L., & Moen, A. (2012). Knowledge development in nursing: Pragmatic, randomized controlled trials as a methodological approach to support evidence-based practice. *Nordic Nursing Research, 2*(3), 233–246.

Ruggeri, M., Lasalvia, A., & Bonetto, C. (2013). A new generation of pragmatic trials of psychosocial interventions is needed. *Epidemiology and Psychiatric Sciences, 20,* 1–7.

Summary of Key Concepts Found at the end of each chapter, these lists compile the most pertinent concepts and information for quick review and later reference.

Summary of Key Concepts

- Summarizing descriptive data is the first step in the analysis of quantitative research data.
- Descriptive data are numbers in a data set that are calculated to represent research variables and do not involve generalization to larger populations.
- Nominal and ordinal data are best represented by frequencies, percentages, and rates.
- Interval- and ratio-level data can be represented by measures of central tendency, variability, and relative position.
- Measures of central tendency include the mean, median, and mode. The mean is easily calculated and interpreted but is influenced by extreme scores. The median represents the midpoint of the data but does not reflect extremes well. The mode is the most frequently occurring value; it is of limited usefulness in descriptive analysis.
- Measures of variability include the variance, standard deviation, and CV, all of which represent how spread out the data values are in relation to the mean.
- Measures of relative position include percentiles and standardized scores, which enable the comparison of values when the scales of measurement are different.
- The relationship between two variables in a sample is represented by the correlation coefficient.
- A frequency distribution enables the researcher to determine the shape of the variable's distribution, which may be normal, skewed, or kurtotic.
- Data must be analyzed using the correct statistical procedure for the level of measurement of a variable.
- The data may be presented numerically and graphically in a way that conveys the most accurate information about the variables in the study.
- Errors in reporting descriptive data include using the wrong statistics for the level of measurement; presenting incomplete, overly complicated, or misleading data; and drawing conclusions that go beyond what the data will support.
- Data must be meticulously collected, entered, checked for quality, and cleaned prior to analysis.

Critical Appraisal Exercises Found at the end of each chapter, these exercises direct readers to apply chapter concepts to a full-length research report.

CRITICAL **APPRAISAL EXERCISE**

Retrieve the following full text article from the Cumulative Index to Nursing and Allied Health Literature or similar search database:

Koli, R., Kohler, K., Tonteri, E., Peltonen, J., Tikkanen, H., & Fogelholm, M. (2015). Dark chocolate and reduced snack consumption in mildly hypertensive adults: An intervention study. *Nutrition Journal, 14*(84), 1–9.

Review the article, looking for information about the research design. Consider the following appraisal questions in your critical review of this element of the research article:

1. What is the specific design chosen for this research? Why is it the most appropriate design for this question?
2. Is the design clearly discernible early in the article? Is it described in such a way that the reader could replicate it?
3. Are the primary variables clearly identified and defined (independent and dependent)?
4. Why did the researchers ask subjects to reduce snack consumption during the study period?
5. Which extraneous effects did the cross-over aspect of this study control? Which others might be present and uncontrolled?
6. What are the strengths of this design for answering the research question? How could the nurse apply these findings in practice?

Skill Builder Found in select chapters, this feature provides practical advice for finding research, reading it critically, and strengthening research skills.

SKILL BUILDER   Develop a Strong Literature Review

It is easy to see the literature search as a task that must be done to get at the "real" work of research. In fact, if it is done well, a thorough review of previous work can actually save the researcher time in the long run. The literature search can help focus the research question, develop the details of a study design, and put the study in a larger context. Doing a literature search requires time and a bit of frustration tolerance—but there are ways to get the most from this critical step.

- Involve a health sciences librarian in the literature search early in the process. Searching the literature is a methodical science, and the expertise a librarian brings can prove invaluable. A health sciences librarian can help locate databases and assist in developing a search strategy, both of which can improve the chances of a successful search.
- Go from general to specific in the search strategy. Look for studies on the overall topic first, and then search for research that is more specific to the unique question.
- Select references to review from the lists of the most relevant studies.
- Resist the urge to look only at full-text databases. Valuable studies may be missed, and the research

may end up with an incomplete literature review if the focus is exclusively on easily accessible articles.
- Use a broad range of sources, including "gray literature" such as conference proceedings, dissertation abstracts, and government reports. Though time consuming, manual searches of the tables of contents of the most relevant journals may reveal studies that were missed in the electronic search.
- Rely on primary sources—in other words, the original studies—instead of quotes or summaries from other articles. Studies may be misquoted and findings reported incorrectly, so the primary source must be evaluated to ensure the findings are reported correctly.

A strong literature review will include studies that both support and refute the researcher's ideas. Any gaps, particular strengths, or evident weaknesses in the current evidence should be revealed. The goal of a literature review is to explore the support for a research project, not to prove a point. The best literature reviews provide direction while reinforcing the need for specialized inquiry.

FOURTH EDITION

NURSING RESEARCH
READING, USING, AND CREATING EVIDENCE

JANET HOUSER, PHD, RN

Provost and Professor

Rueckert-Hartman College for Health Professions

Regis University

Denver, Colorado

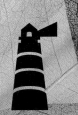

JONES & BARTLETT
LEARNING

World Headquarters
Jones & Bartlett Learning
5 Wall Street
Burlington, MA 01803
978-443-5000
info@jblearning.com
www.jblearning.com

Jones & Bartlett Learning books and products are available through most bookstores and online booksellers. To contact Jones & Bartlett Learning directly, call 800-832-0034, fax 978-443-8000, or visit our website, www.jblearning.com.

Substantial discounts on bulk quantities of Jones & Bartlett Learning publications are available to corporations, professional associations, and other qualified organizations. For details and specific discount information, contact the special sales department at Jones & Bartlett Learning via the above contact information or send an email to specialsales@jblearning.com.

15833-5

Production Credits

VP, Executive Publisher: David D. Cella
Executive Editor: Amanda Martin
Editorial Assistant: Emma Huggard
Senior Production Editor: Amanda Clerkin
Senior Marketing Manager: Jennifer Scherzay
Product Fulfillment Manager: Wendy Kilborn
Composition: S4Carlisle Publishing Services
Cover Design: Scott Moden
Rights & Media Specialist: Wes DeShano
Media Development Editor: Troy Liston
Cover Image: © Valentina Razumova/Shutterstock
Printing and Binding: LSC Communications
Cover Printing: LSC Communications

Library of Congress Cataloging-in-Publication Data
Names: Houser, Janet, 1954- author.
Title: Nursing research : reading, using, and creating evidence / Janet Houser.
Description: Fourth edition. | Burlington, Massachusetts : Jones & Bartlett Learning, [2018] | Includes bibliographical references and index.
Identifiers: LCCN 2016038194 | ISBN 9781284110043
Subjects: | MESH: Clinical Nursing Research--methods | Evidence-Based Nursing | Research Design
Classification: LCC RT81.5 | NLM WY 20.5 | DDC 610.73072--dc23
LC record available at https://lccn.loc.gov/2016038194

6048

Printed in the United States of America
20 19 18 17 16   10 9 8 7 6 5 4 3 2 1

Contents

Preface

This nursing research text is based on the idea that research is essential for nurses as evidence for practice. Its contents are intended to be relevant for nursing students and practicing nurses who must apply evidence to practice. All nurses should be able to read research, determine how to use it appropriately in their practice, and participate in the research process in some way during their careers as professionals. This text is intended to support all these efforts.

Evidence-based practice is one of the most exciting trends in nursing practice to emerge in decades. However, its integration into daily practice requires a solid understanding of the foundations of research design, validity, and application. This text is intended as a reader-friendly approach to a complex topic so that beginners can grasp the fundamentals of appraising research, experienced nurses can use research in practice, and practicing nurses can gain skills to create bedside research projects or participate effectively on research teams.

This text is presented in an uncluttered, straightforward manner. Although it uses many bulleted lists to make the material visually interesting, the sidebars, figures, and tables are limited to those that illustrate truly important concepts. This format allows the reader to grasp the information quickly and to navigate the text efficiently. Margin notes provide definitions of new terms when they first appear, and the Gray Matter features offer information about key concepts that are of particular importance.

This text differs in its approach from traditional texts in that it does not focus primarily on interpreting inferential research; rather, it seeks to impart a fundamental understanding of all types of research that may be used as evidence. It adds depth by considering the use of qualitative research in nursing practice—a natural fit with this holistic profession. This text also addresses contemporary concerns for today's nurses, including ethical and legal issues. Although both ethics and legal issues are mentioned in many research texts, a full chapter is devoted to these topics in this text so that the intricacies of these issues can be thoroughly considered.

The integrated discussion of both the quantitative and the qualitative traditions is another unique facet of this text's coverage of the research process. Most nurse researchers have learned to appreciate the need to consider all paradigms when approaching a research question; separating the two approaches when discussing the fundamental interests of researchers results in a polarized view. Intuitively, nurses know that the lines between quantitative and qualitative designs are not always so clear in practice and that they should consider multiple ways of knowing when evaluating research questions. The planning process covered here helps the novice researcher consider the requirements of both approaches in the context of sampling, measurement, validity, and other crucial issues they share. Detailed descriptions of the procedures for each type of design are given attention in separate chapters.

The chapters are organized around the types of research processes that make up the evidence base for practice. The first section of the text provides information that is applicable to all research traditions, whether descriptive, quantitative, or qualitative. Part I provides an overview of issues relevant to all researchers: understanding the way research and practice are related, the ways that knowledge is generated, and legal and ethical considerations. Part II describes the processes that go into planning research. The chapters in Part III consider the various decisions that must be made in each phase of the research process.

The evidence generated by descriptive, survey, and qualitative designs is placed in the context of both the definition of evidence-based practice and application in practice guidelines. In Parts IV, V, and VI, each major classification of research is explored in depth through review of available designs, guidelines for methods and procedures, and discussion of appropriate analytic processes. Brief examples of each type of research are provided, along with notes explaining the features demonstrated in each case in point. Finally, Part VII details the models and processes used to translate research into clinical practice.

Many chapters begin with a feature called "Voices from the Field" that relates a real-life story of a nurse's experience with the research process, illustrating the way that the material covered in that chapter might come to life. The main content for each chapter is broken into five parts:

- A thorough review of the topic under consideration is presented first. This review lays out the fundamental knowledge related to the topic.
- Next, the nurse is guided to consider the aspects of a study that should be appraised when reading research. All nurses—regardless of their experience—should be able to read research critically and apply it appropriately to practice, and the second section of each chapter addresses this skill. Added features include advice on where to look for the key elements of a research paper, the wording that might be used to describe them, and specific things to look for during the evaluation process. Evaluation checklists support this process.
- The third section of the chapter focuses on using research in practice. This section supports the nurse in determining if and how research findings might be used in his or her practice.
- The fourth section is intended for nurses who may be involved with teams that are charged with creating research or who may plan bedside research projects to improve practice. This section gives practical advice and direction about the design and conduct of a realistic, focused nursing research project.
- The final section of each chapter contains summary points and a critical appraisal exercise so that the nurse can immediately apply the chapter concepts to a real research report.

All of these features are intended to help the reader gain a comprehensive view of the research process as it is used to provide evidence for professional nursing practice. The use of this text as a supportive resource for learning and for ongoing reference in clinical practice has been integrated into the design of each element of the text. The goal is to stimulate nurses to read, use, and participate in the process of improving nursing practice through the systematic use of evidence. Accomplishing this goal improves the profession for all of us.

Acknowledgments

It is a bit misleading to conclude that a text is produced solely by the person whose name appears on the cover. Help and support are needed from many people on both professional and personal fronts to complete a project of this size. The help of editorial staff is always welcome; advice from Amanda Martin was invaluable in merging the interests of writing with those of producing a book that others will want to read. I appreciate Amanda Clerkin's calm and steady approach after our sixth manuscript together, and I've learned a lot from reading Jill Hobbs's edits, which I must begrudgingly admit make my writing much better.

My family—my husband, Floyd; my sisters, Anne and Ande; my niece, Stef; and mini-me, Amanda—provided me with enough encouragement to keep going, even as they reminded me there is life beyond the pages of a book.

I must thank Regis University profusely for providing me with inspirational colleagues and a place that supports my work. Pat Ladewig, as always, provided pragmatic advice and guidance from her impressive experience publishing her own texts. My contributors and reviewers each provided a unique viewpoint and helped me discover the best way to ensure that students "get it."

Writing always makes me realize how much I miss my mom, Marty, who encouraged me to publish from the time she surreptitiously sent one of my poems to *Highlights* magazine when I was 9 years old. She was proud of that poem, framed the issue, and had my grandmother embroider it on a pillow. Seeing this book in print would have impressed her only slightly more, but I know she's smiling.

Contributors

Michael Cahill, MS, CPHQ
Parker Adventist Hospital
Parker, Colorado
Summarizing and Reporting Descriptive Data

Sheila Carlon, PhD, RHIA, FAHIMA
Regis University
Denver, Colorado
Ethical and Legal Considerations in Research

Phyllis Graham-Dickerson, PhD, RN, CNS
Regis University
Denver, Colorado
Qualitative Research Questions and Procedures
Analyzing and Reporting Qualitative Results

LeeAnn Hanna, PhD, RN, CPHQ, FNAHQ
HCA, TriStar Centennial Medical Center
Nashville, Tennessee
Finding Problems and Writing Questions

Kimberly O'Neill, MS, MLIS
Dayton Memorial Library, Regis University
Denver, Colorado
The Successful Literature Search

About the Author

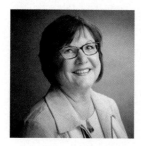

Janet Houser, PhD, RN

Regis University

Dr. Janet Houser is currently Provost at Regis University in Denver, Colorado. Prior to her appointment, she was Dean of the Rueckert-Hartman College for Health Professions and the Vice Provost for Resource Planning.

Dr. Houser has a BSN, an MN in Maternal-Child Health, an MS in healthcare administration, and a PhD in applied statistics and research methods. She has taught nurses, administrators, pharmacists, and physical therapy students from undergraduate through doctoral level, primarily in the subjects of research methods, biostatistics, and quantitative methods. Previous to her position as Dean, Dr. Houser was faculty and Associate Dean for Research and Scholarship.

Dr. Houser spent 20 years in healthcare administration with the Mercy Health System. Her last position was as Regional Director for Professional Practice for Mercy Health Partners in Cincinnati, Ohio, where she was responsible for professional practice and clinical research in 29 facilities.

Dr. Houser has published five books, *Clinical Research in Practice: A Guide for the Bedside Scientist*, *Nursing Research: Reading, Using, and Creating Evidence*, which is in its fourth edition, and *Evidence-Based Practice: An Implementation Guide*. She has more than 30 peer-reviewed publications in journals and has presented her research at regional, national, and international conferences.

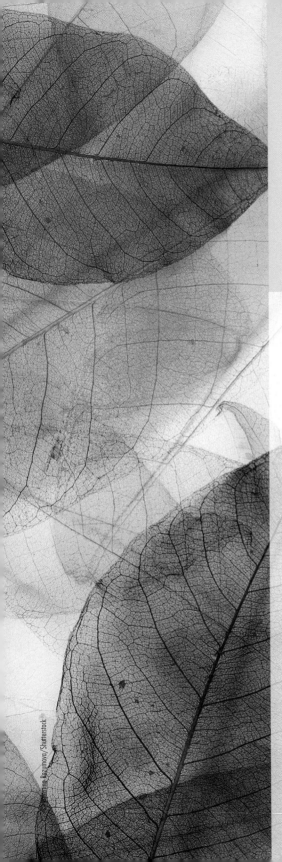

Part I

An Introduction to Research

Chapter 1

The Importance of Research as Evidence in Nursing

CHAPTER OBJECTIVES

The study of this chapter will help the learner to

- Define nursing research and discuss how research is used in nursing practice.
- Describe the evolution of nursing research.
- Investigate the roles that nurses play in research processes.
- Contrast research and other types of problem solving.
- Explore how research is used as evidence guiding the practice of nursing.
- Read research and appraise the credibility of the journal, authors, and publication process.

KEY TERMS

Blinded

Evidence-based practice

Evidence-based practice guideline

External validity

Journal club

Magnet status

National Institute of Nursing Research (NINR)

Nursing process

Nursing research

Outcomes measurement

Peer review

Principal investigator

Quality improvement

Randomized controlled trial

Replication

Systematic review

Research as Evidence for Nursing Practice

The practice of nursing is deeply rooted in nursing knowledge, and nursing knowledge is generated and disseminated through reading, using, and creating nursing research. Professional nurses rely on research findings to inform their practice decisions; they use critical thinking to apply research directly to specific patient care situations. The research process allows nurses to ask and answer questions systematically that will ensure that their decisions are based on sound science and rigorous inquiry. Nursing research helps nurses in a variety of settings answer questions about patient care, education, and administration. It ensures that practices are based on evidence, rather than eloquence or tradition.

VOICES FROM THE FIELD

I was working as the clinical nurse specialist in a busy surgical intensive care unit (ICU) when we received a critically ill patient. He was fresh from cardiac surgery and quite unstable; he needed multiple drugs and an intra-aortic balloon pump just to maintain his perfusion status. The patient was so sick that we were not able to place him on a special bed for pressure relief. For the first 24 hours, we were so busy trying to keep him alive that we did not even get a chance to turn him.

Approximately 36 hours into his ICU admission, he was stable enough to place on a low-air-loss mattress for pressure-ulcer prevention. When we were finally able to turn him, we noted he had a small stage II pressure ulcer on his coccyx. Despite the treatments that we used, the pressure ulcer evolved into a full-thickness wound. The patient recovered from his cardiac surgical procedure but, unfortunately, required surgeries and skin grafts to close the pressure ulcer wound.

The experience I had with this patient prompted me to review the evidence-based practice (EBP) guidelines we had in place to prevent pressure ulcers in critically ill patients. I wanted to make sure we could prevent this kind of incident from happening again, but I had a lot of questions. Could we preventively place high-risk patients on low-air-loss mattresses while they were still in the perioperative service? Did we even know which patients were at risk for pressure ulcers? Which assessment tools did nurses use to assess the patient's risk? When a high-risk patient was identified, which interventions did the nurses use to prevent pressure ulcers? How were the ulcers treated once they appeared?

I was fortunate that my chief nursing officer (CNO) was a strong advocate for EBP, and she encouraged me to initiate an EBP review of pressure ulcer prevention and treatment. Specifically, I wanted to find out which nursing interventions were supported by research evidence when we were trying to prevent pressure ulcers in the surgical ICU. As part of my review, I contacted other inpatient units at the hospital to determine what they were doing.

I discovered that the surgical ICU was no different from the other inpatient units in this regard: There was no standard, evidence-based nursing practice for pressure ulcer prevention. Units were not consistently using the same skin assessment tools, so it was difficult to objectively communicate risk from one unit to another. The tools we were using were not necessarily based on research. It was clear that we needed to identify the best available evidence and devise a protocol.

We started by establishing an evidence-based skin care council for the hospital. This team consisted of bedside nurses from all inpatient units and the perioperative service. Initially the council reviewed the hospital's current nursing skin assessment forms, and we conducted a review of the literature on pressure ulcer prevention and interventions. We discovered the Agency for Healthcare Research and Quality (AHRQ) guidelines on pressure ulcer prevention and treatment—a key source of evidence for healthcare practices.

Over the course of the next year, we revised our nursing policy and procedure, incorporating the AHRQ evidence into a treatment guideline. This guideline included a procedure for skin assessment and nursing documentation, and pressure ulcer assessment and treatment decision algorithms. We reviewed skin-care products and narrowed down the list of products to those that were supported by evidence. One algorithm helped staff make selections between products that maximized prevention and treatment. Another algorithm guided nurses in the use of therapeutic surfaces (e.g., low-air-loss mattresses) to prevent pressure ulcers. To monitor our progress, we began quarterly pressure ulcer prevalence studies. As part of the implementation, we scheduled a skin-care seminar featuring a national expert on skin care.

At the beginning of our EBP skin-care journey, our facility's pressure ulcer prevalence was 9%. Since implementing our EBP skin-care initiatives, it has dropped by two thirds. The EBP skin-care council continues to be active in our hospital. We meet monthly to seek out the best evidence to guide skin- and wound-care product decisions, practice guidelines, protocols, and policies. My initial search for a solution—based on my experience with one patient—led to improvements in practice that have benefited many patients since then.

Mary Beth Flynn Makic, PhD, RN

What Is Nursing Research?

Nursing research is a systematic process of inquiry that uses rigorous guidelines to produce unbiased, trustworthy answers to questions about nursing practice. Research is used as evidence in the evaluation and determination of best nursing practices. Original nursing research aims to generate new knowledge to inform the practice of nursing. More specifically, nurses may use research for the following purposes:

- Synthesize the findings of others into a coherent guide for practice
- Explore and describe phenomena that affect health
- Find solutions to existing and emerging problems
- Test traditional approaches to patient care for continued relevance and effectiveness

Nurse researchers use a variety of methods to generate new knowledge or summarize existing study results. They may measure observable characteristics, solicit perceptions directly from clients, assess words and phrases for underlying meaning, or analyze a group of study findings in aggregate. Nurse researchers have almost limitless options for research design. Moreover, they may assume a variety of roles, ranging from primary investigator for a large, multisite trial to staff nurse in a bedside science project. Nevertheless, the goal is always the same: to generate new knowledge that can be applied to improve nursing practice.

Regardless of the design, research is a rigorous endeavor that is subject to peer review and replication. These two characteristics are essential to ensure that research is unbiased and applicable to the real world. A study is subjected to **peer review** when experts in the field evaluate the quality of the research and determine whether it warrants presentation at a conference or publication in a professional journal. These reviews are generally **blinded**, meaning the reviewer remains unaware of the researcher's identity. In blinded peer review, a research report is subjected to appraisal by a neutral party who is unassociated with the research and unaware of the report's authorship. Reviewers determine whether the study process and outcome are of acceptable quality for communication to the broader professional community. **Replication** ensures that findings can be duplicated in different populations and at different times. This characteristic provides the nurse with confidence that the findings are not limited to a single sample, so that study outcomes will likely be similar in other patient populations.

Research: A Fundamental Nursing Skill

Although many students and practitioners of nursing consider research to be the purview of academics and graduate students, it is actually fundamental to professional nursing

---

Nursing research:
A systematic process of inquiry that uses rigorous guidelines to produce unbiased, trustworthy answers to questions about nursing practice.

Peer review:
The process of subjecting research to the appraisal of a neutral third party. Common processes of peer review include selecting research for conferences and evaluating research manuscripts for publication.

Blinded:
A type of review in which the peer reviewer is unaware of the author's identity, so personal influence is avoided.

Replication:
Repeating a specific study in detail on a different sample. When a study has been replicated several times and similar results are found, the evidence can be used with more confidence.

Magnet status:
A designation for organizations that have characteristics that make them attractive to nurses as workplaces.

practice. There are many reasons why research is critical for the nurse in any role. Nursing is a profession, and along with advanced education and self-regulation, research is one of the central tenets that defines a profession. For nurses to function on healthcare teams as colleagues with therapists, physicians, and other caregivers, they must speak the language of science and use the best available research evidence as the basis for collaborating in planning patient care.

As professionals, nurses are accountable for the outcomes they achieve and the effectiveness of interventions that they apply and recommend to patients. Their accountability is based on a solid understanding and evaluation of the best available evidence as the foundation for decision making and patient counseling. In current healthcare practice, access, cost, and patient safety are all areas that clearly benefit from nursing research.

Consumer demands also require that nurses be held accountable for their practice. Today's consumers and their families are often well informed about the evidence that reveals the effectiveness of care. The Internet has given consumers unprecedented access to health information—some of it questionable, but much of it of high quality—that enables them to evaluate the basis for their own healthcare decisions.

In 2011, the Institute of Medicine issued a seminal report on the future of nursing. In this report, it set a goal that, by 2020, 90% of all clinical decisions would be based on research evidence. Given that the current estimated rate falls far short of that goal, there is an urgent need for healthcare leaders and clinicians to collaborate in designing and implementing effective strategies for research integration into clinical care. In particular, there is a need to enhance the rigor of nursing research studies, and to translate evidence into practice-friendly forms that nurses can use in daily care delivery.

Many nursing organizations are in the process of pursuing or maintaining **Magnet status**, which requires the organization to contribute to new knowledge and innovation in nursing care. Wilson and others (2015) found other benefits from an organization achieving Magnet status: Nurses in Magnet facilities express greater interest in using evidence in practice, report fewer barriers to implementation of EBP, and used EBP with more frequency than nurses in non-Magnet facilities. Integration of evidence into daily practice requires both resources and formalized processes; these assets must be evident and useful in a Magnet organization. To maintain Magnet status, hospitals must show quality outcomes, best practices, and nursing excellence—all of which require development and dissemination of new knowledge (Messmer & Turkel, 2011).

The Evolution of Research in Nursing

Nursing is a relatively young field compared to fields such as philosophy or physics that boast hundreds of years of historical study. Moreover, nursing has not always relied on profession-specific research as a basis for practice. However, as the contemporary nursing literature makes clear, research is taking on fundamental importance as a source of evidence for practice.

More than 150 years ago, Florence Nightingale introduced the concept of scientific inquiry as a basis for nursing practice. Nightingale's work focused on collecting information about factors that affected soldier mortality and morbidity during the Crimean War.

Armed with these scientific data, she was able to instigate changes in nursing practice. Indeed, her work was so impressive that she was inducted into the Statistical Society of London.

The years following Nightingale's breakthroughs were marked by relatively little scientific work in nursing, likely because nursing education was accomplished through apprenticeship rather than scholarly work. As more nursing education moved into university settings in the 1950s, however, research took on greater prominence as a key nursing activity. Journals were founded both in the United States and internationally that focused exclusively on publishing nursing research. More outlets for the publication of nursing research were established in the 1970s and 1980s, leading to the communication of research findings to a broader audience. The creation of the National Center for Research for Nursing within the National Institutes of Health (NIH) in 1986 was a seminal step in recognizing the importance of nursing research. In 1993, the center was given full institute status as the **National Institute of Nursing Research (NINR)**. This move put nursing research on an even footing with medical research and the other health sciences, ensuring financial support and a national audience for disciplined inquiry in the field. The NINR and other national agencies guide the overarching research agenda that focuses nursing research on professional priorities. The mission of the NINR is to support and conduct clinical and basic research on health and illness so as to build the scientific foundation for clinical practice. The ultimate goal is to improve the health of individuals, families, communities, and populations through evidence-based nursing practices (NINR, 2013).

In the 1980s and 1990s, leaders in nursing research met periodically at the Conference on Research Priorities in Nursing Science (CORP) to identify research priorities for the nursing profession. These priorities were established as 5-year agendas. In the 1990s, advances in nursing research were coming so quickly that a more flexible approach was required. The NINR recognized that the issues facing nursing science had evolved as health care had evolved, becoming more complex. The process that the NINR currently uses to develop its research priorities is both expansive and inclusive. The formal process begins with the identification of broad areas of health in which there is the greatest need, and identification of the areas of science in which nursing research could achieve the greatest impact. To maximize the amount and diversity of input into the research priorities, "Scientific Consultation Meetings" are held to bring together individuals from academia, government, industry, and patient advocacy. Experts in science and health care are consulted, and panels of experts discuss current health and research challenges as well as future strategies for research and education. These meetings focus on topics crucial to NINR's future, including the following:

- Preparing the next generation of nurse scientists
- Advancing nursing science through comparative effectiveness research
- Supporting research on end-of-life care
- Forecasting future needs for health promotion and prevention of disease
- Identification of emerging needs in the science of nursing (NINR, 2011)

Some examples of recent NINR nursing research priorities appear in **Table 1.1**.

National Institute of Nursing Research (NINR): A federal agency responsible for the support of nursing research by establishing a national research agenda, funding grants and research awards, and providing training.

GRAY MATTER

Research is critical in nursing for the following reasons:
- The use of research is inherent to the definition of a profession.
- Nurses are accountable for outcomes.
- Consumers are demanding evidence-based care.

Table 1.1 National Institute of Nursing Research's Proposed Strategic Research Investment Areas

Objective	Examples
Enhance health promotion and disease prevention	Develop innovative behavioral interventions Study the behavior of systems that can promote personalized interventions Improve the ways in which individuals change health behaviors Develop models of lifelong health promotion Translate scientific advances into motivation for health behavior change Incorporate partnerships between community agencies and others in healthcare research
Improve quality of life by managing symptoms of acute and chronic illness	Improve knowledge of the biological and genomic mechanisms associated with symptoms Design interventions to improve the assessment and management of symptoms over the course of a disease Study the factors that influence symptom management and use this knowledge to implement personalized interventions Design strategies that help patients manage symptoms over the course of a disease Support individuals and caregivers in managing chronic illness in cost-effective ways
Improve palliative and end-of-life care	Enhance the scientific knowledge of issues and choices underlying end-of life and palliative care Develop and test interventions that provide palliative care across the lifespan Develop strategies to minimize the burden placed on caregivers Determine the impact of provider training on outcomes Create communication strategies to promote end-of-life care
Enhance innovation in science and practice	Develop technologies and informatics-based solutions for health problems Develop and apply technology for disseminating and analyzing health information Examine the use of healthcare technology to support self-management of health, decision making, and access to care Study the use of genetic and genomic technology to understand the biological basis of the symptoms of chronic disease

(continued)

Table 1.1 National Institute of Nursing Research's Proposed Strategic Research Investment Areas (*continued*)

Objective	Examples
Develop the next generation of nurse scientists	Support the development of nurse scientists at all stages of their careers Facilitate the transition of nurses from student to scientist Recruit young nurse investigators, particularly those from diverse backgrounds Mobilize technology to form global partnerships to support research in areas central to NINR's mission

Data from National Institute of Nursing Research. (2011). Bringing science to life: NINR strategic plan. NIH Publication #11-7783, Bethesda, MD: Author.

GRAY MATTER

Nurses may play a variety of roles in research, including the following:
- Informed consumer of research
- Participant in research-related activity, such as journal clubs
- Contributor to a systematic review
- Data collector for a research project
- Principal investigator for a research study

The 1990s and early twenty-first century saw a shift in emphasis from research as an academic activity to research that serves as a basis for nursing practice. The impetus for this shift was partially due to external influences that created demands for accountability, effectiveness, and efficiency. Internal influences in the profession also played a key role in this shift, as nursing professionals strive to create a norm of professional practice that is firmly grounded in best demonstrated practice.

Contemporary Nursing Research Roles

The nurse may be an effective team member on any number of research projects and may take on responsibilities ranging from data collection to research design. The broad number of potential roles in the research setting provides nurses with the chance to participate at their individual comfort level while learning increasingly complex research skills. The professional clinician has both opportunities and responsibilities to use research in a variety of ways to improve practice. **Table 1.2** contains the statement from the American Association of Colleges of Nursing (2006) that describes the expected roles of nurses in research processes.

Most nurses are first exposed to clinical research as informed consumers. The informed consumer of research is able to find appropriate research studies, read them

Journal club:
A formally organized group that meets periodically to share and critique contemporary research in nursing, with a goal of both learning about the research process and finding evidence for practice.

Systematic review:
A highly structured and controlled search of the available literature that minimizes the potential for bias and produces a practice recommendation as an outcome.

Evidence-based practice guideline:
A guide for nursing practice that is the outcome of an unbiased, exhaustive review of the research literature, combined with clinical expert opinion and evaluation of patient preferences. It is generally developed by a team of experts.

Table 1.2 Research Expectations for Nurses

Educational Level	Research Role
Baccalaureate degree	Have a basic understanding of the processes of research. Apply research findings from nursing and other disciplines to practice. Understand the basic elements of evidence-based practice. Work with others to identify research problems. Collaborate on research teams.
Master's degree	Evaluate research findings to develop and implement EBP guidelines. Form and lead teams focused on evidence-based practice. Identify practices and systems that require study. Collaborate with nurse scientists to initiate research.
Practice-based doctorates	Translate scientific knowledge into complex clinical interventions tailored to meet individual, family, and community health and illness needs. Use advanced leadership knowledge and skills to translate research into practice. Collaborate with scientists on new health research opportunities.
Research-focused doctorates	Pursue intellectual inquiry and conduct independent research for the purpose of extending knowledge. Plan and carry out an independent program of research. Seek support for initial phases of a research program. Involve others in research projects and programs.
Postdoctoral programs	Devote oneself fully to establishing a research program and developing as a nurse scientist.

Modified with permission from American Association of Colleges of Nursing. (2006). *AACN position statement on nursing research.* Washington, CD: Author.

critically, evaluate their findings for validity, and use the findings in practice. Nurses may also participate in other types of research-related activities, including journal clubs or groups whose members meet periodically to critique published studies or care standards. Journal clubs are relatively easy to implement and have been demonstrated to be one of the most effective means for sustaining staff nurse enthusiasm for and participation in EBP implementation (Gardner et al., 2016). Attending research presentations and discussing posters at conferences also expose nurses to a variety of research studies.

As the nurse becomes more proficient in the research process, involvement in a systematic review is a logical next step. Conducting a systematic review that results in an evidence-based practice guideline requires the ability to develop research questions methodically, write inclusion criteria, conduct in-depth literature searches, and review the results of many studies critically. Participation in such activities also facilitates changes in clinical practice on a larger scale and requires the nurse to use leadership and communication skills.

Involvement in actual research studies does not require complete control or in-depth design abilities. Indeed, assisting with data collection can take the form of helping measure outcomes on subjects or personally participating as a subject. Clinicians are frequently recruited to participate in studies or collect data directly from patients or their records. Collecting data for the studies of other researchers can give the nurse valuable insight into the methods used to maximize reliability and validity—experience that will help the nurse later if he or she chooses to design an experiment.

Most nurses do not immediately jump into research by undertaking an individual research study, but rather serve on a research team as an initial foray into this area. As part of a team, the nurse can learn the skills needed to conduct research while relying on the time and expertise of a group of individuals, some of whom may be much more experienced researchers. Serving on a team in this way gives the nurse the opportunity to participate in research in a collegial way, collaborating with others to achieve a mutual goal.

A contemporary means for enhancing staff nurse participation in research is through adoption of the clinical scholar or nurse scholar role. Nurse scholar programs typically seek out clinical nurses for specialized training in research and EBP. These nurses are then provided with releases from their usual workloads so that they can identify evidence-based problems, design studies to answer clinical questions, and carry out EBP projects. One study found that a nurse scholar program increased the number of EBP projects by as much as 10 times, led to significant practice improvements, and enhanced the confidence of the clinical nurses who participated in EBP development (Crabtree, Brennan, Davis, & Coyle, 2016).

The most advanced nurses may serve as **principal investigators**, or producers of research, who design and conduct their own research projects. Because individuals are rarely able to accomplish research projects on their own, it is more likely that the nurse will lead a research team. This role requires not only research and analytic skills, but also skills in leading groups, managing projects, and soliciting organizational commitment.

Research Versus Problem Solving

Research is distinct from other problem-solving processes. Many processes involve inquiry. In an organizational setting, **quality improvement**, performance improvement, and **outcomes measurement** all involve systematic processes and an emphasis on data as a basis for decisions. For an individual nurse, the **nursing process** requires that the nurse gather evidence before planning an intervention and subsequently guides the nurse to evaluate the effectiveness of care objectively. Although both organizational and individual problem-solving processes may be systematic and objective, these are not synonymous with research in intent, risks, or outcome (Lee, Johnson, Newhouse, & Warren, 2013). The correct identification of the type of inquiry that is being conducted and reported will help the nurse link the outcome to the appropriate level of practice recommendation (Baker et al., 2014).

The intent of quality improvement is to improve processes for the benefit of patients or customers within an organizational context. Studies in this area are often undertaken

Principal investigator: The individual who is primarily responsible for a research study. The principal investigator is responsible for all elements of the study and is the first author listed on publications or presentations.

Quality improvement: The systematic, data-based monitoring and evaluation of organizational processes with the end goal of continuous improvement. The goal of data collection is internal application rather than external generalization.

Outcomes measurement: Measurement of the end results of nursing care or other interventions; stated in terms of effects on patients' physiological condition, satisfaction, or psychosocial health.

Nursing process: A systematic process used by nurses to identify and address patient problems; includes the stages of assessment, planning, intervention, and evaluation.

to determine if appropriate and existing standards of care are practiced in a specific clinical setting (Baker et al., 2014). Quality improvement is basically a management tool that is used to ensure continuous improvement and a focus on quality. Research, in contrast, has a broader intent. Its goal is to benefit the profession of nursing and to contribute to the knowledge base for practice. Research benefits more people because it is broadly applied; quality improvement is beneficial simply because of its specificity to a single organization.

The risk for a subject who participates in a quality improvement study is not much more than the risk associated with receiving clinical care. Such studies are frequently descriptive or measure relationships that are evidenced by existing data. Often, patients who are the subjects of study for a quality improvement project are unaware they are even part of a study. In contrast, in a research project, subjects are clearly informed at the beginning of the project of the risks and benefits associated with participating in the study, and they are allowed to withdraw their information at any time. Upfront and informed consent is central to the research process.

Finally, the outcomes of a quality improvement study are intended to benefit a specific clinical group and so are reviewed by formal committees and communicated internally to organizational audiences. In contrast, research findings are subjected to rigorous peer review by neutral, external reviewers, and the results are expected to stand up to attempts to replicate them. When quality improvement projects are planned with an expectation of publication, the distinction becomes less clear. Is the goal of publication to share a perspective on a process or to generalize the results to a broader group of patients? If the latter goal is targeted, then quality improvement projects should be subjected to the same rigorous review and control as a research project.

The intent when an individual nurse applies the nursing process for problem solving is even more specific. The nursing process requires an individual nurse to gather data about a patient, draw conclusions about patient needs, and implement measures to address those needs. Data collected from the patient are used to evaluate the effectiveness of care and make modifications to the plan. These steps mirror the research process but take place at an individual level. Research is useful within the nursing process as a source of knowledge about assessment procedures, problem identification, and effective therapeutics, but simply using the nursing process does not constitute research.

GRAY MATTER

The research process is distinct from other problem-solving processes in the following respects:
- Research contributes to the profession of nursing as a whole, not just a single organization or patient.
- Research involves an explicit process of informed consent for subjects.
- Research is subjected to external peer review and replication.

Research as Evidence in Nursing Practice

It would seem a foregone conclusion that effective nursing practice is based on the best possible, most rigorously tested evidence. Yet it is only in the past two decades that an emphasis on evidence as a basis for practice has reached the forefront of professional nursing. Although it may be surprising that the scientific basis for nursing practice has been so slow to be accepted, many reasons exist to explain why evidence-based nursing practice is a relatively recent effort. The past decade has seen unprecedented advances in information technology, making research and other types of evidence widely available to healthcare practitioners. Whereas a nurse practicing in the 1980s might have read one or two professional journals per month and attended perhaps one clinical conference in a year, contemporary nursing professionals have access to an almost unlimited array of professional journal articles and other sources of research evidence via the Internet. Technology supports the communication of best practices and affords consumers open access to healthcare information as well. As a result, EBP is quickly becoming the norm for effective nursing practice.

Evidence-based practice:
The use of the best scientific evidence, integrated with clinical experience and incorporating patient values and preferences in the practice of professional nursing care.

Evidence-Based Practice

What Evidence-Based Practice IS

Evidence-based practice is the use of the best scientific evidence, integrated with clinical experience and incorporating patient values and preferences in the practice of professional nursing care. All three elements in this definition are important. As illustrated in **FIGURE 1.1**, the triad of rigorous evidence, clinical experience, and patient preferences must be balanced to achieve clinical practices that are both scientifically sound and acceptable to the individuals applying and benefiting from them.

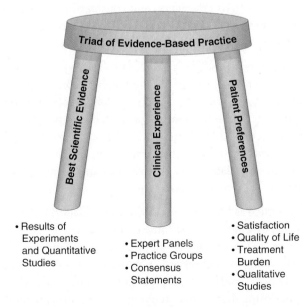

Triad of Evidence-Based Practice

Best Scientific Evidence

Clinical Experience

Patient Preferences

• Results of
  Experiments
  and Quantitative
  Studies

• Expert Panels
• Practice Groups
• Consensus
  Statements

• Satisfaction
• Quality of Life
• Treatment
  Burden
• Qualitative
  Studies

FIGURE 1.1 The Triad of Evidence-Based Practice

Randomized controlled trial:
An experiment in which subjects are randomly assigned to groups, one of which receives an experimental treatment while another serves as a control group. The experiment has high internal validity, so the researcher can draw conclusions regarding the effects of treatments.

Although healthcare practitioners have long used research as a basis for practice, a systematic approach to the translation of research into practice has emerged only in relatively recent times. The impetus for EBP was a 1990 comment by a Canadian physician on the need to "bring critical appraisal to the bedside." The first documented use of the term *evidence-based practice* appeared more than two decades ago, when a clinical epidemiology text (Sackett, Haynes, Guyatt, & Tugwell, 1991) used the term to describe the way students in medical school were taught to develop an attitude of "enlightened skepticism" toward the routine application of diagnostic technologies and clinical interventions in their daily practice. The authors described how effective practitioners rigorously review published studies to inform clinical decisions. The goal, as stated in this publication, was to achieve an awareness of the evidence on which professional practice is based and a critical assessment of the soundness of that evidence.

The term entered the U.S. literature in 1993 when an article in the *Journal of the American Medical Association* described the need for an established scientific basis for healthcare decisions (Oxman, Sackett, & Guyatt, 1993). The authors of the article noted that the goal of EBP is to help practitioners translate the results of research into clinical practice, and they recognized that the scientific practice of health care required sifting through and appraising evidence to make appropriate decisions.

EBP has rapidly evolved into an international standard for all healthcare practitioners. Using the best scientific evidence as a basis for practice makes intuitive sense and places nursing in the company of the other science-based health professions in using evidence as a foundation for clinical decision making.

What Evidence-Based Practice Is NOT

A wide range of activities contributes to EBP. Many of these activities—such as reviewing research, consulting expert colleagues, and considering patient preferences—are common in nursing practice. Even so, many such activities are not considered EBP, but rather other forms of decision making used to solve problems.

Evidence-Based Practice Is Not Clinical Problem Solving

Although EBP serves as a mechanism for solving clinical problems and making decisions about interventions, it remains distinct from traditional problem-solving approaches in health care. Conventional decision making about clinical practices relied on expert opinion—sometimes achieved by consensus, but rarely through experimentation—combined with standard practice. EBP, by comparison, is a systematic process of critically reviewing the best available research evidence and then incorporating clinical experience and patient preferences into the mix.

Evidence-Based Practice Is Not Solely Randomized Controlled Trials

EBP does not mean choosing only those interventions supported by randomized controlled trials—although these studies are clearly important in providing guidance for effective practices. A somewhat tongue-in-cheek article by Smith and Pell (2006) suggested that we did not need a randomized trial to inform practitioners of the importance of a parachute as a measure of preventing death when jumping from an airplane (and, in fact, noted the difficulty in recruiting a control group for such a trial!). EBP does not rely solely on one type of evidence, but rather is founded on a hierarchy of evidence, with individual studies rated on a scale from "strongest" to "weakest" based on the type of design and quality of execution. Evidence can come from many different types of studies in addition to randomized trials.

Evidence-Based Practice Is Not "Cookbook Medicine"

The existence of guidelines based on the best available evidence does not mean the practitioner has an edict to practice in a single way. In fact, evidence alone is never sufficient to make a specific clinical decision about a specific patient. The nurse needs evidence plus good judgment, clinical skill, and knowledge of the patient's unique needs to apply evidence to a specific patient care situation. The definition of EBP, in fact, holds evidence as only one element of the triad of decision making; that is, clinical judgment and patient values must also be considered when applying the evidence to a particular situation.

Evidence Is Not the Same as Theory

Theoretical effects must be tested and retested before therapies can be determined to be effective. As late as the early twentieth century, physicians still believed that blood-letting was an effective treatment for a host of disorders. This belief was based on the empirical observation that a patient's pulse rate slowed when he or she was bled and the theory that a slower pulse reduced irritation and inflammation. Although the empirical observations were accurate—the patient's pulse would certainly slow when bloodletting was performed, but due to impending hypovolemic shock—the theoretical relationship to a therapeutic response was ill founded. Many contemporary healthcare interventions are, unfortunately, based on similar theoretical relationships that have been untested for years. Recent research has refuted many of these theoretical assumptions, including the protective value of hormone-replacement therapy, the use of rubbing alcohol to prevent infection in a neonate's umbilical cord, and the use of heat to treat acute inflammation, among many others.

Evidence-Based Nursing Is Not Evidence-Based Medicine

The nature and processes of research are likely to be unique for any given profession. In the health realm, medicine and nursing have different philosophical roots and approaches to patient care. Medicine relies on an extensive scientific knowledge base that is primarily concerned with the cause of disease and effects of treatment. The evidence for medical care, by necessity, focuses on scientific studies that quantify these effects. Nevertheless, medical evidence has been criticized for its sometimes artificial nature. It is a research paradox that the more an experiment is controlled, the less applicability the results will have in the real world. Randomized controlled trials, then, may provide the most rigorous scientific evidence, but that evidence may not apply very well to individual patients with a broad range of physical, psychological, and behavioral conditions.

   Nursing, in contrast, requires a holistic approach to the care of individuals with physical, psychosocial, and/or spiritual needs. This care is founded on the nurse–patient relationship and the nurse's appreciation for the patient's unique needs. The evidence for nursing care, then, requires a broad range of methodologies as a basis for care. This is not to imply that these sources of evidence are not subjected to healthy skepticism and systematic inquiry, but rather that a broader range of evidence is considered as a basis for practice.

The Importance of Evidence-Based Practice in Nursing

EBP is important to the nurse for many reasons. At the top of this list is the contribution of evidence to the effective care of patients. Studies have supported the contention that patient outcomes are substantially improved when health care is based on evidence from well-designed studies versus tradition or clinical expertise alone. Evidence has been shown to be effective in supporting practices that achieve optimal outcomes in a range of behavioral, physiological, and psychosocial outcomes. In one recent meta-analysis, Leufer and Cleary-Holdforth (2009) aggregated outcomes studies related to EBP changes. A wide range of effects was found in multiple specialties including orthopedic, cardiovascular, respiratory, and obstetric outcomes. EBPs in obstetrics and neonatal care reduced morbidity and mortality, sometimes dramatically. The use of corticosteroids in premature labor, for example, reduced the risk of premature infant death by 20%. In another study, Deighton et al. (2016) demonstrated an association between EBPs and mental health outcomes, particularly for interventions related to the treatment of emotional disorders. The linkage between EBPs and outcomes is an important one, and determining the scientific support for a practice prior to its implementation makes intuitive sense.

Today's healthcare providers operate in an era of accountability, in which quality issues, patient safety, and cost concerns are primary drivers of patient care processes (Markon, Crowe, & Lemyre, 2013). Practices that are unnecessary are eliminated; ineffective practices are replaced with practices that result in desired outcomes.

Existing practices may even be unintentionally harming patients (as was found in the hormone-replacement studies), so it is ethically unjustified to continue using untested interventions. Evidence can help healthcare professionals avoid errors in decision making relative to patient care. Using research decreases the need for trial and error, which is time consuming and may prove counterproductive. In any case, time is not wasted on practices that may be ineffective or unnecessarily time intensive.

Today's consumers are well informed about their options for personal health care and often resist the traditional, paternalistic approach to health interventions. The public expects that care will be based on scientific evidence and believes that care processes should routinely lead to high-quality outcomes that are physically and mentally desirable. Healthcare professionals, in turn, must be able to respond to their patients' questions about the scientific merit of interventions and about the relative benefit of treatment options.

GRAY MATTER

EBP is important in nursing practice because research has shown that
- Patient outcomes are better when evidence is used as a basis for practice.
- Nursing care is more efficient when ineffective processes are replaced.
- Errors in decision making become less frequent with EBP.
- Consumers want evidence-based information to make decisions.

Evidence can take a variety of forms—journal articles, policies, guidelines, professional consensus statements, and standards of practice as well as formalized research. Although EBP implies scientific evidence, the words *relevant* and *rigorous* might be better adjectives to describe the kind of evidence needed by healthcare professionals. Critical skills include the ability to judge both the *type of evidence* that is needed and the *value of that evidence*.

Healthcare practitioners do not practice in professional isolation, but rather explore what works and does not work using empirical methods. An increased emphasis on EBP can be viewed as a response to these broader forces influencing the context of healthcare delivery and as a logical progression toward the utilization of research as a basis for patient care decisions.

How Can Evidence Be Used in Health Care?

At its best, evidence provides the basis for effective, efficient patient care practices. At a minimum, an evidence-based approach can enhance practice by encouraging reflection on what we know about almost every aspect of daily patient care. The EBP process need not be onerous, because it basically entails just six elements: (1) Ask a relevant clinical question, (2) search for the best evidence in the literature, (3) critically appraise the evidence, (4) integrate the evidence with clinical experience and client preferences, (5) evaluate the outcome of the practice change, and (6) disseminate the outcome (Facchiano & Snyder, 2012). The original question can come from a variety of sources in a healthcare setting; likewise, evidence can improve outcomes for a wide range of organizational processes.

Evidence as a Basis for Healthcare Processes

Evidence can be incorporated into virtually every phase of the healthcare process. For example, evidence exists for best practices in the following areas:

- Assessment of patient conditions
- Diagnosis of patient problems
- Planning of patient care
- Interventions to improve the patient's function or condition, or to prevent complications
- Evaluation of patient responses to intervention

Evidence as a Basis for Policies and Procedures

Although healthcare professionals from different educational programs, backgrounds, and experience may have different ways of delivering patient care, few can argue with the need for best practices. EBP provides the foundation for policies and procedures that are tested and found effective, as opposed to "the way we've always done it."

Evidence as a Basis for Patient Care Management Tools

The evidence that is revealed through systematic review of research and other sources provides an excellent basis for patient care management tools such as care maps, critical paths, protocols, and standard order sets. A major benefit of using patient care management tools is reduction of variability in practices, and evidence serves as a rational basis for standardized practices.

Evidence as a Basis for Care of the Individual

The complexity of patients who need care in the healthcare system can make the clinician wonder if evidence can ever be applied to an individual patient. It is easy to consider the question, "Is my patient so different from those in the research that results will not help me make a treatment decision?" This question, more than any other, may stand in the way of applying evidence to individual patient care situations. In fact, one study found that the more familiar a patient was to a practitioner, the *less likely* the clinician was to use evidence as a basis for that person's care (Summerskill & Pope, 2002).

As practitioners, we must ask whether these assumptions about the uniqueness of patients are in their best interests when it comes to clinical care. Uncertainty is inherent in the healthcare process; evidence helps to quantify that uncertainty. Concern for the uniqueness of the individual patient is not a reason to ignore the evidence, but rather an impetus to learn to apply the evidence both critically and appropriately. Evidence is not intended to be rigid, but rather—as our definition makes explicit—to be *integrated* with clinical experience and a patient's unique values to arrive at optimal outcomes.

Evidence in clinical practice is not solely limited to patient care, however. Healthcare professionals might be interested in evidence as it relates to team functioning, the best way to communicate change, organizational models for research utilization, or even the effects of insurance on healthcare usage. Evidence in health care abounds on a variety of topics, and research utilization can improve patient care in a multitude of ways.

GRAY MATTER

Evidence can be used as a basis for the following aspects of nursing practice:
- Nursing care processes such as assessment, diagnosis, treatment, and evaluation
- Policies and procedures that guide nursing practice within an organization
- Patient care management tools such as care maps, standard order sets, and critical paths
- Care decisions regarding individual patient needs

Strategies for Implementing Evidence-Based Practice

Considering the benefits of basing clinical nursing practice on evidence, it would make sense for evidence-based nursing practice to be the norm. Unfortunately, this is not the case. In an integrative review conducted by Saunders and Julkunen (2016), the vast majority of nurses were found to *believe* in the value of EBP in improving care quality and patient outcomes. Even so, most of the nurses considered their own knowledge and skills insufficient for employing EBP, and did not believe they were using evidence as a basis for their own practice.

Many reasons can be cited to explain why EBPs are the exception rather than the rule, including limitations created by EBP systems themselves. Some barriers are related to human factors, whereas others are related to the organizations within which nursing care is delivered. Table 1.3 lists some of the common barriers to using evidence as a basis for practice.

Organizations do not commonly have systems in place to support clinicians in the development of EBP tools. Although more resources have become available to practitioners who want to participate in the development of practice guidelines, few operational models exist to guide healthcare organizations that want to implement pervasive EBP (Houser & Oman, 2011). Even when nurses are motivated and competent in the creation and use of EBPs, barriers in the organizational culture may hinder their ability to increase the use of EBP in the workplace (Williams, Perillo, & Brown, 2015). The impact of culture is a strong one; in Williams et al.'s study, nurses reported that their colleagues' lack of support for changing practice was one of the most formidable barriers to EBP. A collaborative workplace where questioning of current practices is encouraged is needed for wide-scale adoption of EBPs, yet it remains the exception rather than the rule.

Table 1.3 Barriers to Using Evidence in Clinical Practice

Limitations in evidence-based practice systems	Overwhelming amount of information in the literature Sometimes contradictory findings in the research
Human factors that create barriers	Lack of knowledge about evidence-based practice Lack of skill in finding and/or appraising research studies Negative attitudes about research and evidence-based care Perception that research is for medicine, not nursing Patient expectations (e.g., demanding antibiotics)
Organizational factors that create barriers	Hierarchical structures that do not encourage autonomous decision making Lack of authority for clinicians to make changes in practice Colleagues' lack of support for practice change Demanding workloads with no time for research activities Conflict in priorities between unit work and research Lack of administrative support or incentives

The complexities of changing practice based on evidence are daunting indeed. Majid and colleagues (2011) studied the barriers to and facilitators of EBP as perceived by more than 2000 nurses in organizational settings. Although the nurses in this study generally held positive views about the value of EBP, they also described several barriers to its implementation:

- Not enough time to keep up with evidence review given their workload
- Lack of adequate training and educational support for appraisal of evidence
- Inability to understand statistical and research terminology
- Inadequate organizational and leadership support
- Lack of access to databases and search strategies

An additional barrier identified in the study by Williams et al. (2015) was the lack of authority to change practices in a hierarchical organization. These researchers found that top-down organizations and those in which nurses had little autonomy were the least likely to have a widespread EBP culture. To implement EBP effectively, nurses must believe that their inputs and ideas are valued, and must perceive that they have a level of power appropriate to enact changes within their practices.

An updated review of the literature from 2010 to 2015 conducted by Mallion and Brooke (2016) yielded more heartening findings. These researchers discovered that the traditional barriers of lack of time, knowledge, and skill continue to affect the wholesale adoption of EBPs, but that nurses' attitudes toward EBP had changed over time. While still acknowledging the difficulty inherent in continuously adopting EBP, the nurses in these studies included in Mallion and Brooke's literature review valued evidence and had positive impressions of their ability to improve practice.

Strategies for Overcoming Barriers

Although little can be done to reduce the complexity of contemporary clinical care, some strategies can be undertaken to improve the rate at which healthcare professionals utilize research as a basis for their practice.

Begin the process by specifically *identifying the facilitators of and barriers to evidence-based practices*. Use of a self-assessment tool such as that tested by Gale and Schaffer (2009) can help identify organizational strengths and limitations in preparation for an EBP effort.

Education and training can improve knowledge and strengthen practitioners' beliefs about the benefits of EBP. Clinicians may fear they will appear to lack competence if they engage in EBP, and greater knowledge will give them confidence in determining an evidence base for their practice.

One of the most helpful—and difficult—strategies is to *create an environment that encourages an inquisitive approach* about clinical care. The first step in identifying opportunities for best practices is questioning current practice. This can be accomplished by creating a culture in which EBPs is valued, supported, and expected, and in which nurses have the authority and autonomy to change practices within their scope of care.

Florczak (2016) has even more basic recommendations for improving research uptake: Nurse researchers, first and foremost, need to conduct studies that are of high quality, especially in terms of sampling methods and controls. Nurses will not be confident about incorporating evidence into practice unless that evidence is strong and convincing. Studies chosen by nurse researchers should focus on outcomes relevant to practice, in which considerations related to patient response, nurse burden, and costs are addressed in addition to effectiveness. Researchers are well advised to collaborate with practitioners and patients in the design of studies and recommendations intended for application to practice.

Despite the barriers inherent in implementing EBP in clinical practice, it is imperative that nurses create structures and processes that reduce these obstacles. Regardless of the system within which the clinician practices, a systematic approach can be employed to find and document the best possible evidence for practice. This process involves defining a clinical question, identifying and appraising the best possible evidence, and drawing conclusions about best practice.

Reading Research for Evidence-Based Practice

Reading research as evidence requires that the professional nurse have a basic understanding of research processes and can apply that understanding to the critical appraisal of individual studies. This systematic process of assessing the reliability, validity, and trustworthiness of studies is explored in detail throughout this text. The appraisal process begins by determining whether the journal, authors, and publication process are credible.

Consider the following key issues when assessing credibility:

- Does the author have the appropriate clinical and educational credentials for the research study? If not, have team members been recruited who have the requisite knowledge and skill? Teams strengthen the results of a research project by providing a diversity of perspectives and enlarging the expertise that is accessible to the team members.
- Is there evidence of a conflict of interest that might introduce bias into the study? For example, does the financial sponsor of the study have something to gain from positive or negative results? Sponsors may unintentionally impose their own expectations on a study and a researcher that may introduce bias into the study. Do the authors have an association with any of the entities in the study? If the authors are employed by an agency being tested in the study, then researcher bias might potentially influence the interpretation of data or the selective reporting of findings.
- Is the journal unbiased? In other words, does the publication have anything to gain by publishing positive or negative results? The publication should have an external editorial board and a cadre of reviewers who are not associated financially with the publication. The names and credentials of the editorial board should be accessible in the publication.
- Has the research study undergone blinded peer review? Blinded peer review enables a critical appraisal of the research study by a neutral party who is not influenced by the stature (or lack of it) of the authors.
- Has the study been published within a reasonable time frame? Health care is characterized by a rapidly changing clinical environment, and studies whose publication is delayed may be outdated before they reach print. Many journals note the date on which a manuscript was received and the length of time until it was reviewed and accepted. This type of notice enables the reader to determine if the information in the study is contemporary or subject to historical effects.

It is sometimes difficult to determine whether a journal is peer reviewed. This policy may be explicitly stated in the front of the journal, but the absence of such a description does not mean the journal is not a scholarly one. The reader may have to scrutinize the front matter of a journal (the masthead and publication information) or a journal webpage to determine the nature of the publication.

The front matter should also include the names of the external editorial board. The existence of an external editorial board means there is objective oversight of the content and quality of material published in the journal. The names of actual reviewers are rarely published, however; the peer review process is more likely a blinded one, meaning that article authors do not know the identity of the manuscript reviewer, and the reviewer does not know the identity of the authors.

If it is not clear whether the journal is peer reviewed, or if an article has been retrieved electronically and the journal's front matter is not available, some hints may indicate whether a journal is a scholarly one. Characteristically, peer-reviewed journal issues are identified by volume and number, and the pages are numbered sequentially through the entire year instead of starting over with each issue. An article published in October, therefore, would likely have page numbers in the hundreds. The first page may also specify the date on which a manuscript was received, reviewed, and subsequently published. This information would confirm that a journal article has been peer reviewed.

The first page of the article should describe the author's credentials and place of employment, along with contact information. Any potential conflicts of interest should be identified here as well. Funding sources for research studies might appear in the credentials section or at the end of the article. Ideally, the journal will also identify any potential conflicts of interest—such as companies owned by the journal's parent company—that might introduce bias into the publication's selection process.

Reading research, much like any nursing skill, becomes easier with practice. As a practicing nurse reads, studies, and engages in research projects, this process becomes more efficient and informative. The process of evaluating research, which may initially require a great deal of focus and effort, eventually becomes second nature. As the appraisal of research becomes part of the nurse's routine, the ability to select studies for application to practice allows the nurse to ensure that his or her practice is based on sound evidence.

Using Research in Evidence-Based Practice

Research is a key EBP. Scientific, rigorous, peer-reviewed studies are the foundation of evidence for professional nursing practice. Selecting, reviewing, and incorporating research findings into practice lie at the heart of professional nursing care delivery; however, EBP does not eliminate the need for professional clinical judgment. The application of a specific EBP guideline to a specific patient situation is based on the nurse's assessment of the situation and an appraisal of the interventions that are most likely to be successful. The clinician remains responsible for combining evidence with clinical expertise and patient values in managing individual patients and achieving optimal outcomes.

Where to Begin?

The process of applying research to EBP begins by identifying a problem that will be best addressed by a review of the evidence. The choice of a subject to study may be driven by a variety of factors. Newell-Stokes (2004) classifies three general categories that may uncover the need for EBP.

The first category includes problem-focused factors. These factors are generally clinical problems that are identified through quality improvement processes, benchmarking studies, regulatory agency feedback, practicing clinicians, or administrative data. For example, a hospital may identify a problem with skin breakdown through nurse observation, quality data indicating an increase in pressure ulcer rates, analysis indicating pressure ulcer rates that are higher than those in comparable hospital units, or data that demonstrate higher costs for patients with skin breakdown.

The second category includes factors related to nursing knowledge. A knowledge deficit may be evident, or new knowledge may emerge through research studies. In addition, a new professional association or new national guideline presents opportunities for incorporating evidence-based changes into practice. A practice change often has a better chance of implementation if users perceive the existence of a solid base of evidence for that practice change. For example, a nurse who attends a national conference may find that hydrotherapy is an evidence-based treatment for pressure ulcers and use the information to motivate a change in nursing practice.

The third category includes factors such as new equipment, technology, or products that become available to the nurse. All of these new developments present opportunities to use evidence in practice to improve outcomes.

Once the need is identified for a change in practice, the way the research is gathered and used may take a variety of forms.

CHECKLIST FOR EVALUATING THE CREDIBILITY OF A RESEARCH ARTICLE

- ❏ The authors have the appropriate clinical and educational credentials for this research study.
- ❏ There is no evidence of any conflict of interest for the authors that might introduce bias into the way the study is designed or the way the results are viewed.
- ❏ There is evidence that this journal is peer reviewed (at least one of these):
  - • Pages are sequentially numbered for the entire year.
  - • Issues are identified by volume and number.
  - • The journal has an external editorial board.
  - • The article indicates a review date.
- ❏ The publication has no financial connection to positive or negative results from the study.
- ❏ The study has been published in a reasonable time frame (i.e., a reasonable interval from the date of study to the date of publication).

Processes for Linking Evidence to Practice

Evidence can be incorporated into practice through several processes. For example, an individual nurse may appraise research studies and share findings with colleagues. Also, a specific question may be answered by reviewing the literature or attending research presentations at conferences.

Although reviewing research studies is a good beginning for establishing evidence for nursing practice, it is possible to introduce bias into the selection of the articles to review. Nurses may consciously or unconsciously select only those articles that support their point of view while ignoring studies that challenge their beliefs. Engaging in a systematic review process will control the potential for such bias to occur. A systematic review process is a structured approach to a comprehensive research review. It begins by establishing objective criteria for finding and selecting research articles, combined with documentation of the rationale for eliminating any study from the review.

Research studies that are selected for inclusion in the review should be subjected to careful and thorough appraisal of study quality and validity. They are graded based on the strength of evidence they provide as well as their design and quality criteria. Several different rating scales may be used to evaluate a research study's strength as evidence, but it is important to recognize that one rating system is not necessarily better than another. Individual values, the nature of the practice question, and the kind of knowledge needed drive the choice of a rating system. Most grading systems include between four and six levels. Table 1.4 depicts a rating system for levels of evidence that is a composite of the work of Armola et al. (2009), Ahrens (2005), and Rice (2008).

Table 1.4 Rating Systems for Grading Levels of Evidence

Level of Rating	Type of Study
Level I	Multiple randomized controlled trials (RCTs) reported as meta-analysis, systematic review, or meta-synthesis, with results that consistently support a specific intervention or treatment
	Randomized trials with large sample sizes and large effect sizes
Level II	Evidence from well-designed controlled studies, either randomized or nonrandomized, with results that consistently support a specific intervention or treatment
Level III	Evidence from studies of intact groups Ex-post-facto and causal-comparative studies Case-control or cohort studies Evidence obtained from time series with and without an intervention Single experimental or quasi-experimental studies with dramatic effect sizes
Level IV	Evidence from integrative reviews Systematic reviews of qualitative or descriptive studies Theory-based evidence and expert opinion Peer-reviewed professional organization standards with supporting clinical studies

Using this scale, for example, a randomized trial of the use of aromatherapy in a post-anesthesia care unit to reduce nausea would be classified as the strongest level of evidence if the findings came from a large study with definitive results or if the results were successfully replicated several times at several sites. The same study conducted in a single setting with a small sample of convenience would provide evidence that was less authoritative. Weaker still would be evidence that was generated through observation or expert opinions.

These strength-of-evidence rating scales apply primarily to the evaluation of treatments, interventions, or the effectiveness of therapies. Recall the definition of EBP: practice based on the best demonstrated evidence combined with clinical experience and patient preferences. The hierarchy of evidence may look quite different depending on the nature of the practice under study.

Review and rating of the evidence should result in recommendations for practice, with the strength of these recommendations being commensurate with the level of evidence and the quality of the study. The link between the strength of the evidence and the strength of the resulting recommendation is the way in which varying levels of evidence are incorporated into a single practice guideline. Table 1.5 depicts the way that the American Academy of Pediatrics (2004) recommends that evidence be linked to a subsequent system of recommendations. Based on the strength of the evidence and the preponderance of benefit or harm, recommendations are generated that are classified as strongly recommended, optional, or recommended. Some evidence results in no recommendation because a conclusion cannot be definitively drawn. Some evidence that shows harm to the patient may result in "not recommended" status.

The systematic review process is complex and time consuming, and should be undertaken only when no other EBP guidelines exist. The effort is warranted, though, when

Table 1.5 The Link Between Evidence and Recommendations for Practice

Type of Evidence	Clear Evidence of Benefit or Harm	Benefit and Harm Are Balanced
Well-designed, randomized controlled trials (RCTs) or reports of multiple RCTs	Strong recommendation for or against the intervention.	Action is optional.
RCTs with limitations of quasi-experimental studies	Recommendation for or against the intervention.	Action is optional.
Observational and descriptive studies, case controls, and cohort designs	Recommendation for or against the intervention.	Action is optional.
Expert opinion, case studies	Action is optional.	No recommendation for or against the intervention.

Reproduced with permission from American Academy of Pediatrics. (2004). American Academy of Pediatrics policy statement: Classifying recommendations for clinical practice guidelines. *Pediatrics, 114,* 874–877. Copyright © 2004 by the AAP.

no clear guidance exists for specific practices, or when the development of a guideline is likely to be affected by practitioner bias.

Creating Evidence for Practice

Nurses commonly serve as the primary investigators in studies that focus on the needs of patients and the effectiveness of nursing interventions. When a nurse conceives of, designs, and implements a research project, he or she is designated as a primary investigator. The primary investigator is responsible for all aspects of a research study's conduct and outcome, even if a team is involved. The primary investigator also has the right to be the first author noted on a research publication.

Designing a research study is an advanced and complex skill that requires experience in the clinical processes under study as well as an understanding of the complexity of research design and analysis. That is not to say that the professional nurse cannot gain the skill and experience needed to be a primary investigator—only that becoming a nurse researcher is an evolutionary process that occurs over time. It is the rare nurse who is able to design and conduct a brilliant study on the first attempt. More commonly, a nurse learns the process by becoming involved in the research of others in some way—either in data collection, through team participation, or even as a subject. Only gradually does he or she gain the ability to conceive of and lead a research project.

Creating nursing research is a systematic, rigorous process. The remainder of this text will guide the nurse as he or she gains the foundation needed to read, use, and create evidence.

Future Directions for Nursing Research

It is clear that nursing research will continue to assume a prominent role in supporting the professional practice of nursing. The future of nursing research is exciting and requires that all nurses accept responsibility for seeking and using evidence as a basis for practice. As part of nursing's future, research will likely evolve into a routine and integral part of the professional nursing practice environment. This requires the engagement of nurses in disciplined inquiry on some level, whether as informed consumers or as primary investigators and team leaders. Nurses must be involved in the promotion of research in support of nursing practices. As such, they must become adept at planning and implementing change in nursing practices. An open mind and adaptability are key characteristics for ensuring adoption of EBPs.

Collaboration with physicians and members of other disciplines in the design and implementation of patient-centered research will continue to elevate nurses to the level expected of all of the health science professions. Participation on a research team encourages other professions to treat nurses as respected colleagues and valued members of the healthcare team.

The future of nursing requires an emphasis on increasing the contribution of research to the knowledge of nursing based on a strategic research agenda. This includes a broadening of the opportunities for dissemination of nursing research findings through research conferences, clinical groups, electronic formats, and publication.

Summary of Key Concepts

- The practice of nursing is founded on nursing knowledge, and nursing knowledge is generated and disseminated through reading, using, and creating nursing research.
- Nursing research is a systematic process of inquiry that uses rigorous, systematic approaches to produce answers to questions and solutions to problems in nursing practice. Research is designed so that it is free of bias and results are trustworthy. The hallmarks of solid, well-respected research are peer review and replication.
- Nurses may use research to synthesize the findings of others, explore and describe phenomena, find solutions to problems, or test traditional approaches for efficacy.
- Research is fundamental to nursing practice because conduct of research is characteristic of a profession and nurses are accountable for the care they deliver. Consumers and external agencies are demanding that healthcare professionals provide evidence for the effectiveness of the interventions they propose and implement.
- Nursing is a relatively young profession, but its practitioners have a proud history of disciplined inquiry. The NINR gives nursing research national stature and financial support and also establishes a national agenda of priorities for nursing research.
- Nurses may fulfill a variety of roles in contemporary nursing research practice, ranging from informed consumers to data collectors to primary investigators. As they become more proficient in nursing research, their roles may broaden and involve projects of increasing complexity.
- Research is not synonymous with problem solving; it is intended to benefit the profession as a whole. A systematic approach and upfront, informed consent of subjects are hallmarks of the research process.
- The benefit of research to nurses lies in its use as evidence for practice. EBP entails the use of the best scientific evidence integrated with clinical experience and incorporating patient values and preferences in the practice of professional nursing care. Numerous types of research are required to accomplish this goal.
- EBP is important in nursing because outcomes are improved, care is more efficient and effective, and errors are reduced when practitioners use evidence as a standard of care. Consumers are also asking for evidence to help them make decisions about their treatment options, and nurses are in a unique position to provide them with appropriate evidence.
- Evidence can be used as a basis for nursing practice in assessing the patient's condition, diagnosing patient problems, planning patient care, evaluating interventions, and evaluating patient responses.
- Barriers to using evidence as a basis for nursing practice may be related to the nature of evidence in practice, individual issues, or organizational constraints. Nurses must identify barriers to the use of evidence in practice and implement strategies to overcome them.
- Translation of research into practice is based on a careful evaluation of the characteristics of a patient population, matched with an assessment of the credibility and **external validity** of studies relative to patient needs.

External validity: The ability to generalize the findings from a research study to other populations, places, and situations.

- Future directions in nursing research include focusing on research as an integral part of nursing practice in a collaborative environment. Collaboration with other healthcare team members in research enhances the value of the profession as a whole and garners respect for its practitioners.

For More Depth and Detail

For a more in-depth look at the concepts in this chapter, try these references:

Bowers, L., Pithouse, A., & Hooton, S. (2012). How to establish evidence-based change in acute care settings. *Mental Health Practice, 16*(4), 22–25.

Fitzsimmons, E., & Cooper, J. (2012). Embedding a culture of evidence-based practice. *Nursing Management, 19*(7), 14–21.

Foster, M., & Shurtz, S. (2013). Making the critical appraisal for summaries of evidence (CASE) for evidence-based medicine: Critical appraisal summaries of evidence. *Journal of the Medical Library Association, 101*(3), 192–198.

Sandstrom, B., Borglin, B., Nilsson, R., & Willman, A. (2011). Promoting the implementation of evidence-based practice: A literature review focusing on the role of nursing leadership. *Worldviews on Evidence-Based Nursing, 4,* 212–225.

Sullivan, D. (2013). A science perspective to guide evidence-based practice. *International Journal of Childbirth Education, 28*(1), 51–56.

Upton, P., Scurlock-Evans, L., Stephens, D., & Upton, D. (2012). The adoption and implementation of evidence-based practice (EBP) among allied health professions. *International Journal of Therapy and Rehabilitation, 19*(9), 497–505.

CRITICAL APPRAISAL EXERCISE

Retrieve the following full-text article from the Cumulative Index to Nursing and Allied Health Literature, or a similar search database:

Ortiz, J., McGilligan, K., & Kelly, P. (2004). Duration of breast milk expression among working mothers enrolled in an employer-sponsored lactation program. *Pediatric Nursing, 30*(2), 111–118.

Review the article, including information about the authors and sponsors of the study. Consider the following appraisal questions in your critical review of this research article:

1. Do the authors have the appropriate clinical and educational credentials for this research study? What are the strengths and weaknesses of this research team?
2. Is there evidence of any conflict of interest that might introduce bias into the way the study is designed or the way the results are viewed? Do the authors have any potential to realize a financial gain from the results of this study?
3. What is the evidence that this journal is peer-reviewed? Find the home page of this journal on the Web. Does the journal have an editorial board?
4. Does the journal have anything to gain by publishing positive or negative results from this study?
5. Is there evidence of bias in the way the study was designed or implemented? If so, how does it affect the nurses' use of these data in the practice setting?
6. Appraise the level of evidence this research study provides the nurse and the strength of the recommendation for practice provided by the results.

References

Ahrens, T. (2005). Evidence-based practice: Priorities and implementation strategies. *AACN Clinical Issues, 16*(1), 36–42.

American Academy of Pediatrics. (2004). Policy statement: Classifying recommendations for clinical practice guidelines. *Pediatrics, 114*(3), 874–877.

American Association of Colleges of Nursing. (2006). AACN position statement on nursing research. Retrieved from http://www.aacn.nche.edu/publications/position/nursing-research

Armola, R., Bourgault, A., Halm, M., Board, R., Bucher, L., Harrington, L., . . . Medina, J. (2009). AACN's levels of evidence: What's new? *Critical Care Nurse, 29*(4), 70–73.

Baker, K., Clark, P., Henderson, D., Wolf, L., Carman, M., Manton, A., & Zavotsky, K. (2014). Identifying the differences between quality improvement, evidence-based practice, and original research. *Journal of Emergency Nursing, 40*(2), 195–198.

Crabtree, E., Brennan, E., Davis, A., & Coyle, A. (2016). Improving patient care through nursing engagement in evidence-based practice. *Worldviews on Evidence-Based Nursing, 13*(2), 172–175.

Deighton, J., Argent, R., Francesco, D., Edbrooke-Childs, J., Jacob, J., Fleming, I., . . . Wolpert, M. (2016). Associations between evidence-based practice and mental health outcomes in child and adolescent mental health services. *Clinical Child Psychology and Psychiatry, 21*(2), 287–296.

Facchiano, L., & Snyder, C. (2012). Evidence-based practice for the busy nurse practitioner: Part one: Relevance to clinical practice and clinical inquiry process. *Journal of the American Academy of Nurse Practitioners, 24,* 579–586.

Florczak, K. (2016). Evidence-based practice: What's new is old. *Nursing Science Quarterly, 29*(2), 108–112.

Gale, B., & Schaffer, M. (2009). Organizational readiness for evidence-based practice. *Journal of Nursing Administration, 39*(2), 91–97.

Gardner, K., Kanaskie, M., Knehans, A., Salisbury, S., Doheny, K., & Schirm, V. (2016). Implementing and sustaining evidence-based practice through a nursing journal club. *Applied Nursing Research, 31,* 139–145.

Houser, J., & Oman, K. (2011). *Evidence-based practice: An implementation guide for healthcare organizations.* Sudbury, MA: Jones & Bartlett Learning.

Institute of Medicine (IOM). (2011). *The future of nursing: Leading change, advancing health.* Prepared by Robert Wood Johnson Foundation Committee Initiative on the Future of Nursing. Washington, DC: National Academies Press.

Lee, M., Johnson, K., Newhouse, R., & Warren, J. (2013). Evidence-based practice process quality assessment: EPQA guidelines. *Worldviews on Evidence-Based Nursing, 10*(3), 140–149.

Leufer, T., & Cleary-Holdforth, J. (2009). Evidence-based practice: Improving patient outcomes. *Nursing Standard, 23*(32), 35–39.

Majid, S., Foo, S., Luyt, B., Zhang, X., Theng, Y., Yun-Ke, C., & Mokhtar, I. (2011). Adopting evidence-based practice in clinical decision-making: Nurses' perceptions, knowledge, and barriers. *Journal of the Medical Library Association, 99*(3), 229–236.

Mallion, J., & Brooke, J. (2016). Community- and hospital-based nurses' implementation of evidence-based practice: Are there any differences? *British Journal of Community Nursing, 21*(3), 148–154.

Markon, M., Crowe, J., & Lemyre, L. (2013). Examining uncertainties in government risk communication: Citizens' expectations. *Health, Risk & Society, 15*(4), 313–332.

Messmer, P., & Turkel, M. (2011). Magnetism and the nursing workforce. In *Annual review of nursing research* (pp. 233–252). New York, NY: Springer.

National Institute of Nursing Research (NINR). (2011). *Bringing science to life: NINR strategic plan.* NIH Publication #11-7783. Bethesda, MD: Author.

National Institute of Nursing Research (NINR). (2013, March). NINR mission and strategic plan. Retrieved from http://www.ninr.nih.gov/aboutninr/ninr-mission-and-strategic-plan#right-content

Newell-Stokes, G. (2004). Applying evidence-based practice: A place to start. *Journal of Infusion Nursing, 27*(6), 381–385.

Oxman, A., Sackett, D., & Guyatt, G. (1993). Users' guides to the medical literature: I. How to get started. *Journal of the American Medical Association, 270,* 2093–2095.

Rice, M. (2008). Evidence-based practice in psychiatric care: Defining levels of evidence. *Journal of the American Psychiatric Nurses Association, 14*(3), 181–187.

Sackett, D., Haynes, R., Guyatt, G., & Tugwell, P. (1991). *Clinical epidemiology: A basic science for clinical medicine* (2nd ed.). Boston, MA: Little, Brown.

Saunders, H., & Julkunen, K. (2016). The state of readiness for evidence-based practice among nurses: an integrative review. *International Journal of Nursing Studies, 56,* 128–140.

Smith, G., & Pell, J. (2006). Parachute use to prevent death and major trauma related to gravitational challenge: Systematic review of randomized controlled trials. *International Journal of Prosthodontics, 19*(2), 126–128.

Summerskill, W., & Pope, C. (2002). An exploratory qualitative study of the barriers to secondary prevention in the management of coronary heart disease. *Family Practitioner, 19,* 605–610.

Williams, B., Perillo, S., & Brown, T. (2015). What are the factors of organizational culture in health care settings that act as barriers to the implementation of evidence-based practice? A scoping review. *Nurse Education Today, 35,* e34–e41.

Wilson, M., Sleutel, M., Newcomb, P., Behan, D., Walsh, J., Wells, J., & Baldwin, K. (2015). Empowering nurses with evidence-based practice environments: Surveying Magnet, Pathway to Excellence, and non-Magnet facilities in one healthcare system. *Worldviews on Evidence-Based Nursing, 12*(1), 12–21.

Chapter 2

The Research Process and Ways of Knowing

© Valentina Razumova/Shutterstock

CHAPTER OBJECTIVES

The study of this chapter will help the learner to

- Discuss the philosophical orientations that influence the choice of a research design.
- Contrast the characteristics of quantitative and qualitative research.
- Review the steps involved in the research process.
- Determine the way that a design is linked to the research question.
- Classify research based on characteristics related to intent, type, and time.
- Evaluate which kind of evidence is best provided by quantitative and qualitative research.

KEY TERMS

Applied research	Longitudinal studies	Qualitative research
Basic research	Mixed methods	Quantitative research
Cross-sectional methods	Paradigm	Quasi-experimental studies
Experimental research	Prospective studies	Retrospective studies

Introduction

What is the nature of truth? It is hard to think of a more difficult question to answer. This fundamental question must be considered, however, to ensure that the research process is successful in providing evidence for practice. Research is about the search for truth. There are, however, multiple approaches to determining and describing truth. The successful researcher understands which approach is effective for the particular problem to be solved. The key is to consider assumptions about the nature of the world, the question to be answered, and the intent of the researcher.

The most fundamental questions to be answered in the beginning of a research process are philosophical but necessary ones: What constitutes knowledge? What is the nature of the world, and how can this research reflect that nature? The researcher should carefully consider these issues before proceeding with the design of the inquiry.

It is a mistake to jump straight from research question to design without considering the philosophical foundation on which the study will be built.

These philosophical considerations must represent more than the researcher's view of the world. That is, they must be carefully matched to a design that will address the specific nature of the research question. The goal is to produce knowledge that is relevant and applicable to the body of nursing knowledge and that becomes evidence for practice.

VOICES FROM THE FIELD

When I started my doctorate, I was sure I wanted to do a straightforward quantitative experiment. I like numbers and statistics, so this kind of study seemed to be a natural extension of my interests. My subject, however, was a bit novel: I was trying to build a comprehensive model to measure inpatient nurse workload. I had always worked in hospitals and used patient acuity systems (systems used to measure the intensity of a patient's care needs) to assess the nursing workload, but a nurse said something that intrigued me: "If all I had to do was take care of my patients, I'd be fine." I set out to find out what all those other demands were, and how they affected the nurse's perception of workload.

I found out just how novel this topic was when I tried to do a literature review and discovered that I could not find any relevant literature. There were lots of opinion articles about measuring workload, and plenty of published quantitative studies focused on patient acuity, but none tried to look at workload holistically. Reluctantly, I concluded that I needed to utilize a mixed-methods design—that is, I needed first to figure out what the forces affecting the nurse's workload were, and then to measure how much impact they had on the nurse's day.

I conducted a series of focus groups with nurses, observed them during their regular workdays, and interviewed quite a few individually. I found that I could describe many nonpatient demands—equipment needed repair, supplies were missing, and other therapists and technicians interrupted patient care. In addition, there were some macro issues at play: Nurses said that strong teams were able to accomplish more work, but weak teams actually created more pressure. All of the nurses mentioned the effects of good leadership on recruitment and retention, and subsequently on the stability of the nursing staff, which helped build teams.

After theme analysis and triangulating the data from my focus groups, observations, and interviews, I developed a model of the demands on a nurse's time. This preparation seemed to take forever, but when I finally began to test the model quantitatively, the work went quickly. I was able to determine the elements that directly affected workload and those that had an indirect effect. I figured out that teamwork, leadership, and retention were central to efficient unit operations. Demonstrating caring, communicating with team members, and entering information into the health record also consumed a lot of time. I discovered that "hunting for things" is a legitimate time drain.

This study was a classic case in which answering the research question required both quantitative and qualitative methods. The qualitative phase helped me determine the fundamental things that frustrate a nurse, and the quantitative phase let me demonstrate whether those influences were real and strong.

Janet Houser, PhD, RN

The Research Process

Regardless of the philosophical assumptions made in a specific study, some characteristics are universal to all research studies. Research by its very nature is systematic and rigorous; it is about a disciplined search for truth. "Systematic" implies that decisions are carefully considered, options weighed, and a rational basis documented to support the choices that are made. Those decisions and choices help form the foundation for and build a research study. They also make up phases of study that are more or less completed in sequence. These phases are depicted in **FIGURE 2.1**:

- *Define a research problem:* Identify a gap in the knowledge of nursing practice that can be effectively addressed with evidence.
- *Scan the literature:* Complete a systematic review of the literature to determine basic knowledge about the problem, so as to identify relevant evidence and a potential theoretical framework.
- *Determine an appropriate design:* Select a design that is appropriate for the philosophical assumption, the nature of the question, the intent of the researcher, and the time dimension.
- *Define a sampling strategy:* Design a sampling plan that details both how subjects will be recruited and assigned to groups, if appropriate, and how many subjects will be needed.
- *Collect data:* Gather the data using appropriate data collection protocols and reliable, valid methods.
- *Analyze data:* Apply analytic techniques that are appropriate for the type of data collected and that will answer the question.
- *Communicate the findings:* Disseminate the findings to the appropriate audiences through conferences and publication.
- *Use the findings to support practice:* Promote the uptake of the research by linking it to specific guidelines for nursing practice.

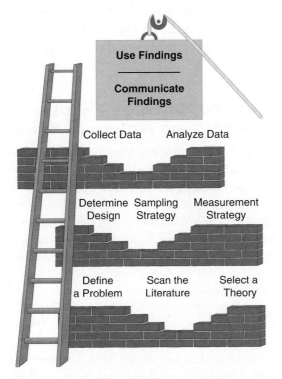

FIGURE 2.1 The Research Process: Building a Study

Paradigm:
An overall belief system or way of viewing the nature of reality and the basis of knowledge.

Quantitative research:
A traditional approach to research in which variables are identified and measured in a reliable and valid way.

These phases may look as if they make up steps, with the end of one phase leading directly to the beginning of another. It is, however, misleading to call the research process a series of steps. Such a description implies that the tasks are done in a particular sequence and that the components are distinct and mutually exclusive. In reality, the design of a research study is a fluid process, one that may be considered a work in progress until the final plan is complete. The process may resemble an elaborate game of Chutes and Ladders more than anything else. In this game, progress is made until the player reaches a chute, which will take the player back to a lower level. In research, several things may happen more or less at the same time—for example, the search for a theoretical framework, the literature review, and construction of the research question. Although the researcher may complete most of these tasks and move on to the design of the study, occasionally a situation will arise that prompts the researcher to reconsider the phrasing of the question, or new literature may be published. As a consequence, the phases may be conducted out of sequence, or the researcher may go back and forth between phases. The phases may overlap, or some phases may not be visited at all. So many varieties of research are possible that any depiction of the research process must come with the caveat that it is a general guide that is adapted to the particular situation at hand.

In quantitative research, decisions are usually finalized before data collection begins, although emergent issues may, even then, require adaptation of the research plan. In contrast, in qualitative research, the research plan is adapted based on both the data generated by the respondents and the nature of those data. Qualitative design decisions may not be completed until the final report is written.

In general, the way the research process emerges and the particular phases that are implemented in a research study are based on many characteristics of both the research problem and the researcher. These characteristics and assumptions lend themselves to several general classifications of research. The choice of an overall research classification is the first step in determining the specifics of a research design.

Classification of Research by Philosophical Assumptions About the Nature of the World

The philosophical assumptions that drive the design of a study are rooted in the paradigms of those who are doing the studying. A **paradigm** is an overall belief system, a view of the world that strives to make sense of the nature of reality and the basis of knowledge. The disciplined study of nursing phenomena is rooted in two broad paradigms, both of which are relevant for nursing research. These two broad paradigms reflect methods that are primarily quantitative (based on the measurement of observable phenomena) or qualitative (based on the analysis of the meaning of events as depicted in the words and actions of others).

Quantitative Research

Quantitative research is the traditional approach to scientific research. It is rooted in the philosophical assumptions of positivism and determinism. Positivism assumes that features of the environment have an objective reality; the world is viewed as something available for study in a more or less unchanging form. A related assumption underlying the scientific method is determinism: a belief that events are not random, but rather have antecedent causes. In the face of these beliefs—the existence of an objective reality, in which events can be linked to an associated cause—the researcher's challenge is to understand the relationships among human phenomena. The task of positivist scientific inquiry, then, is to make unbiased observations of the natural and social world.

Quantitative research involves identifying the variables that represent characteristics of interest and then measuring them in a reliable, valid way. This type of research is characterized by a tightly controlled context that enables the researcher to rule out extraneous effects. Both the way subjects are selected and the protocols for the study are designed to eliminate bias. Statistical analysis is used to establish the level of confidence in the results and to rule out the effects of random error. These conclusions, then, constitute the contribution to scientific knowledge.

There is no doubt that the scientific study of cause and effect in nursing practice is necessary and important for evidence-based practice; quantitative approaches are particularly well suited for answering questions about the nursing actions that can influence outcomes. These studies produce some of the strongest evidence for the benefits of an intervention. Nevertheless, nurses pose many questions that are not adequately addressed by a strict adherence to measurement of an objective reality. In turn, the single adherence to a positivist view has drawn considerable criticism from nurse researchers, and many of these criticisms are legitimate. The nature of nursing care involves helping others attain their health goals, many of which are defined by the individual, not the nurse. Perceptions of quality of life, the meaning of a life event, and the willingness to endure side effects for a therapeutic result are all based on the patient's construction of reality, not the nurse's perceptions. In turn, many related questions are better addressed with a process of naturalistic inquiry.

Qualitative research:
A naturalistic approach to research in which the focus is on understanding the meaning of an experience from the individual's perspective.

Qualitative Research

Qualitative research is based on a naturalistic paradigm. This belief system is represented by a view of reality that is constructed by the individual, not the researcher. In the naturalistic view, reality is not a fixed entity, but rather exists in the context of what the research participant believes it to be. Qualitative researchers believe that many different views of reality are possible, and all of them are right. An associated belief for the naturalistic researcher is relativism, or the belief that there are always multiple interpretations of reality, and that these interpretations can exist only within an individual. The qualitative researcher, then, believes there is no process in which the ultimate basis for a singular truth can be identified.

Qualitative methods focus on an understanding of the meaning of an experience from the individual's perspective. Extended observation of participants, in-depth interviews or focus groups, case studies, and studies of social interaction are examples of qualitative methods. The inquiry process focuses on verbal descriptions and observable behaviors as a basis for analysis and conclusions.

Qualitative methods are appropriate for addressing questions in which the meaning of the patient's experience is central to understanding the best therapeutic approach. Issues of behavior change, motivation, compliance with a regimen, and tolerance of a treatment are all examples of topics in which the patient's perception is central to assisting the patient to a healthy state. The analysis of themes that describe the meaning of the experience for the patient is based on words and observations, rather than on measurable phenomena. The researcher establishes a relationship with the subject, and bias is considered an inherent part of the research process. The findings from qualitative studies are used to enhance evidence-based practice by incorporating the patient's preferences and values into guides for nursing practice.

The differences in philosophy, roles, and methods between quantitative and qualitative research are depicted in **Table 2.1**. These contrasts are made to help the student understand the variations between these two overall approaches. In reality, both types of research have many characteristics in common:

- A disciplined, rigorous approach based on external evidence
- Methods that require samples and the cooperation of individuals
- A focus on the rights of human subjects and ethical guidelines
- An ultimate aim of discovering new knowledge that can be used to improve nursing practice

Table 2.1 Quantitative Versus Qualitative Characteristics

Element	Quantitative	Qualitative
View of reality	Reality is objective and can be seen and measured.	Reality is constructed by the individual.
View of time	Reality is relatively constant.	Reality is continuously constructed.
Context	Reality can be separated from its context.	Reality is embedded in its context.
Researcher approach	Objective, detached.	Personally involved.
Populations studied	Samples that represent overall populations as subjects.	Individual cases, represented as informants.
Measures	Human behavior or other observable phenomena.	Study the meanings that individuals create.
Observations	Analyze reality as definable variables.	Make holistic observations of the total context.
Design	Preconceived and highly controlled.	Emergent and fluid, adaptable to informants' views.
Analysis	Descriptive and inferential statistics.	Analytic induction to determine meaning.
Generalization	Use inference to generalize from a sample to a defined population.	Transfer knowledge from case analysis to similar cases.
Reports	Objective, impersonal reports in which the researcher's opinions are undetectable.	Interpretive reports that reflect the researcher's reconstruction of the meaning of the data.

Many nurse researchers assume they must select only one approach and carry out the study in a pure and inflexible way. In fact, it is the rare study that relies on just one approach or the other. The choices made in research design are probably less about a solely qualitative approach versus a solely quantitative approach, and more about selection from a continuum of choices that may overlap from one approach to the other. Many quantitative studies involve asking the subjects to respond to questions or give opinions in which the participants' words are later analyzed to enhance the statistical findings. Experimental researchers may rate subject behaviors using scales that contain subjective elements, or they may record their own observations of behaviors. Conversely, many qualitative studies use measurement to determine the reliability of multiple raters in determining themes and to verify the trustworthiness of conclusions. A basic qualitative validation method is triangulation, or the search for multiple sources to confirm the same finding, in which numbers are often retrieved to confirm verbal data. There are many situations in which a blend of methods is appropriate, and these mixed methods designs are becoming more common.

Mixed methods:
A research approach that combines quantitative and qualitative elements; it involves the description of the measurable state of a phenomenon and the individual's subjective response to it.

Mixed Methods

Mixed methods are becoming an important tool in nursing research, particularly in evaluation research. Evaluation research is the application of research methods to the study of programs, projects, or phenomena. Increasingly, the question is not whether mixed methods are appropriate, but rather how they should be used.

Mixed-method designs can provide pragmatic advantages when exploring novel or complex nursing problems (McCusker & Gunaydin, 2015). The qualitative data provide a deep understanding of the human experience, while the quantitative data enable the researcher to identify and measure relationships. Research that draws on the strengths of both paradigms is increasingly recognized as essential in all fields—including in medicine, where it is needed to support effective patient care guidelines.

Mixed methods are often applied in an ad hoc way, meaning the researcher initiates the study by using a primarily quantitative or qualitative method, and then integrates elements of the alternative approach as an afterthought. The most effective use of mixed methods, however, occurs when they are employed in a systematic way (Kettles, Creswell, & Zhange, 2011). Mixed methods are commonly used in descriptive studies, where they may be used to describe both the measurable state of a phenomenon and the individual responses to it. For example, mixed methods might be used for the following purposes:

- Describe the rate of hand washing on a nursing unit (quantitative) as well as the nurses' perceptions about the importance of hand washing (qualitative)
- Measure the presence of bacteria on a nurse's hands after washing (quantitative) and observe the hand-washing steps the nurse used (qualitative)
- Count the number of times a nurse washed his or her hands between patients (quantitative) and record the nurse's report on the convenience of hand-washing facilities (qualitative)

Choosing a Design

Many considerations go into the choice of a general approach to research design. The philosophical orientation of the researcher is just one element. The nature of the research question, the skills and abilities of the researcher, and access to resources and samples all are important elements to consider prior to choosing the research methodology.

Of primary importance to the selection of an approach is the nature of the research question. Research questions that focus on the effectiveness of an intervention require a scientific approach (assuming effectiveness is defined as an objectively measured outcome). For example, the effectiveness of a skin-care regimen in preventing pressure ulcers is best studied by applying the proposed regimen to one group of patients, applying a standard regimen to another group of patients, and then measuring the rate of pressure ulcer development in both groups. If the regimen is effective, then the subjects getting the new regimen will have a lower pressure ulcer rate than those with the standard regimen. This is the traditional experiment, and it is still one of the most common research designs in health care.

In contrast, research questions that focus on the acceptability of an intervention may require a qualitative approach. The new regimen may be effective, but it may be painful, have an unpleasant smell, or consist of a cream that sticks to clothing. Assessment of these attributes, which will almost certainly affect whether a patient complies with the skin-care regimen, requires asking the patients about their preferences for the treatment and whether the outcome outweighs the unpleasant side effects.

Some of the considerations when choosing an approach are researcher driven. Many researchers have a personal preference for one approach over another. When the research question may be answered in several different ways, or when various aspects of a phenomenon require study before evidence can be deduced, then the researcher's personal preference may drive the selection of an approach. The skills that are required for quantitative research include the capacity to define variables, recruit subjects, use random assignment methods, create reliable and valid measurements, and analyze results with statistical techniques. The skills that are required for qualitative researchers are quite different. They include the ability to find and select those subjects who can best inform the question, observe and record actions and interactions in detail, skillfully interview subjects or focus groups, and distill

GRAY MATTER

Consider the following elements prior to choosing a research design:
- Philosophical orientation of the researcher
- Nature of the research question or problem
- Skills, abilities, and preferences of the researcher
- Resources and sample access

GRAY MATTER

The following skills are required for quantitative research:
- Defining variables
- Recruiting subjects
- Using random assignment methods
- Creating reliable and valid measurements
- Analyzing results with statistical techniques

GRAY MATTER

The following skills are required for qualitative research:
- Finding and selecting subjects appropriate for the question
- Observing and recording actions and interactions in detail
- Interviewing subjects skillfully
- Distilling meaning from large amounts of word-based data

meaning from large amounts of word-based data. Both skill sets can require years to develop and hone. It is natural, then, that most researchers find themselves specializing in one approach or the other.

A host of practical considerations must be addressed when selecting an approach. Quantitative methods require measurement tools, subjects who are willing to undergo experimental treatments (or the risk of no treatment), statistical software, and access to individuals knowledgeable in statistical analysis and interpretation. Qualitative methods need less in the way of tools and software, but they require informants who are willing to be observed or interviewed, often for extended periods of time. The particular individuals who are accessible as well as the material resources required may drive the selection of a feasible research approach.

Theoretical considerations may also influence the selection of a specific design. The researcher may start the design process by deciding which concepts are of interest. The way these concepts interact with each other and create a framework is called a theory. Theoretical models are commonly tested with both quantitative and qualitative designs, and they provide a roadmap for future research. Theoretical and conceptual frameworks are the necessary backbone of a research study. Using a well-founded and well-referenced framework lends credence to the study, but, even more importantly, allows for comparisons across studies as well as building from or between studies. Basing a study on a sound theoretical framework is one way to ensure the research will be systematically designed.

Basic research:
Theoretical, pure, fundamental, or bench research done to advance knowledge in a given subject area.

Applied research:
Research conducted to gain knowledge that has a practical application and contributes in some way to a modification of practice.

A Note About Using Theoretical Frameworks in Nursing Research

Theory is an attempt to explain the world around us. Nurses become part of the world of health care through an understanding of theories about nursing, which attempt to explain why nurses do what they do. Nursing care is a complex process, and explanations of human actions and interactions can be complicated and difficult to understand without a road map. Theory is a method of mapping these complex processes of human action and interaction that affect patient care and understanding their interrelationship.

The word *theory* comes from the Greek *theoria,* which means "vision." Nurse scientists use theories to explain their visions of reality. Theories are not facts; instead, they are methods of posing what might be reality. Just as there are many visions of reality, so there are many theories that attempt to explain that reality. These theories often form the basis for research studies, in that many aspects of a conceptual model might potentially be the subject of study.

Nurse researchers also use theory as a *framework* for their studies. Developing a conceptual foundation involves a series of steps that focus on the selection and definition of concepts, concept analysis, relational statements, and conceptual models of action and interaction. In this way, theoretical frameworks form the backbone of a research study. Using a strong framework lends credence to the study's results, but more importantly allows for the replication of the study and the synthesis of its outcomes into guidelines.

Myriad thoughtful decisions must be made to choose the right approach for a particular research problem. The key word is *thoughtful.* These decisions should be based on a sound rationale, and the researcher should be able to articulate the basis for these decisions.

Classifications of Research by the Intent of the Researcher

Research is classified by the basic belief system that drives its design features, but it must also reflect the intent of the researcher. There are two kinds of goals for research: (1) to provide new knowledge for the foundation of nursing and (2) to provide knowledge that can be immediately applied to the practice of nursing. The first of these is referred to as *basic research*; the latter is termed *applied research.*

Basic research is commonly referred to as theoretical, pure, fundamental, or bench research. One might think of the work done by scientists in laboratories as basic research. It is used to test theories and to build the body of knowledge that forms the foundation for practice, but it does not directly apply to the practice setting. Examples of basic research include measuring neuromuscular responses to stimuli and studying the effects of circulatory volume on neonatal cardiac function.

Applied research is undertaken with the single goal of improving nursing practice. The findings from such research are intended to contribute in some way to a modification of nursing practice. Examples of applied research include investigating the effects of topical drugs on phlebitis and determining the efficacy of specific counseling techniques after the death of a spouse.

Both basic and applied research may be conducted by using quantitative, qualitative, or mixed methods. Most clinical nursing research is considered applied research, and the findings that are generated as evidence for practice are exclusively of an applied nature. This is not to imply that basic research is not valuable. Indeed, one must have a clear understanding of the underlying theoretical and physiological basis for a given nursing practice to understand its mechanisms of effect.

Classifications of Research by the Nature of the Design

Another classification of research is associated with the nature of the design. Experimental research refers to studies of cause and effect, which are usually undertaken to determine the effectiveness of an intervention. In an experimental design, some type of randomization method is employed to select subjects or assign them to groups according to how well they represent the population of interest. The researcher manipulates some aspect of the patient's treatment in a highly controlled setting and compares the outcomes to those for a group that has received no treatment or a standard treatment. If the outcomes are different, the researcher assumes the difference is a result of the treatment because all other variables have been controlled. Experimental designs are characterized by highly structured protocols for sample selection and assignment, intervention, measurement, and analysis. Such designs aim to eliminate bias and control for rival explanations for the outcome.

Nonexperimental designs cover a broad range of studies that do not share these characteristics and, therefore, cannot test cause and effect. Quasi-experimental studies mimic experimental designs in most ways except for the selection and assignment of subjects. Such studies often use convenience samples or existing groups to test interventions. For example, a quasi-experimental study might test an intervention by selecting populations in two different nursing homes, where one group gets the treatment and the other does not. However, subjects are not assigned to the nursing homes randomly.

Other nonexperimental designs include descriptive research, correlation research, and predictive research. *Descriptive* research involves the study of a particular situation or event that already exists. The researcher does not manipulate any variables, although the study itself is systematic and thorough. *Correlation* research focuses on the existing relationships between variables. Such a study might, for example, search for a relationship between a single variable in two populations (e.g., do teens with mothers who had teen pregnancies have a higher teen pregnancy rate themselves?). Correlation studies might also search for relationships between two variables in the same sample (e.g., do overweight teens have higher pregnancy rates?). *Predictive* research takes the correlation aspect one step further, searching for relationships in which the values of one variable can be used to predict the values of another (e.g., do certain family characteristics predict the risk of a teen pregnancy?). Predictive research is particularly helpful in public health studies and research involving the determination of whether a risk factor will lead to a particular health condition.

Experimental research: Highly structured studies of cause and effect, usually applied to determine the effectiveness of an intervention. Subjects are selected and randomly assigned to groups to represent the population of interest.

Quasi-experimental studies: Studies of cause and effect similar to experimental design but using convenience samples or existing groups to test interventions.

Classifications of Research by the Time Dimension

Retrospective studies:
Studies conducted using data that have already been collected about events that have already happened. Such secondary data were originally collected for a purpose other than the current research.

A final classification of research studies is by the time dimension chosen for the studies. These investigations may focus on the past or the future, referred to as retrospective and prospective studies, respectively.

Retrospective studies are conducted using data that have already been collected about events that have already happened. For nursing research, these data often come from chart review. In such a study, the researcher is unable to control most aspects of variable definition and data collection because those steps were performed before the study was conceived. The researcher conducting a retrospective study relies on the accuracy and completeness of these secondary data, or data that were originally collected for a purpose other than the research study. For example, a nurse might conduct a retrospective study to determine differences in the rate of ventilator-associated pneumonia between patients who received oral care every 4 hours and those who did not. The diagnosis of ventilator-associated pneumonia and the timing of oral care could both be retrieved from patient charts—a convenient source of reliable data. However, in this case, the nurse researcher is dependent upon the staff nurses' documentation of the timing and extent of oral care. If the chart does not have a record of oral care in a 4-hour period, is it because such care was not provided or because it was not recorded? If oral care is recorded, was the care rendered according to current standards? The nurse researcher must balance the convenience of secondary data with the risks of inaccuracy and incompleteness of the data set.

Prospective studies:
Studies planned by the researcher for collection of primary data for the specific study and implemented in the future.

Prospective studies are those conducted by the researcher. This approach enables the researcher to control most aspects of research design and implementation, and primary data are collected (that is, data are collected by the researcher directly from subjects for the specific study at hand). Prospective studies are generally more reliable than retrospective studies due to the greater control afforded to the researcher. For example, a nurse might conduct a prospective study of oral care and ventilator-associated pneumonia by experimenting with different time periods, methods, or durations of oral care and measuring the rate of ventilator-associated pneumonia in the patients participating in the study. In this case, the procedures can be highly controlled and the outcomes reliably measured and recorded accurately. Such a study would be difficult to design and carry out, however, because of the need to address ethical questions, sampling challenges, and substantial time demands. The accuracy and completeness of data would be realized at the expense of considerable complexity and effort.

Longitudinal studies:
Studies conducted by following subjects over a period of time, with data collection occurring at prescribed intervals.

Studies may also be characterized based on whether they are conducted over time or at a single point in time. Such studies are referred to as longitudinal and cross-sectional studies, respectively.

Longitudinal studies are conducted over time—often very long time periods—to study the emergence of disease or the long-term effects of treatments. Subjects are followed over a period of time, with data collection occurring at prescribed intervals during that period. An advantage of longitudinal studies is their ability to determine the effects of risk factors or interventions over time. A disadvantage is the potential for attrition as subjects are lost to the study over its duration. There may also be effects from the act of repeatedly measuring the same individuals over time. An example of a longitudinal study would be monitoring the children of smokers over time to measure the emergence of pulmonary disease.

Cross-sectional methods focus on collecting data at a single point in time. No follow-up is intended or built into the design. The result is a comprehensive picture of the existence of a phenomenon in the present, without concern for how it will look in the future. Cross-sectional methods often examine a single phenomenon across multiple populations at a single point in time. These methods have the advantage that they are completed in a limited amount of time and may yield valuable information about how different populations respond to the same disease or treatment. Their primary disadvantage is that the effects of time are not evaluated and cannot be analyzed. An example of a cross-sectional study would be determining the prevalence and distribution of pulmonary diseases in a sample of children who have a parent smoker in the home at a given point in time.

Longitudinal and cross-sectional studies are frequently used in public health and epidemiology to study the distribution and determinants of disease over time or across populations. These methods can also be used in nursing research to study the effects of risk factors, interventions, or nursing practice changes as they unfold at different times and for different people.

> **Cross-sectional methods:**
> Studies conducted by looking at a single phenomenon across multiple populations at a single point in time, with no intention for follow-up in the design.

Reading Research for Evidence-Based Practice

Although it is relatively easy to categorize research by its approach, type, time dimension, and other distinctions in a research textbook, in reality these distinctions are not quite so tidy or clear-cut. Reading a research study while trying to classify its characteristics often results in frustration. Just as the research process must be viewed as a fluid process that articulates decisions made on a continuum, so reading a research study challenges the nurse not to determine whether the right design has been selected, but whether the researcher has made the right choices.

Often, in the introduction of a study, qualitative researchers will make explicit their reasons for choosing a particular design. In general, a qualitative study will state that it is a qualitative approach somewhere in the abstract, introduction, or initial methods sections. This is not usually the case with quantitative research. Instead, it is often up to the reader to determine the specific decisions the researcher made and to try to deduce the reasoning behind those decisions.

The reader can pick up some hints early in the abstract and the methods section that will provide clues about the time dimension of the study. Comments about the use of "secondary data" or "using data collected for another study" will indicate the study is retrospective. In this case, the critical reader should be looking for evidence that the researchers accounted for the lack of accuracy and specificity that accompanies retrospective studies, or at least acknowledged its existence. Researchers will rarely identify primary data explicitly as such, but the inclusion of an intervention protocol or a measurement procedure indicates that the data were prospectively gathered.

It is usually relatively easy to determine whether a study is longitudinal or cross-sectional. The reader can look for measures that were collected repeatedly on the same individuals as a clue that a study is longitudinal. The researcher might use terms such as *paired sample, dependent data,* or *repeated measures* to indicate that data were collected over time from the same subjects. If it is clear that data were collected once from individuals at a single point in time, then the study is a cross-sectional one.

It is important to categorize the type of study before using it as evidence. The hierarchy of evidence encompasses a variety of research designs, but the connection to the strength of a practice recommendation is based, to a great extent, on the type of study. Listed here are some of the points to appraise when reading a research study to determine whether the authors used the appropriate approach:

- Does the research question match the specific approach that was chosen?
- If an intervention was tested, was a quantitative approach used?
- If patient preferences and values were assessed, was a qualitative method or a mixed method used?
- Does the researcher articulate a rationale for decisions about the research approach?
- Does the author provide logical reasoning for the specific design selected? If not, can it be deduced from the characteristics of the study?

The initial review of a research study for its approach, type, and time dimension is useful in determining the level of evidence that its findings represent. This assessment ensures that the nurse will use the research results appropriately in supporting evidence-based nursing practice.

Using Research in Evidence-Based Practice

Although it would seem obvious that applied research is the most helpful for evidence-based practice, basic research may also be used for this purpose. The hierarchy of evidence considers basic research about physiology and pathophysiology to be legitimate considerations in making practice decisions, on par with professional expert opinion and descriptive research. When developing a research-based practice guideline, a good starting place is a basic foundation of the existing knowledge about the physiological and psychological forces that may be in play in a given nursing practice situation.

The results of both quantitative and qualitative research are useful in evidence-based practice. Although randomized controlled trials (experimental designs)—both singularly and in aggregate—clearly provide the strongest evidence for practice, they do not provide the only evidence for practice. Well-designed quasi-experimental, descriptive, correlation, and predictive designs can provide evidence that can be used to determine whether an action can be designated as recommended, optional, or not recommended.

Qualitative and mixed methods are primarily useful in determining the preferences and values of the patient. They may, however, be used to theorize which interventions might be effective, particularly when little research is found or when the research topic deals with behavioral, psychological, or spiritual issues. Exploratory studies often give rise to theories that subsequently can be tested with quantitative methods, improving on the evidence for practice. The best practice guidelines are those that incorporate a variety of research studies and methods into a single guideline so the needs of patients can be addressed in a comprehensive, evidence-based manner.

Creating Evidence for Practice

Given all these approaches, types, and dimensions of research, outlining a specific research study may seem daunting. A systematic approach to making the decisions that are required, however, helps narrow the choices relatively quickly and makes the process a manageable one. Using criteria for each step in the decision-making and design process can help ensure that the right choices are made for the right reasons.

Criteria for Selecting an Approach

The primary consideration when selecting an approach is ensuring a match between the problem and the approach chosen to provide a solution. If the question is one that relates to the effectiveness of an intervention, identifies factors that influence a patient's outcome, or finds the best predictors for a patient's condition, then clearly a quantitative approach is needed. If the problem is one that requires an in-depth understanding of the patient's experience and the meaning of a phenomenon, then qualitative research is required. Either approach may be used for exploratory research or when there is little existing research. However, a qualitative or descriptive study is often a good way to start an exploration of a phenomenon for which little or no existing literature is available.

Mixed methods are the best way to capture the outcomes of both approaches. Mixed methods are complex, however, and require that the researcher have a command of both quantitative and qualitative research skills. It is rare that a novice researcher would undertake a mixed-method study to address a single problem. Instead, mixed methods are often reserved for evaluation of complex issues or for developing and testing models of action and interaction.

A careful self-assessment of personal experiences and abilities will also help the researcher arrive at a feasible study method. Time devoted to reflection about one's propensity toward quantitative or qualitative methods is time well spent in preparing for a research study. Using a method that is not compatible with the researcher's nature can be frustrating and result in poorly executed research. If a researcher knows that a particular approach is difficult for him or her to apply, then the nurse may want to join a research team to learn more about the process and to gain the mentorship and support that comes from individuals who are competent in and passionate about the approach. A pragmatic self-assessment of available time, software, resources, and competency is also useful before arriving at a conclusion about a study design.

Finally, the nurse researcher should consider the expectations of the audience he or she is trying to reach. That audience may include fellow nurses, healthcare team members, or administrators. The nurse researcher would also do well to consider other audiences that must be addressed to communicate the results effectively, such as journal editors, conference attendees, graduate committees, or professors. The needs and interests of these audiences may be as important as those of fellow practitioners when it comes to ensuring that the research results are communicated broadly enough to be used in practice.

Summary of Key Concepts

- Research is about the search for truth, but there are multiple ways to determine and describe truth. The key to a successful research process is to understand which approach is appropriate for the particular problem to be solved.
- The research process is a fluid, dynamic one that includes multiple processes. These processes may occur in sequence, or they may overlap; some phases may even be skipped. The phases in the research process include defining the research problem, scanning the literature, selecting a theoretical framework, determining an appropriate design, defining a sampling strategy, collecting and analyzing data, communicating the findings, and using the findings to support practice.
- Philosophical assumptions drive the fundamental design of a study and are rooted in the paradigms of quantitative or qualitative methods. Quantitative studies employ measurement to produce an objective representation of relationships and effects. Qualitative studies use verbal reports and observations to arrive at an interpretation of the meaning of a phenomenon.
- Mixed methods may involve elements of both quantitative and qualitative research, but the standards for both approaches must be met. Mixed methods are most effective for evaluation research and for developing and testing models of action and interaction.
- A design should be chosen based on the nature of the research question and the preferences and skills of the researcher, as well as practical considerations such as access to subjects, software, and other resources.
- Research can be classified by the intent of the researcher. Basic research reflects an intent to contribute to the fundamental body of knowledge that is nursing. Applied research reflects the sole intention of providing evidence that can be directly applied to the practice of nursing.
- The nature of research design can be categorized as experimental or nonexperimental. Experimental designs are highly controlled, with a goal of testing cause and effect. Nonexperimental designs can be descriptive, correlative, or predictive. Both types of designs provide evidence for nursing practice, but the recommendations from experimental designs are considered stronger.
- Research can be categorized by its time dimension as retrospective or prospective. Retrospective studies use secondary data that have already been collected. Prospective studies use real-time processes to collect primary data explicitly for the study.
- Studies can also be classified as longitudinal or cross-sectional. Longitudinal studies measure some aspect of the same subjects over time, whereas cross-sectional studies measure a characteristic from multiple populations at a single point in time.

For More Depth and Detail

For a more in-depth look at the concepts in this chapter, try these references:

Creswell, J. (2013). *Research design: Qualitative, quantitative, and mixed methods approaches.* Thousand Oaks, CA: Sage.

Lee, S., & Smith, C. (2012). Criteria for quantitative and qualitative data integration: Mixed methods research methodology. *CIN: Computers, Informatics, Nursing, 30*(5), 251–256.

Merriam, S., & Tisdell, E. (2015). *Qualitative research: A guide to design and implementation* (4th ed.). San Francisco, CA: Jossey-Bass.

Patton, M. (2014). *Qualitative research and evaluation methods: Integrating theory and practice.* Thousand Oaks, CA: Sage.

Perreault, K. (2011). Research design: Qualitative, quantitative, and mixed methods approaches. *Manual Therapy, 16*(1), 103.

Vogt, W., Gardner, D., & Haeffele, L. (2012). *When to use what research design.* New York, NY: Guilford Press.

Walsh, K. (2011). Quantitative vs qualitative research: A false dichotomy. *Journal of Research in Nursing, 17*(1), 9–11.

CRITICAL **APPRAISAL EXERCISE**

Retrieve the following full-text article from the Cumulative Index to Nursing and Allied Health Literature or similar search database:

Kolehmainen, N., Ransay, C., McKee, L., Missiuna, C., Owen, C., & Francis. J. (2015). Participation in physical play and leisure in children with motor impairments: Mixed-methods study to generate evidence for developing an intervention. *Physical Therapy, 95*(10), 1374–1386.

Review the article, focusing on the design of the study. Consider the following appraisal questions in your critical review of this research article:

1. What is the author's rationale for using mixed methods for the study of this subject?
2. Discuss the link between the purpose of the study and this specific design.
3. Classify this study with respect to each of the following dimensions:
   a. The intent of the researcher
   b. The type of study
   c. The time dimension of the study
4. Which characteristics did this study possess that were quantitative in nature?
5. Which characteristics did this study possess that were qualitative in nature?
6. Describe the reasons you think a mixed-methods approach was the most appropriate for this population and research goals.

References

Kettles, A., Creswell, J., & Zhange, W. (2011). Mixed methods research in mental health nursing. *Journal of Psychiatric and Mental Health Nursing, 18*, 535–542.

McCusker, K., & Gunaydin, S. (2015). Research using qualitative, quantitative or mixed methods and choice based on the research. *Perfusion, 30*(7), 537–542.

Chapter 3

Ethical and Legal Considerations in Research

CHAPTER OBJECTIVES

The study of this chapter will help the learner to

- Describe fundamental ethical concepts applicable to human subjects research.
- Discuss the historical development of ethical issues in research.
- Describe the components of valid informed consent.
- Identify the features of populations that make them vulnerable in a research context.
- Discuss statutes and regulations related to conducting clinical research.
- Describe the history, functions, and processes related to the institutional review board.
- Identify the three levels of review conducted by institutional review boards.
- Relate protections for human subjects to guidelines for animal welfare in research.
- Discuss the major provisions of the privacy rule (HIPAA) that affect data collection for research.

KEY TERMS

A priori

Beneficence

Ethics

Exempt review

Expedited review

Full disclosure

Full review

Health Insurance Portability and
    Accountability Act (HIPAA)

Informed consent

Institutional review board (IRB)

Justice

Nontherapeutic research

Respect for persons

Right of privacy

Therapeutic research

Vulnerable populations

Introduction

Ethics is the study of right and wrong. It explores what one might do when confronted with a situation where values, rights, personal beliefs, or societal norms may be in conflict. In everyday life, we are often faced with ethical situations when we must ask a key question: What is the right thing to do in this particular situation?

Ethics:
A type of philosophy that studies right and wrong.

Ethical considerations tell us *how* we should conduct research. These directives for the ethical conduct of nursing research are guided by the researcher's integrity and applied through personal decision making. Legal guidelines, in contrast, tell us how we are *required* to conduct research. These guidelines are found in laws and regulations that are provided by agencies external to the nurse researcher. Ethics and legal considerations are often inextricably intertwined. In the end, it does not matter if an ethical guideline or a legal regulation provides guidance to the nurse researcher: They are equally important for quality research.

Researchers face ethical and legal situations in almost every step of the research process, from selecting participants to collecting data to reporting findings at the conclusion of the study. The ethics of human subjects research and international and federal control over such research, however, have evolved since the mid-twentieth century. Professional organizations and international associations alike have developed codes of ethics that apply to research involving human subjects. In this chapter, the ethical foundation of research is examined, considering both recent and remote examples of scientific transgressions that helped form current research practices. What society has legislatively imposed in the context of research regulation is discussed as well.

Learning from the Past, Protecting the Future

When humans participate as subjects in research studies, care must be taken to preserve their rights: their right to be informed of the study process and potential risks, their right to be treated in a fair and transparent manner, and their right to withdraw from a study at any time for any reason without question or negative consequences (Franklin, Rowland, Fox, & Nicolson, 2012).

Unfortunately, breaches of ethical conduct have a long history. In the aftermath of World War II, disclosure of Nazi experimentation on prison camp detainees revealed the need for consideration of basic human rights in research involving human subjects. In the United States, the revelation of the deception and nontreatment of men of color with syphilis during the Tuskegee syphilis study (1932–1972) led to long-lasting mistrust of the medical research community, and has limited researchers' ability to recruit diverse populations for medical studies. The Willowbrook Study (1963–1966) engendered particular outrage because its subjects were mentally handicapped children; it led to improved protections for children and other vulnerable populations within the research context. Unfortunately, ethical breaches are not solely of historical interest: The Gelsinger case at the University of Pennsylvania and the Roche case at Johns Hopkins Asthma and Allergy Center occurred long after healthcare organizations had enacted standards for ethics in research. These cases (discussed later in this chapter) illuminate the fact that any research involving human subjects always requires careful consideration of the rights of those subjects.

Although the primary investigators for these research activities were physicians, evidence suggests that nurses were aware of deceit in recruitment and delivery of nontherapeutic treatment, at least during the Tuskegee syphilis study. Why are these events historically important to nurses? Reflection and careful thought about the roles of nurses in research—from observer to data collector to principal investigator—and the responsibility nurses have to humankind mandate that we learn from the past and, in doing so, protect the future.

VOICES FROM THE FIELD

As soon as I identify an idea for a research project, I start thinking about the legal implications of this study or how this study will look in the eyes of our institutional review board (IRB). When I was a novice researcher, the IRB seemed like a big hurdle to overcome. Now that I am an experienced researcher, I view it as a significant asset to the research process.

The IRB is made up of a wide variety of professionals who evaluate a study from their area of expertise. There is a lot of research experience on the IRB. Its members pay particular attention to the risks and benefits of each study, and it is clear their focus is on protecting the rights of subjects. But they can also give you excellent advice and suggestions to make your study stronger and ensure it is ethical. They also give good feedback about the soundness of the overall study design and the ability of the study team to perform this particular research.

This became very clear to me when I had to consider the legal implications of a recent study that I helped design. The study itself seemed quite benign. The research question was, "Do two 15-minute foot massages done on two consecutive days decrease anxiety in inpatient cancer patients?" We chose to answer this question using a randomized controlled trial (RCT) study design. The two co-primary investigators (PIs) were bedside nurses on our inpatient cancer unit who cared deeply about their patients and wanted to do a study on ways to help lessen the stress of being hospitalized. The study team included an oncologist who was also the chief of oncology services, several clinical nurse specialists, the unit director, an experienced massage therapist, and me in my role as medical epidemiologist and nurse researcher. As a team, we designed a study that we felt adequately addressed our study question.

The IRB saw it differently. They were concerned that we had not adequately addressed the risks of a foot massage; although rare, they still needed to be expressed in both the protocol and the consent process. We needed to inform potential subjects that there was a risk of dislodging a clot, causing severe pain or discomfort, or irritating or damaging the skin. Further, the board suggested that our control group (no massage) would be a better comparison group if we offered some type of therapeutic nurse interaction for the same amount of time as our foot massage. This would help overcome any placebo effect from the treatment. They had concerns about our measurement tools and our enrollment methods as well. Our simple little study suddenly wasn't so simple—and we had to admit their suggested changes would improve the study in a lot of ways.

Instead of becoming discouraged, we took the IRB's recommendations to heart and began to redesign our study. We realized we needed to better communicate how we had identified and addressed risks in our IRB documents, so we rewrote our consent form. We asked for advice from a variety of sources and wrote a better protocol that included a comparison therapy. We identified a stronger instrument and cleaned up our sampling procedure. In retrospect, I'm relieved we were stopped when we were—we honestly hadn't considered the risks carefully enough, and the IRB made us do that.

In retrospect, we should have asked for feedback from clinical and scientific colleagues outside of our team before submitting our project for IRB review—a lesson learned. Even though it was small and seemingly benign, we needed to be more aware of the risks involved.

Joanna Bokovoy, RN, DrPH
Medical Epidemiologist

Nazi Medical Experimentation

From 1933 until 1945 and the liberation of the death camps in Europe, atrocities were inflicted on World War II concentration camp detainees in the name of science. As part of the goal of advancing the Third Reich in Europe, the Nazis conducted medical experiments whose results were intended to be used to produce a race of pure Aryans who would rule the world.

Under the guise of benefiting soldiers of the Third Reich, Nazi physicians carried out experiments to test the limits of human endurance. For example, prisoners were submerged for days at a time in a tank of cold water. The intent was to test how long German pilots, who had to parachute into the cold North Sea, would survive. Different types of clothing were tested, as well as different methods for resuscitating the experimental subjects who survived. Other prisoners were burned with phosphorus to track wound healing. Surgery was performed without anesthesia to gauge pain levels, in utero surgery was carried out to determine fetal growth and development during stages of pregnancy, and surgical gender changes were accomplished. Many of the subjects of these experiments did not survive.

These experiments were not randomly carried out by only a few scientists; instead, they were regarded as fulfillment of governmental policy in support of the war effort. These atrocities in the name of scientific experimentation made it clear that international oversight of the rights of human subjects in research was necessary.

The Tuskegee Study

It is tempting to consider the Nazi studies to be examples of outrageous acts that could not occur in our own society. Unfortunately, the U.S. Public Health Service has its own record of egregious treatment of experimental subjects.

In 1932, the Public Health Service initiated a study to determine the natural history of syphilis. Called the "Tuskegee Study of Untreated Syphilis in the Negro Male," the study initially involved 600 black men—399 with syphilis and 201 without. The study was conducted without obtaining the informed consent of the subjects. While the subjects were led to believe they were being treated for a blood disorder, in reality the progress of their syphilis was allowed to unfold without treatment. Although originally projected to last 6 months, the study went on for 40 years. In 1972, a news story about the study caused a public outcry that led the government to appoint an ad hoc advisory panel to investigate the study. The panel concluded that the Tuskegee Study was "ethically unjustified" and ordered reparations for the men and their families (Centers for Disease Control and Prevention, 2011).

The Willowbrook Study

Lest we rationalize these examples of inhumane treatment of research subjects as affecting only adults, the Willowbrook study, conducted from 1963 to 1966, provides an example of research in which children were the target. The study's conduct was doubly egregious because these children—residents of a state-run school for children with learning disabilities—were also mentally compromised. The stated purpose of the study was to determine the course of untreated hepatitis. At the time, the school was supposedly not accepting new students, but it admitted additional children whose parents were willing to enroll them in the study. This policy introduced an added element of influence: If the school accepted only children whose parents agreed to their participation in the study, it may have put pressure on those parents who had few options for caring for their children and were desperate for state assistance.

Reports allege that the children in the Willowbrook study were deliberately infected with the hepatitis virus—some by being fed extracts of stools from known infected children, and later by injection. After a period of observation during which the children were untreated, a vaccine was tested on the subjects.

In some circles, the value of this study is still heavily debated. On the one hand, it did, indeed, result in development of the hepatitis vaccine used today. On the other hand, highly vulnerable children were infected with hepatitis, and the voluntary nature of their parents' consent is questionable (Hardicre, 2014).

All of these episodes raised concerns about the need to protect the rights of human subjects. As a result of these violations of basic human rights, both international and national guidelines for the ethical treatment of research subjects were developed.

International Guides for the Researcher

Two major international codes and reports guide researchers in carrying out ethical research: the Nuremberg Code and the Declaration of Helsinki.

The Nuremberg war crimes trials, which were held from 1945 to 1947, focused on crimes against humanity. They were presided over by judges from the four Allied powers—the United States, Great Britain, France, and the Soviet Union. The city of Nuremberg, Germany, was purposely chosen as the site for the trials because, after 11 Allied air strikes during the war, the city was declared 90% dead. During the trials, a large-scale prosecution of Nazi officials took place, many of whom presented as a defense the notion that they were simply following their superiors' orders. Their crimes included inhumane acts on civilians, initiating and waging aggressive acts of war, murder, near extermination of a race, slavery, ill treatment of prisoners, plunder, and destruction.

In response to the revelations in these trials, the Nuremberg Code was developed in 1949. This code contained guidelines requiring voluntary, informed consent to participate in medical experimentation. It further specified that the research must serve a worthy purpose, that the desired knowledge must be unobtainable by other means, and that the anticipated result must justify the performance of the experiment. All unnecessary physical and mental suffering was to be avoided. A little known fact is that the Nuremberg Code led to the notion of substituting animal experimentation in advance of or in lieu of human experimentation. This later raised concerns about the humane treatment of animals, a topic discussed later in this chapter.

The Nuremberg Code further guaranteed that no experiments were to be permitted when death or disability was an expected outcome, "except, perhaps, in those experiments where the experimental physicians also serve as subjects." Risks were to be commensurate with the importance of the problem, and human subjects were to be protected from even a remote possibility of harm. Experiments were to be conducted only by properly qualified scientists, and the subject had the right to stop the experiment at any time. Further, the scientist in charge was obligated to stop the experiment if injury, disability,

Therapeutic research:
Studies in which the subject can be expected to receive a potentially beneficial treatment.

Nontherapeutic research:
Studies that are carried out for the purpose of generating knowledge. They are not expected to benefit the research subject, but may lead to improved treatment in the future.

or death was likely to result. The code may be viewed online at https://ori.hhs.gov/chapter-3-The-Protection-of-Human-Subjects-nuremberg-code-directives-human-experimentation.

GRAY MATTER

The Nuremberg Code, developed in 1949, contains research guidelines stipulating that:
* Consent is voluntary and informed for subjects who participate in medical experimentation.
* The research serves a worthy purpose.
* The knowledge gained is unobtainable by any other means.
* The anticipated results justify performance of the experiment.
* Unnecessary physical and mental suffering or harm is avoided.
* Death or disability is not an expected outcome.
* Properly qualified scientists conduct the experiments.

The Declaration of Helsinki—an extension of the Nuremberg Code—was adopted in 1964 by the World Medical Association and amended and updated most recently in 2008. The Declaration of Helsinki expanded the principles of the Nuremberg Code to differentiate between therapeutic research and nontherapeutic research. Therapeutic research is expected to confer on the study subject an opportunity to receive a treatment that might be beneficial. Nontherapeutic research is carried out for the purpose of generating knowledge and is not expected to benefit the study subject, but might lead to improved treatment in the future.

Similar to the Nuremberg Code, the Declaration of Helsinki requires informed consent for ethical research, while allowing for surrogate consent when the prospective research subject is incompetent, physically or mentally incapable of providing consent, or a minor. Furthermore, the Declaration of Helsinki states that research within these groups should be conducted only when this research is necessary to promote the health of the representative group and when this research cannot otherwise be performed on competent persons.

National Guidelines for the Nurse Researcher

In 1974, Congress passed the National Research Act, which resulted in the formation of the National Commission for the Protection of Human Subjects of Biomedical and Behavioral Research. As part of their work, members of the national commission wrote the *Ethical Principles and Guidelines for the Protection of Human Subjects of Research* report. Commonly known as the Belmont Report, this document, which was published in 1978, has become the cornerstone statement of ethical principles on which regulations for protection of human subjects are based (U.S. Department of Health, Education, and Welfare [HEW], 1978).

The Belmont Report (which can be viewed online at http://www.hhs.gov/ohrp/humansubjects/guidance/belmont.html) begins by stating, "Scientific research has produced substantial social benefits. It has also posed some troubling ethical questions.

Public attention was drawn to these questions by reported abuses of human subjects in biomedical experiments. . ." (HEW, 1978, p. 1). As a result, state and national regulations, as well as international and professional codes, have been developed to guide researchers. These rules are based on broader ethical principles that provide a framework to evaluate investigators' judgment when designing and carrying out their research. Three foundational ethical principles relevant to the ethics of human subjects are described in the Belmont Report: respect for persons, beneficence, and justice.

Respect for Persons

Respect for persons, the first principle, incorporates two ethical convictions: that individuals should be treated as autonomous beings capable of making their own decisions, and that persons with diminished autonomy or those not capable of making their own decisions should be protected. The extent of protection afforded to those incapable of self-determination will depend on the risks, harms, and benefits of the study. Consequently, the principle of respect for persons is divided into two separate moral requirements: the requirement to acknowledge a person's autonomy and the requirement to protect those individuals with diminished autonomy.

Persons with diminished autonomy sometimes are regarded as vulnerable or as a member of a **vulnerable population**. These groups may contain some individuals who possess limited autonomy (that is, they cannot fully participate in the consent process)—for example, children, individuals with dementia and other cognitive disorders, prisoners, and pregnant women. Some ethicists regard older persons, terminally ill persons, and other hospitalized persons, as well as those who are homeless, students, or transgender, as also deserving of special consideration by researchers. Researchers have a special obligation to ensure a study involving vulnerable populations is ethical. However, Lange, Rogers, and Dodds (2013) argue that a description of the features that makes a group vulnerable is more helpful than labeling actual population groups. These authors offer a simple standard for identifying such individuals: Vulnerable subjects are those who are especially prone to harm or exploitation.

Under this definition, identifying vulnerable populations becomes a much broader task. For example, refugees, the bereaved, persons with dementia, alcoholics, persons with disabilities, and persons diagnosed with mental illness could all be considered vulnerable and deserving of special protection. The challenge is to illuminate the needs of these vulnerable patients—many of whom could benefit greatly from population-specific research—while respecting their integrity and minimizing their risks from participating in such research (Nordentoft & Kappel, 2011).

Special consideration for research studies that may include vulnerable populations involve ensuring the following protections:

- The risks of participating would be acceptable to volunteers in the general public.
- Selection of subjects is fair and unbiased.
- The written consent form is understandable given the subject's expected level of function and comprehension.
- Adequate follow-up is provided (Juritzen, Grimen, & Heggen, 2011).

Respect for persons: A basic principle of ethics stating that individuals should be treated as autonomous beings who are capable of making their own decisions. Persons who have limited autonomy or who are not capable of making their own decisions should be protected.

Vulnerable populations: Groups of people with diminished autonomy who cannot participate fully in the consent process. Such groups may include children, individuals with cognitive disorders, prisoners, and pregnant women.

Beneficence:
A basic principle of ethics that states that persons should have their decisions respected, be protected from harm, and have steps taken to ensure their well-being.

Justice:
A basic principle of ethics that incorporates a participant's right to fair treatment and fairness in distribution of benefit and burden.

Beneficence

One of the most fundamental ethical principles in research is **beneficence**—that is, "do no harm." According to the Belmont Report, "Persons are treated in an ethical manner not only by respecting their decisions and protecting them from harm, but also by making efforts to secure their well-being. Two general rules have been formulated as complementary expressions of beneficent actions: (1) do no harm and (2) maximize possible benefits and minimize possible harms" (HEW, 1978, §B.2).

Human subjects can be harmed in a variety of ways, including physical harm (e.g., injury), psychological harm (e.g., worry, stress, and fear), social harm (e.g., loss of friends or one's place in society), and economic harm (e.g., loss of employment). Researchers must strive to minimize harm and to achieve the best possible balance between the benefits to be gained from participation and the risks of being a participant.

The Belmont Report tells us that the assessment of the risks and benefits of a study presents an opportunity to gather comprehensive information about the proposed research. The investigator strives to design a study that will answer a meaningful question. A review committee will determine whether risks inherent in participation are justified. Prospective subjects will make an assessment, based on their understanding of risks and benefits, as to whether to participate in the study.

Justice

The third broad principle found in the Belmont Report is **justice**. The principle of justice incorporates participants' right to fair treatment and fairness in distribution of benefit and burden. According to the report, an injustice would occur when a benefit to which a person is entitled is denied or when some burden is unduly imposed. For example, the selection of research subjects needs to be closely scrutinized to determine whether some subjects (e.g., welfare recipients, racial and ethnic minorities, or persons confined to institutions) are being systematically selected because of their easy accessibility or because of their compromised position. The application of justice also requires that research should not unduly involve persons from groups unlikely to be beneficiaries of the results of the research. However, members of diverse groups also should be included, and not excluded, without a prior knowledge of their suitability to participate.

GRAY MATTER

During research, human subjects can suffer harm in the following ways:
- Physically (injury)
- Psychologically (worry, stress, or fear)
- Socially (loss of friends or place in society)
- Economically (loss of employment)

Certain diverse groups, such as minorities, the economically disadvantaged, the homeless, the very sick, and those persons who have a compromised ability to provide consent, should be protected against the danger of being recruited for a study solely for

Table 3.1 Ethical Principles and Research Design	
This Ethical Principle	**Is Managed with This Design Principle**
Respect for persons	Informed consent process Subject selection process Adequacy of follow-up systems
Beneficence	Assessment of risk and benefit
Justice	Subject selection process

the researcher's convenience. In short, this means that researchers may not take advantage of underprivileged persons so as to benefit those who are privileged.

Table 3.1 links the ethical principles to the elements of research design. In addition to these ethical principles, some values are recognized as fundamental to the scientific enterprise as a whole. These concepts go beyond the ethical treatment of subjects and address the ethical behavior of the researcher. The primary values that are the focus of the entire research process include truthfulness, trust, and best interests. Related values include carefulness, openness, freedom, credit, education, social responsibility, legality, opportunity, and mutual respect (Horner & Minifie, 2011a).

The ethical nurse researcher considers all these principles as a research study is being designed and adheres to these values as the research is being carried out. The failure to identify and resolve ethical issues can place both the conduct and the results of a research study in jeopardy (Milton, 2013).

The Ethical Researcher

Bad behavior in the name of science has given rise to the need for laws, regulations, and safeguards. The public's perception of research, its benefits, and its risks is shaped by the way research is conducted and by the way results are reported. Researchers, then, should abide by the ethical guidelines cited in the Nuremberg Code, the Belmont Report, and the Helsinki Declaration. Additionally, other guidelines have been developed that are specific to research funded by the federal government or foundations.

Table 3.2 summarizes the responsibilities of an ethical nurse researcher. Such researchers abide by ethical guidelines so as to uphold the public's confidence in research and its contribution to knowledge for the greater good. These guidelines declare that the ethical researcher should honor the following criteria:

- Adhere to principles of beneficence by doing no harm, maximizing benefits, and minimizing possible harms
- Respect the autonomy of the participants in the consent process
- Employ the principle of justice in subject selection
- Explain the research procedures to the participants
- Obtain proper and informed consent

Informed consent:
A process of information exchange in which participants are provided with understandable information needed to make a participation decision, full disclosure of the risks and benefits, and the assurance that withdrawal is possible at any time without consequences. This process begins with recruitment and ends with a signed agreement document.

Table 3.2 Responsibilities of an Ethical Nurse Researcher
To respect individuals' autonomy in consenting to participate in research
To protect those prospective subjects for whom decisional capacity is limited
To minimize potential harm and to maximize possible benefits for all subjects enrolled
To ensure that benefits and burdens associated with the research protocol are distributed equally when identifying prospective subjects
To protect privacy, to ensure confidentiality, and to guarantee anonymity when promised
To notify institutional officials of breaches of research protocols and incidents of scientific misconduct
To maintain competence in one's identified area of research
To maintain proficiency in research methods

- Ensure the confidentiality of participants
- Maintain appropriate documentation of the research process
- Adhere to research protocols
- Report results in a fair and factual manner (National Academy of Sciences, 2009)

One way to ensure that the researcher conducting a study meets these criteria is to select the most appropriate participants for the study. The study subjects must also understand their role in the research. The most important aspect of this process is to secure the participants' informed consent.

Informed Consent

Informed consent encompasses much more than just a form or a signature; rather, it is a process of information exchange that includes recruitment materials, verbal dialogue, presentation of written materials, questions and answers, and an agreement that is documented by a signature. According to the Belmont Report, the consent process contains three components: information, comprehension, and voluntariness. Participants should be able to ask questions, understand the risks and benefits, and be assured that if they choose to participate they may withdraw at any time without consequences.

To judge how much information should be disclosed to a prospective subject, the "reasonable subject" standard should be used. This standard requires that the extent and nature of the information provided be sufficient for a reasonable person to decide whether to participate (Odeh, 2013).

Organization of the Informed Consent

Prospective subjects who are fully informed about the nature of the research and its associated risks and benefits are positioned to make an educated decision about whether to participate. Essential content for informed consent in research can be found in the U.S. Department of Health and Human Services' Code of Federal Regulations (CFR 45, Part 46.106). Information that is essential for informed consent can be found in Table 3.3.

Table 3.3 Elements of the Informed Consent Form

Title of study and name(s) of investigator(s)

Introduction and invitation to participate

Basis for selection

Explanation of study purpose and procedures

Duration of participation

Reasonably foreseeable risks/unforeseen risks

Benefits of participation/cost of participation

Appropriate alternatives to participation

Voluntary withdrawal from study

Payments/compensation

Confidentiality of records

Contact person

Funding statement/conflict of interest statement

Statement of voluntary participation

Signature lines

Full disclosure: Reporting as much information about the research as is known at the time without threatening the validity of the study. This practice allows the subject to make an informed decision as to whether to participate.

Deception or Incomplete Disclosure

When explaining the research procedures to the prospective subject, the researcher must explain all information that is known about risks and benefits. The subject needs to know if the treatment, drug, or procedure used in the study is not necessary for his or her care and if it may have outcomes that are questionable or not completely understood. **Full disclosure**, or reporting as much information as is known at the time, is crucial so the participant can make an informed decision as to whether to participate.

Some participants may not be informed of some aspects of the research because having such knowledge would likely impair the validity of the research. This threat to validity—called the Hawthorne effect, treatment effects, or placebo effect—may lead subjects to behave differently simply because they are being treated. Such an outcome might happen in a study involving experimental drugs or complementary therapies, for example. Balancing the expectations of participants for the care they will receive with the purpose of the research may be challenging. This issue is most often addressed by using vague, rather than deceptive, language. However, incomplete disclosure is generally allowable only when all of the following conditions are met:

1. No other nondeceptive method exists to study the phenomenon of interest.
2. The study will make a substantial contribution to the body of knowledge.
3. The deception is not expected to cause significant harm or emotional distress.
4. Participants are debriefed about the deception as soon as possible (Boynton, Portnoy, & Johnson, 2013).

Incomplete disclosure should never be used to enroll participants in a study or to elicit cooperation and participation from reluctant subjects by masking or minimizing potential risks.

Comprehension

Because a person's informed consent to participate is based on his or her understanding of the benefits and risks, in addition to the overall importance of the area under study, the researcher acts as a communicator and evaluator when ensuring that the prospective subject understands the intent of the study. When developing the informed consent form, the investigator may use institutional boilerplate templates to communicate all necessary information in an organized fashion. It is important to avoid the use of healthcare jargon and technical terms, and instead to use simple language. For participants from a general population (for example, hospitalized patients), the wording of the consent form should be at a seventh- or eighth-grade reading level. Readability formulas, based on length of sentences and number of syllables per word, can be found in Microsoft Word, or reading level can be calculated directly with any number of free, Internet-based instruments.

Case in Point: Jesse Gelsinger

Gene therapy is viewed as having the potential to produce highly impressive advances in medical treatment. In 1992, an investigator with an excellent reputation as a genetic researcher founded a company with the intention of commercializing successful gene therapies. Corporate investors contributed millions of dollars to the company. Following the establishment of the business venture, the investigator designed a clinical trial in which a genetically engineered cold virus was used to deliver genes to correct a genetic liver disorder. This virus had been tested in animals, but not yet in humans, prior to the beginning of this trial.

The investigator's original proposal involved testing the gene therapy on terminally ill newborns, but this plan was rejected by the institutional bioethicist. Following this setback, the investigator modified the proposed research protocol and decided to test the gene therapy on stable patients with the previously identified genetic liver disorder. Institutional approval was provided in 1995, and the trial commenced at multiple study sites. In 1999, Jesse Gelsinger, an 18-year-old subject who had the genetic liver disorder, but who was asymptomatic and living a normal life, was enrolled in this gene therapy clinical trial at the University of Pennsylvania.

At the same time, researchers from other study sites began to contact the investigator, expressing concern about the safety of using the cold virus. The trial continued, however, and Gelsinger—the next-to-last patient enrolled in the clinical trial—received a dose that was 300 times the dose received by the first patient. Gelsinger died from a massive immune system response to the gene therapy. The Food and Drug Administration (FDA) immediately shut down all gene therapy research at the University of Pennsylvania. After Gelsinger's death, 921 adverse events in this and other gene therapy trials were reported to the FDA and to the National Institutes of Health (NIH) (Parascandola, 2004).

> **Questions Raised by the Death of Jesse Gelsinger**
> - Should high-risk research be conducted on "healthy, stable" persons?
> - Was this particular research protocol ready for human trials?
> - Were the adverse events ignored? Misinterpreted? Apparent only in retrospect?
> - Did a financial conflict of interest (the investigator owned the gene therapy company) bias the researcher's judgment?

A priori:
Conceived or formulated before an investigation.

Research Integrity

All types of research, but particularly research involving human subjects, should be conducted under strict ethical guidelines. Research integrity involves more than meeting basic ethical principles for the treatment of human subjects. The researcher's work must demonstrate integrity in all phases of the research process—from design to analysis through reporting and follow-up.

A well-designed study may be ethical by plan but manipulated during implementation. For this reason, most analysis decisions should be made *a priori*, meaning before data have been collected. Otherwise, it may be possible to manipulate the data to mislead the reader or to selectively report findings that are supportive of the researcher's point of view. This manipulation of data can be accomplished in statistical analysis by changing the significance level or by making erroneous assumptions to make the results seem more conclusive (Wasserman, 2013). Data in graphs can be manipulated by changing the distance between the values on the axes to make the results appear more significant than they are. **FIGURE 3.1** demonstrates how the same data may be presented two different ways to mislead the reader. In these examples, the vertical axis has been altered to make

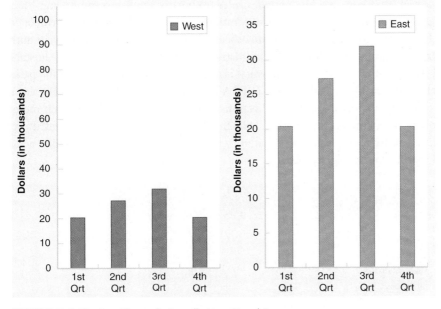

FIGURE 3.1 The Two Hospitals Actually Have Equal Revenues

it appear as if one hospital is making more money when, in fact, the hospitals have identical revenue figures.

Completing a training course in research protocols is one of the best ways to ensure that research is conducted under the most ethical guidelines. The NIH requires ethics training for anyone involved with NIH grants or anyone who conducts research in NIH facilities. The areas typically covered in this type of training include data acquisition and management, publication practices, research misconduct, and responsible authorship, among others. Those new to the research process should participate in some type of training on the responsible conduct of research, whether or not the study is federally sponsored.

Legal and Regulatory Guidelines for Conducting Research

Ethics and law are intimately intertwined; in fact, they might be considered different points on the same continuum. Obeying the law (the minimum standard) is at one end of the continuum, and acting ethically (above the expected minimum behavior) is at the opposite end. This duality of law and ethics also exists in research. The nurse researcher can think of the law as a minimum standard and ethics as a higher standard. Law can also be thought of as a means of conflict resolution. Although most people do the right thing ethically, if they do not, the law is there to resolve the situation. The good researcher maximizes both the legal and ethical protections afforded to subjects in a study.

Brief Overview of Laws Related to Research

The four sources of law that may affect researchers are common law, administrative law, statutory law, and tort law. *Common law* is derived from judicial decisions made during a trial (case law) and often applies rules from early English common law. Medical malpractice lawsuits are an example of common law. *Administrative law* is formulated by the federal and state governments and other regulatory agencies and obtains its authority from Congress. An example of administrative law is the Health Insurance Portability and Accountability Act (HIPAA), which is a federal regulation governing the patient's right to privacy and confidentiality. HIPAA has had dramatic effects on data collection for research purposes, and its implications extend to cutting-edge research methods involving social media, the Internet, and "Big Data" resources. Most laws that affect the clinical researcher are statutes or statutory laws. *Statutory laws* are enacted, amended, and repealed by the legislature.

GRAY MATTER

Four categories of law:
- Common
- Administrative
- Statutory
- Tort

A fourth category of legal issues has its roots in tort law. Torts are civil wrongs committed against individuals or their property. Examples of tort law include negligence, malpractice, assault, battery, false imprisonment, invasion of privacy, and causing mental or emotional distress. Although these last allegations are unlikely in a clinical research project, they can happen and may subsequently provoke a malpractice claim. Most claims are brought when a subject believes he or she has been harmed due to negligence on the part of the researcher. Examples of negligence in clinical research include using an instrument known to be defective, using equipment that is not functioning properly, denying a patient reasonable treatment so as to obtain a control group, or not following a specified research protocol so that a patient's safety is compromised. All of these circumstances may cause injury to the participant and result in a claim of negligence. Under federal regulations, no informed consent form can include language through which the subject waives or even appears to waive any legal rights. In other words, obtaining informed consent from a study participant does not release the investigator from liability for negligence (U.S. Department of Health and Human Services, CFR 45, Part 46.116).

A researcher could also be accused of defamation (a false and harmful oral statement) or libel (a false and harmful published statement) as a result of the way he or she presents information in the written account of the research. Truthful researchers need not fear either of these outcomes; both require the intent to distribute information that is known to be incorrect. Reporting the truth is the best defense against accusations of defamation and libel. To further protect the legal rights of subjects, the researcher should guard against referring to individuals' identity in any written research reports.

The researcher must also guard against inflicting mental or emotional distress. In a research design that involves sensitive topics, the participant may experience painful emotions such as grief, despair, or shame. Most research protocols, therefore, include in the consent form statements such as "potential emotional distress may occur as a result of this research" so that the subject may make a fully informed decision about participation.

A new source of legal issues is the challenge of determining individuals' rights to their cells as property—a problem that arises when tissue is used to develop cell lines that may potentially be sold for millions of dollars. The global expansion of biobanks of human tissue has raised a wide range of bioethical concerns related to consent, privacy, control, ownership, and disclosure issues (Nisbet & Fahy, 2013). In large part, the debate focuses on whether tissue is the tissue donor's property, and whether researchers need to obtain informed consent to use tissue from a living donor in research. Other concerns relate to the welfare of vulnerable study participants, oversight of such programs, and donor compensation.

The right to the tissues stored in biobanks is not a clear-cut question of ownership. From a legal standpoint, tissues removed for therapeutic or diagnostic purposes are considered "abandoned," and their use for research purposes does not require consent. Patients may not even be aware they have contributed their cells to research. Generic consent forms signed during medical procedures often grant practitioners the right to dispose of tissues as they see fit, which may include donating the tissues for research. In case of tissue sample donation, if donors have consented to those samples' use in research and no longer possess the tissues, they have transferred the right of ownership, including the right to obtain compensation or share in profits from the tissues' subsequent sale

Right of privacy:
A person's right to have his or her health information kept confidential and released only to authorized individuals and to have his or her body shielded from public view.

(Moore & McSherry, 2013). The debate continues as to the ethical implications of such a transaction, particularly when the researcher stands to gain financially from the research.

The **right of privacy** is the right to be left alone. Patients and research participants have a right to the confidentiality of their health records and the release of that information only to those parties whom they have authorized. The right to privacy covers the right both to physical privacy of the person's body and to the privacy of one's health information.

Privacy is also about human dignity and the privacy of one's own person. Accusations of invasion of privacy have been brought against personnel for uncovering patients' bodies unnecessarily or performing examinations in front of others. This practice may be particularly problematic when the research protocol calls for multiple data collectors to check interrater reliability.

Invasion of privacy may also involve the written word. Patients have a right to privacy of their health information throughout the research process, whether they disclose such information verbally or it is retrieved from an electronic or written record. In the field of clinical research, breaches of this right invoke HIPAA sanctions. In cases of breaches of confidentiality or invasion of privacy, the patient or participant need not prove damages, making it easier for the patient or subject to initiate a lawsuit.

To avoid accusations of discrimination in the population under study, researchers must be careful when choosing the populations to exclude from the research. Valid reasons to exclude a particular population, such as pregnant women, members of certain age groups, or patients with certain diagnoses, must be specifically documented. These exclusion criteria are necessary both for good design and to ensure that subjects are selected without bias. Proper selection of the research population is a primary consideration when researchers are studying potentially life-saving treatments.

The key to avoiding any of these accusations is the accurate documentation of all research steps in addition to following the ethical principles discussed earlier in this chapter. Following these guidelines will minimize the threat of any legal action by a research participant and reassure the researcher that he or she is doing the right thing.

Legal Issues Surrounding Informed Consent

Signing a consent form to participate in research has the same purpose and carries the same value as does signing the consent form for treatment in healthcare facilities. Requirements governing what should be included in an informed consent form are the same for legal purposes and for ethical purposes. However, legal issues have been raised about who can provide consent for participation in a research study. If the individual cannot legally consent to participate in the research (for example, if the individual is a minor, has been judged incompetent, or is a member of a vulnerable population), the researcher must ensure that the person's interests are protected. Consent must be obtained from the subject, if possible, as well as from the legal guardian. In some cases, formal consent is obtained from the legal guardian, and simultaneously assent is provided by the participant. For example, a child should agree that he or she is willing to participate in a study (assent) even though the legal consent is required from the parents.

If the research involves human subject participation, in addition to consent, the researcher should obtain an authorization that allows the researcher access to the

Table 3.4 Participant Authorization for Release of Information

Full Name: _____   Record Identifier: _____

Date of Birth: _____

Address: _____

City, State, Zip Code: _____

Other Contact Information: _____

Select One Option Below:

1. _____ I authorize the following person(s) or agencies access to my personal health information for a period not to exceed 90 days from the date of signature below.

2. _____ I decline authorization for any and all requests for release of my personal health information.

_____   _____

Patient/Participant/Date   Researcher/Agency/Date

participant's medical information. This authorization for access to medical information may be incorporated into the consent form. **Table 3.4** provides an example of an authorization for release of information.

Emerging Issues: Ethical Use of Social Media

Increasingly, health researchers are using personal communication devices and social media to facilitate communication with potential research participants and to gather data. Social media, like any method that blurs the line between the public and private spheres, could qualify as an ethically risky research space (Nind, Wiles, Bengry-Howell, & Crow, 2012). The principles that apply to human subjects in face-to-face research should likewise be applied to the use of any intermediary technology used in a study, such as the Internet. Specifically, the researcher should clearly demonstrate the ethical principles of respect, integrity, and beneficence when utilizing such means of communication.

To date, a few guidelines for the use of social media in research have emerged, but no standard set of rules has been adopted as yet by any research oversight group. Respect in this setting can be demonstrated by letting the subject control the interaction with the researcher. Integrity can be maintained by focusing on the privacy of the subject while being cognizant of the potential for personal information to be taken out of context. To prevent this possibility, a specific research project page should be created, and subjects should be allowed to control which data are uploaded. When the study's project page is linked to an individual's social media page, the public should be unable to determine which data are being used for the research. Using a specific project page can also protect participants against the public exposure of their identities. To practice beneficence, the researcher should be proficient in the functions of the social media being used, particularly the privacy settings. The consent to participate should include specific language that differentiates between materials that can be submitted privately and those that may be revealed publicly—for example, a private message versus a public post (Lunnay, Borlagdan, McNaughton, & Ward, 2015).

Institutional Review Boards

Research that involves human subjects in some way—as opposed to retrieving data from records or databases—requires a higher level of oversight. This oversight is provided by legal entities that also are charged with maintaining ethical standards in research. These entities, called **institutional review boards (IRBs)**, are required by law in any organization that allows the conduct of research involving people.

The roots of IRBs can be traced back to the National Commission for the Protection of Human Subjects of Biomedical and Behavioral Research, which was established in 1974. This commission advised the U.S. Department of Health and Human Services on policies related to research. It was also instrumental in the adoption of the recommendations of the Belmont Report of 1978.

The U.S. Department of Health and Human Services, acting on these recommendations, developed new regulations governing research and human subjects of research under the Code of Federal Regulations (CFR). These new regulations called for the creation of IRBs, also known as human subjects committees, as safeguards against the inhumane treatment of individuals that had, in the past, been inflicted in the name of science. Part 46 of CFR 45 requires that any research conducted on human subjects be approved by an IRB. According to requirements in Part 46, the mission of the IRB is "to ensure that research is ethically acceptable and that the welfare and rights of research participants are protected."

Case in Point: Nicole Wan

Nicole Wan was a 19-year-old sophomore pre-med student at the University of Rochester in 1996 when she volunteered for a study on the effects of environmental air quality. This pollution research project was funded by a Massachusetts Institute of Technology (MIT) grant from the National Institute of Environmental Health Sciences (NIEHS). Wan was one of 200 participants enrolled in an arm of the study at the University of Rochester Medical Center. Participants were paid $150 to undergo a bronchoscopy to examine and collect lung cells.

A medical resident, who was functioning in the role of investigator, administered aerosolized lidocaine, a local anesthetic, to prevent Wan from gagging and to allow for easier passage of the bronchoscope into the patient's lower airway. Because Wan had discomfort during placement of the bronchoscope, additional lidocaine spray was administered. After completion of the study protocol, she left the medical center and went to a friend's apartment, where she suffered a cardiac arrest 3 hours later. Although Wan was resuscitated by emergency personnel and admitted to an intensive care unit (ICU) at the medical center, she suffered irreversible pulmonary and neurological damage and died 2 days later. The county medical examiner ruled Wan's death to be an accident due to acute lung toxicity. On autopsy, her serum levels of lidocaine were found to be four times the maximum levels (McGuire, 1996).

Questions Raised by the Death of Nicole Wan

- Is participation in a clinical trial appropriate for a 19-year-old college student? Should parents be notified when students enroll in such studies?
- What is the "age of reason" for participation in a clinical trial that may carry risk?
- Why did a medical resident, rather than the principal investigator, administer the study protocol?

The Review Process

Research studies that involve human subjects must be reviewed by the IRB. The IRB helps the researcher determine whether there is a potential for a legal or ethical breach and ensures that safeguards are in place to avoid this risk.

There are three categories of research review by an IRB:

- Exempt review
- Expedited review
- Full review

An **exempt review** covers proposals that do not require review by the IRB. (The IRB determines whether a study is exempt; this is not the researcher's decision.) This category is limited to studies that pose no risk for the subjects. Such a designation is common when the researcher employs surveys, noninvasive procedures, secondary data or documents, or other methods where it would be impossible to identify any research subject individually. The exemption only refers to the fact that the IRB does not need to review the study proposal; it does not exempt the researcher from the same ethical principles that govern all research.

An **expedited review** is used for research that poses only minimal risk to the participants or for those studies that use drugs that do not require FDA approval. Minimal risk means that the probability or magnitude of discomfort anticipated in the research is not greater than what is ordinarily encountered in daily life. It may also be considered no more risky than what would be encountered during the performance of routine physical or psychological examinations or tests. Expedited review research studies are usually reviewed by one or two members of the IRB, who may consult with other board members as necessary.

A **full review** is necessary for all research that poses more than minimal risk to the subjects and for research that does not qualify for exempt status. These studies are reviewed by the full committee, with particular attention being paid to the methods, consent process, and selection of the subjects. Studies that require direct access to participants, use personally identifiable medical information, and involve more than minimal risk are subject to full review by the committee. Additional review by a privacy board may be required if personal health information (PHI) is needed for the study. This committee may or may not be part of an IRB and will determine whether patient authorization is required, whether a disclosure notice is required, or whether a waiver can be issued to the researcher that exempts him or her from the consent process. A waiver means the research can be conducted using the methods described in the research protocol and that patient authorizations and disclosures documenting record access are not required. Disclosure forms are discussed in more detail later in this chapter.

Researchers should not make assumptions based on these descriptions that their research may be exempt or expedited. No aspect of a study should commence without approval from the appropriate committee or review board. It is the IRB that tells the researcher whether a study is exempt or qualifies for expedited review—not the other way around.

Exempt review:
A review of study proposals that pose no risk to subjects; the full IRB is not required to participate.

Expedited review:
A review of study proposals that pose minimal risk to subjects; one or two IRB members participate.

Full review:
A review of study proposals that pose more than minimal risk to subjects, that do not qualify for exempt status, and in which the full IRB committee participates.

GRAY MATTER

Full IRB review must be done under the following conditions:
- Studies require direct access to participants.
- Human subjects are put at more than minimal risk.
- Protected health information is required.
- Federal funds are received.
- Publication is anticipated.

Quality improvement studies are exempt from IRB review. Such studies are typically conducted for the purpose of internal organizational improvement, and there is no expectation of publication or generalization of the results to larger groups. Occasionally, though, quality improvement may be conducted with the idea of publishing a report on the study; in such a case, IRB oversight is appropriate. **FIGURE 3.2** lists a set of questions that can help a study designer determine whether a proposed project is solely focused on quality improvement—and therefore requires no IRB oversight—or whether it constitutes research.

When preparing the IRB/Human Subjects Approval Form, the researcher must clearly describe the following eight required elements (CFR 45, Part 46):

1. The research project, the subjects, and how they will be selected and informed
2. The methods and procedures to be used; the subjects should understand their level of participation, what is required, and for how long
3. Risks to the participants, particularly if drugs or treatments are used
4. Benefits to participants
5. How confidentiality and anonymity will be maintained
6. Contact information for questions of participants
7. Explanation of any compensation
8. Statement about voluntary participation

The IRB is more than a safety net for subjects; it also has the capacity to advise, mentor, and develop new researchers. A tremendous amount of research expertise is available to the researcher via the members of the IRB. Consulting with them early and often in a study can help strengthen the study design. Although much is made of the regulatory authority of the IRB, just as much can be said for its capacity to provide an additional critical evaluation of the research as it is designed. The IRB serves as another safeguard to help the researcher design a strong, ethical, and legal research study. Doing the right thing from the beginning of a study is the best way to avoid legal and ethical accusations.

RESEARCH VS. QUALITY CHECKLIST

Quality Improvement activities are exempt from IRB (Institutional Review Board) review while Research activities are not. However, sometimes it is not clear as to whether the activity should be categorized as "quality improvement" or "research". By completing this checklist, you can determine if you need to contact the IRB Manager for further direction.

Contact the IRB Manager (ext. 77972) if your activity involves patients, employees, and/or lab specimens (from human subjects), and you answer yes/unsure to any of the following:	Yes/unsure	No
1. It **does** assign people or lab specimens to groups for simultaneous comparison		
2. It **is** being conducted in hopes of contributing to generalizable knowledge in the area of study (and not for the sole purpose of improving PVHS processes)		
3. The initial intent **is** to publish the results*		
4. It **does** involve patient /subjects undergoing procedures that normally would not be done for their disease/problem (i.e. beyond the normal standard of care or for employees—their work day)		
5. It **does** involve increased risk or burden to the participants (e.g. additional blood draws, fatigue, embarrassment, or giving personal information)		
6. It **does** involve interactions or observations that don't routinely occur in patient care (for patients) or everyday life		
7. It **does** involve releasing protected health information (PHI) or personal information to individuals/entities other than for regulatory/accreditation purposes		

*If the initial intent was not to publish results, but it is later determined that the results will be published, then the IRB Manager needs to be contacted.

Kimberly Woods-McCormick RN MS
IRB Manager
Poudre Valley Health System

FIGURE 3.2 Checklist to Differentiate Research from Quality Improvement Studies
Used with permission of University of Colorado Health. North IRB, Fort Collins, CO 80526.

Case in Point: **Ellen Roche**

In April 2001, Ellen Roche, a healthy 24-year-old laboratory employee at Johns Hopkins Asthma and Allergy Center, was recruited as a normal volunteer to participate in an NIH-funded research study at her workplace. The aim of this study was to determine factors leading to airway irritation in asthma patients. The protocol required the use of inhaled hexamethonium to induce asthma-like effects. The pulmonary toxicity associated with oral, intramuscular, or subcutaneous hexamethonium administration for hypertension was first reported in 1953. Between that time and 1960, 11 articles that included individual case reports and a small series of autopsied cases were published. In 1970, a review article on the use of hexamethonium listed six references from the 1950s.

Johns Hopkins used a stronger concentration of hexamethonium than that cited in the case reports from the 1950s and 1960s. The first volunteer developed a cough; the second volunteer experienced no ill effects. Roche, the third volunteer, developed irreversible lung damage after receiving 1 gram of hexamethonium by inhalation, and died approximately 1 month later. Even as Roche was being treated in the ICU, the trial continued, with six additional volunteers being enrolled. However, none of these six volunteers reached the point in the protocol when hexamethonium would be inhaled. The study was stopped when Roche died.

Later, it was found that this specific study had not been part of the original grant application to NIH, but was mentioned as a planned study in continuation applications. A representative from NIH stated that the hexamethonium study was felt to be consistent with the original goals of the funded primary study and, therefore, was not otherwise scientifically reviewed (Becker & Levy, 2001).

Questions Raised by the Death of Ellen Roche

- Did the investigators have sufficient experience with the agent?
- Did the IRB do a thorough review of this study protocol?
- Was there any coercion involved in enrolling a subject who was an employee of the Asthma and Allergy Center?

Research Involving Animals

Research that may benefit humans is often first conducted on animal subjects. The reason for using animals in research is to advance scientific knowledge while confining unknown risks to nonhuman subjects (Horner & Minifie, 2011a). In recent times, however, the use of animals in research studies has become the subject of considerable debate. Those who advocate on behalf of animals' welfare recognize the value of testing interventions first on animals, but campaign for the humane treatment and care of these subjects. Some who advocate for animal rights go even further, insisting that animal research should be abolished altogether. Both groups base their stance on studies that demonstrate animal sentience (that is, the ability to experience pain in both vertebrate and invertebrate animals) and a philosophical analysis of the moral status of animals (Ferdowsian & Gluck, 2015).

The NIH's Office of Laboratory Animal Welfare (2002) stipulates that applications for Public Health Service grants must include procedures designed to ensure that discomfort and injury to animals used in experimentation will be limited to only unavoidable levels. Furthermore, it requires that analgesic, anesthetic, and tranquilizing drugs be used to minimize the pain and discomfort caused by experiments. Research facilities must be accredited by the Association for Assessment and Accreditation of Laboratory Animal Care International; alternatively, they may be evaluated by an institutional animal care and use committee (IACUC), a review committee analogous to the IRB for human subjects.

Multiple guidelines exist to guide researchers in the ethical and humane use of animals in research. In essence, these regulations and guidelines hold researchers accountable for the humane care and treatment of animals used in research through the "three R's":

- *Reduce* the number of animals used in experiments.
- *Refine* experimental procedures to minimize animal pain and suffering.
- *Replace* animal subjects with nonanimal alternatives when scientifically feasible (Ibrahim, 2006).

In June of 2013, the NIH announced its decision to significantly reduce the use of chimpanzees in agency-supported biomedical research. It retained fewer than 50 captive chimpanzees for future biomedical research. The number of research studies involving these primates plummeted. In June of 2015 the U.S. Fish and Wildlife Service announced it had classified captive chimpanzees as "endangered." The ability to conduct research on any endangered species is very difficult, and in November of that year, Dr. Francis Collins, the Director of the NIH, made the decision to send its colony of chimpanzees to a sanctuary equipped to care for them.

Even with this national example, the debate continues as to whether research on animals is sufficiently humane. The research literature identifies the need for evidence-based guidelines for laboratory animal care and treatment, and broad-based education regarding such guidelines' application is needed. Also needed are studies to determine the relative benefits of animal testing when realistic alternatives are emerging, such as interactive computer simulations, cadavers, and lifelike manikins (Mangan, 2007). Animal experimentation, much like human experimentation, raises concerns about necessity, purpose, design, risks, and benefits, as well as their relation not to whether the subject is human, but whether the subject has the capacity for suffering.

Research Misconduct

Obtaining the necessary approvals of the IRB and privacy committee does not guarantee that the researcher is then free from accusations of battery, negligence, or invasion of privacy. It is up to the researcher to carry out the research in an ethical, legal, and moral manner and to document the procedures and results accurately.

Research misconduct, as defined by the federal government, includes fabrication, falsification, and plagiarism. Fabrication is the intentional misrepresentation or "making up" of data or results by the researcher. Falsification occurs when the researcher falsifies or manipulates the results, changes the procedures, omits data, or accepts subjects into the study who were not in the original inclusion criteria. This may seem like a rare occurrence, but in 2015, all 14 incidents of research misconduct documented on the Office of Research Integrity webpage (ORI.hhs.gov/case_summary, retrieved August 17, 2016) by the U.S. Department of Health and Human Services were related to falsifying data, and

Health Insurance Portability and Accountability Act (HIPAA): Legislation passed by Congress in 1996, which protects the privacy of personal health information.

all cases were serious enough to result in imposed sanctions. Plagiarism usually arises from the written account of the research, when ideas, statements, results, or words are not attributed to the appropriate person but rather are represented as the writer's own work.

Other sources of research misconduct can involve undisclosed conflicts of interest, misleading authorship, data acquisition and ownership, and duplicate publication practices. Research misconduct affects the cost of research overall by increasing the oversight required and by diminishing the confidence and respect of the public regarding the results of scientific research. The public may begin to grow skeptical of research results if such behaviors become commonplace (Horner & Minifie, 2011b).

The key factor in determining if research misconduct took place is whether the researcher intentionally misrepresented the data. Research misconduct has not occurred if a researcher made honest mistakes. Misconduct also has not occurred if researchers simply have differences of opinion. This is an important distinction. Good researchers take calculated and controlled risks. As long as the researcher takes the time to carefully plan a strong study, gains the approval of the necessary IRB and privacy committees, and maintains inflexible ethical standards during the implementation of the study, the researcher has fulfilled his or her obligation as an accountable steward of the study.

The HIPAA Privacy Rule

> What I may see or hear in the course of the treatment or even outside of the treatment in regard to the life of men, which on no account one must spread abroad, I will keep to myself, holding such things shameful to be spoken about.
>
> —Hippocratic Oath (Edelstein, 1943)

Since April 14, 2003, the effective date of the U.S. privacy rule, otherwise known as HIPAA, organizations have more tightly scrutinized research proposals, especially those that involve the use of patient data and human subjects.

Reacting to the increasing accessibility of electronic data specific to individuals, Congress passed the **Health Insurance Portability and Accountability Act (HIPAA)** in 1996. Aimed mostly at electronic health record (EHR) initiatives, one of HIPAA's main elements is a requirement for the protection of PHI. This rule protects all elements considered protected health information—a broad range of information that varies from telephone numbers to diagnoses. **Table 3.5** lists the information that is considered identifiable PHI.

The introduction of HIPAA's privacy rule resulted in changes from the way healthcare organizations traditionally handled patients and their information. Healthcare workers now are given access to only the PHI that is necessary to perform the assigned work at hand. For example, those personnel working in ancillary departments receive only a diagnosis that enables them to process the tests or bills. Therefore, the researcher cannot automatically assume that access to all the information required to complete research will be provided, even if the researcher is employed by the facility.

Failure to comply with the rule can be very costly to both the researcher and the organization. The privacy rule specifically states that any employee who fails to comply with the privacy policy will be subject to corrective action, termination of employment,

Table 3.5 Identifiable Personal Health Information

Name

Past, present, or future health conditions

Description of health care provided to the patient

Telephone numbers

Fax number

Email address

Social Security number

Medical record number

Health plan beneficiary number or account number

Past, present, or future payment for provision of health care

Medical device identifier

Internet Protocol (IP) address

Biometric identifiers, including finger and voice print

Full-face photographic images and any comparable image

Any other unique identifying number, characteristic, or code

and possibly prosecution by the Office of Civil Rights. Heavy fines accompany proven violations of the rule. These potential consequences have given organizations pause when requests for access to PHI are made.

In turn, researchers must not assume that simply because they work in a healthcare facility, they will have ready access to that facility's patient data, databases, or diagnostic information or even limited data sets. The provisions of the privacy rule provide additional safeguards for study participants, which can make it difficult, though not impossible, to do research in healthcare facilities. The researcher should determine well in advance of the start of the study as to whether access to certain data elements and health information can be obtained and how.

If the researcher requires access to the medical records of the patient or study participant, signed consent forms should be obtained that authorize the researcher to access the information. The research consent form should include an authorization for access to records. If that provision is not included, the researcher must document how access to the information will be obtained. Retrospective studies that involve the use of patient data from electronic sources or the medical record may require the researcher to supply a disclosure statement to document access. Alternatively, the IRB may grant a waiver that exempts the researcher from obtaining authorization, although disclosure statements may still be required. Table 3.6 provides an example of a disclosure statement.

While healthcare providers concede that sharing health data is crucial for the development of population health programs and public policy, ethical guidelines for

Table 3.6 Sample Disclosure Statement for Research Records

Disclosure for Research Purposes

Date: _____   IRB/Approval # _____

Patient Name: _____   Medical Record # _____

Researcher: _____

The above-named patient's record was accessed by the researcher for purposes of data collection in a research study approved by this organization.

Information used from this record will not disclose any individually identifiable health information and will be kept confidential as described in the research protocol on file with the organization's research review board.

the use of data from large clinical data warehouses are unclear. Technological advances have outpaced the ability to develop and gain wide agreement on ethical, legal, and social issues regarding the use of shared PHI and the reuse of data for research. On the one hand, use of data housed in large databases has enabled translational research projects that have been used to improve practice on a grand scale. On the other hand, there are no universal guidelines for transparency, trust, and security (Lamas, Barh, Brown, & Jaulent, 2015). The use of information drawn from large data warehouses raises questions about the reuse of data collected for one purpose for an entirely different purpose—in this case, research. Some of the issues under debate include patients' right to information about use of their data and their right to consent, researchers' agreements for data sharing, rights to access data warehouses in public institutions (e.g., the Medicare program), means to optimize data confidentiality, and considerations of the common good.

Reading Research for Evidence-Based Practice

Most studies will not explicitly describe the ethical or legal issues they faced unless those issues were unusual or difficult to resolve. This is not a weakness, but rather reflects the reality that ethical and legal compliance are a given when planning any research study. Ethical and regulatory guidelines are not negotiable, so it may be simply stated that the study underwent IRB review. When such a statement is made, it is safe to assume the study was reviewed by an objective panel and met basic ethical and legal requirements.

If explicit reference to the IRB is not made, then the nurse reader will need to scrutinize the methods section to determine whether a breach of ethical or legal requirements might have occurred. Particular attention should be paid to the methods for selecting the sample, obtaining informed consent, assigning subjects to treatment groups, and accessing their medical data. All of these procedures should reflect a fundamental respect for the ethical principles described in this chapter. The reader should be especially concerned if there were significant risks associated with the study, or if data were collected from medical records without a description of how privacy was protected. However, the absence of any mention of procedures to safeguard subjects does not mean these safeguards were not in place.

CHECKLIST FOR EVALUATING THE ETHICAL ISSUES IN A STUDY

❏ Adequate protections are in place to protect subjects from any potential harm.

❏ The authors document approval from the IRB.

❏ It is clearly indicated that subjects underwent informed consent.

❏ If vulnerable populations were involved, special consideration was given to informed consent and study procedures.

❏ Steps were taken to protect the anonymity, confidentiality, and privacy of subjects.

❏ There was no evidence of any type of coercion (implied or otherwise) to motivate participants to agree to the study.

❏ The researchers provided full disclosure to potential subjects. If deception was necessary to achieve the goals of the study, participants were debriefed about the experience.

❏ The benefits of the study outweighed the risks for individual subjects; a risk/benefit assessment was considered.

❏ Subjects were recruited, selected, and assigned to groups in an equitable way.

Using Research in Nursing Practice

The nurse should be hesitant to use the results of research in practice if he or she suspects the study was conducted unethically or in some way breached the legal protections of subjects. The nurse should be aware that research misconduct can occur, and that studies that are the result of such misconduct cannot be trusted. Ethical and legal constraints also help ensure research quality and validity of findings; results that were generated through deception or duress will likely not represent the population well. In other words, if the researcher cannot be trusted, then the research findings cannot be trusted either.

Creating Evidence for Practice

The nurse researcher can best deal with the potential ethical and legal issues in a research study by focusing on strong designs that answer the research question with a minimum of disruption in subjects' lives. If the nurse researcher focuses on doing the right thing, it is rare that an ethical or legal issue will arise.

The researcher must keep in mind, however, that compliance with ethical and regulatory issues is not confined to the design period. Some problems may arise during the implementation of a research study. Adherence to the principles that guide the legal and ethical treatment of subjects—whether in preparation for an IRB review or for actual data collection—should be ongoing throughout the study. Inadvertent problems and unforeseen issues may arise during research. The careful researcher considers these fundamental guidelines as a basis for decisions about the entire research process, not just the IRB application.

New ethical challenges may emerge when investigators are conducting research on the Internet. Through this medium, researchers can access subjects worldwide, from settings that are rarely represented in studies. Yet, gathering data on the Internet requires attention to additional ethical standards:

- Ensure subjects have a safe, private space to respond.
- Support the ethical acquisition of web addresses; ensure that the list owner has endorsed the study.

- Assess the potential risk of harm to participants and the intrusiveness of the study.
- Evaluate the vulnerability of the subjects.
- Implement a process to ensure subjects are of legal age to participate (Williams, 2012).

Research contributes knowledge to a field. The public relies on this knowledge to determine future courses of action, whether it is to decide on a course of medical treatment or merely to keep abreast of trends and current data. All research, then, must always be conducted with integrity, honesty, and respect for all parties involved, and with the utmost attention to ethical guidelines and regulatory limits.

Summary of Key Concepts

- When humans participate as subjects in research studies, care must be taken to preserve their rights.
- Subjects have the right to be informed of the study processes and potential risks, to be treated in a fair manner, and to withdraw from the study at any time.
- The Nuremberg Code and the Declaration of Helsinki are international guidelines for the conduct of ethical research; the United States also has the Belmont Report to guide researchers' behavior.
- Therapeutic research, in which the subject can be expected to receive a potentially beneficial treatment, differs from nontherapeutic research, which contributes to the body of knowledge but not to an individual's health.
- The foundational ethical principles that guide researchers in the treatment of human subjects are respect for persons, beneficence, and justice.
- The basic values that guide the research process include truthfulness, trust, and the best interests of the participants.
- Vulnerable populations include those groups with limited autonomy or capacity to make decisions. These populations are subject to special protections to ensure they are not exploited in research.
- Informed consent is a process of information exchange that begins with subject recruitment. Full disclosure of risks and benefits and the provision of understandable information needed to make a participation decision are hallmarks of a strong informed consent process.
- Deception or incomplete disclosure should be avoided in research. When it is necessary, there should be a strong rationale and subjects must be fully debriefed after the experience.
- Informed consent documents should be prepared in the most comprehensible way possible so that subjects are fully aware of the particulars of the study.
- Research integrity extends beyond subject rights to the way data are collected, analyzed, and reported.
- The nurse researcher advocates for the participants in research studies and must protect their autonomy and confidentiality at all times.

- IRB requirements have their origin in federal regulations and require varying levels of involvement in the approval process, depending on whether they involve expedited, exempt, or full board review.
- The IRB was established in response to the inhumane treatment of subjects, and the protection of individuals who are asked to participate in research remains the IRB's primary concern. The IRB is also a helpful group in providing critical feedback that can improve the design and strength of a study.
- Animal experimentation, much like human experimentation, raises concerns about necessity, purpose, design, risks, and benefits. Guidelines in this area focus on reducing the number of animals used in experiments, refining experimental procedures to minimize animal pain and suffering, and replacing animal subjects with nonanimal alternatives when scientifically feasible.
- HIPAA provides another layer of protection by guaranteeing the subject's right to protection of PHI. The researcher must plan carefully to ensure that all legal requirements are met, particularly because violations can carry with them serious consequences.

For More Depth and Detail

For a more in-depth look at the concepts in this chapter, try these references:

Anderson, E., & DuBois, J. (2012). IRB decision making with imperfect knowledge: A framework for evidence-based research ethics review. *Journal of Law, Medicine, & Ethics, 40*(4), 951–969.

Bradford, W., Hurdle, J., LaSalle, B., & Facelli, J. (2013). Development of a HIPAA-compliant environment for translational research data and analytics. *Journal of the American Medical Informatics Association, 21*, 185–189.

Cseko, G., & Tremaine, W. (2013). The role of the institutional review board in the oversight of the ethical aspects of human studies research. *Nutrition in Clinical Practice.* doi: 10.1177/0884533612474042

Dereli, T., Coskun, Y., Kolker, E., Guner, O., Agirbasli, M., & Ozdemir, V. (2014). Big data and ethics review for health systems research in LMIC's: Understanding risk, uncertainty, and ignorance—and catching the black swans? *American Journal of Bioethics, 14*(2), 48–50.

Greaney, A., Sheehy, A., Heffernan, C., Murphy, J., Mhaolrúnaigh, S., Heffernan, E., & Brown, G. (2012). Research ethics application: A guide for the novice researcher. *British Journal of Nursing, 21*(1), 38–43.

Hudgins, C., Rose, S., Fifield, P., & Arnault, S. (2013). Navigating the legal and ethical foundations of informed consent and confidentiality in integrated primary care. *Families, Systems, and Health, 31*(1), 9–19.

McKee, R. (2013). Ethical issues in using social media for health and health care research. *Health Policy, 110*, 298–301.

Milton, C. (2013). The ethics of research. *Nursing Science Quarterly, 26*(1), 20–23.

Vayena, E., Mastroianni, A., & Kahn, J. (2012). Ethical issues in health research with novel online sources. *American Journal of Public Health, 102*(12), 2225–2230.

Williams, S. (2012). The ethics of Internet research. *Online Journal of Nursing Informatics, 16*(2). Retrieved from http://ojni.org/issues/?p=1708

CRITICAL **APPRAISAL EXERCISE**

Retrieve the following full text article from the Cumulative Index to Nursing and Allied Health Literature or similar search database:

DeGrazia, M., Giambanco, D., Hamn, G., Ditzel, A., Tucker, L., & Gauvreau, K. (2015). Prevention of deformational plagiocephaly in hospitalized infants using a new orthotic device. *Journal of Obstetric, Gynecologic & Neonatal Nursing, 44*(1), 28–41.

Review the article, looking for evidence of any ethical or legal issues that arose in the study and how the researchers dealt with them. Consider the following appraisal questions in your critical review of this research article:

1. In which ways are the subjects in this study vulnerable? Which protections should be put in place to protect these subjects from harm?
2. Identify the potential risks inherent in this study for the subjects. What should specifically be included in the informed consent for this study?
3. What evidence is provided by the authors that the study was reviewed by the IRB and that appropriate informed consent was obtained?
4. How do the authors minimize the risks to the subjects?
5. In your opinion, do the potential benefits of this treatment outweigh the potential risks to the infant? Why or why not?

References

Becker, K., & Levy, M. (2001). Ensuring patient safety in clinical trials for treatment of acute stroke. *Journal of the American Medical Association, 286*(21), 2718–2719.

Boynton, M., Portnoy, D., & Johnson, B. (2013). Exploring the ethics and psychological impact of deception in psychological research. *IRB: Ethics & Human Research, 18*(2), 7–13.

Centers for Disease Control and Prevention. (2011). U.S. Public Health Service syphilis study at Tuskegee. Retrieved from http://www.cdc.gov/tuskegee/timeline.htm

Edelstein, L. (Trans.). (1943). *The Hippocratic oath: Text, translation and interpretation.* Baltimore, MD: Johns Hopkins University Press.

Ferdowsian, H., & Gluck, J. (2015). The ethical challenges of animal research. *Cambridge Quarterly of Healthcare Ethics, 24,* 391–406.

Franklin, P., Rowland, E., Fox, R., & Nicolson, P. (2012). Research ethics in accessing hospital staff and securing informed consent. *Qualitative Health Research, 22*(12), 1727–1738.

Hardicre, J. (2014). An overview of research ethics and learning from the past. *British Journal of Nursing, 23*(9), 483–486.

Horner, J., & Minifie, F. (2011a). Research ethics 1: Responsible conduct of research (RCR)—historical and contemporary issues pertaining to human and animal experimentation. *Journal of Speech, Language, and Hearing Research, 54,* S303–S329.

Horner, J., & Minifie, F. (2011b). Research ethics III: Publication practices and authorship, conflicts of interest, and research misconduct. *Journal of Speech, Language, and Hearing Research, 54,* S346–S362.

Ibrahim, D. (2006). Reduce, refine, replace: The failure of the three R's and the future of animal experimentation. *University of Chicago Legal Forum,* 195–220.

Juritzen, T., Grimen, H., & Heggen, K. (2011). Protecting vulnerable research participants: A Foucault-inspired analysis of ethics committees. *Nursing Ethics, 18*(5), 640–650.

Lamas, E., Barh, A., Brown, D., & Jaulent, M. (2015). Ethical, legal and social issues related to the health data-warehouses: Re-using health data in the research and public health research. *Digital Healthcare Empowering Europeans.* doi: 10.3233/978-1-61499-512-8-719

Lange, M., Rogers, W., & Dodds, S. (2013). Vulnerability in research ethics: A way forward. *Bioethics, 27*(6), 333–340.

Lunnay, B., Borlagdan, J., McNaughton, D., & Ward, P. (2015). Ethical use of social media to facilitate qualitative research. *Qualitative Health Research, 25*(1), 99–109.

Mangan, K. (October 12, 2007). Medical schools stop using dogs and pigs in teaching. *Chronicle of Higher Education,* A12.

McGuire, D. (1996, April 9). Rochester death halts MIT-funded study. *The Tech.* Retrieved from http://www-tech.mit.edu/V116/N17/rochester.17n.html

Milton, C. (2013). The ethics of research. *Nursing Science Quarterly, 26*(1), 20–23.

Moore, H., & McSherry, W. (2013). Ethical implications of consent in translational research. *Cancer Nursing Practice, 12*(10), 22–26.

National Academy of Sciences. (2009). *On being a scientist: Responsible conduct in research* (3rd ed.). Washington, DC: National Academies Press.

National Institutes of Health. (2015). NIH will no longer support biomedical research on chimpanzees. Bethesda, MD. https://www.nih.gov/about-nih/who-we-are/nih-director/statements/nih-will-no-longer-support-biomedical-research-chimpanzees

Nind, M., Wiles, R., Bengry-Howell, A., & Crow, G. (2012). Methodological innovation and research ethics: Forces in tension or forces in harmony? *Qualitative Research, 13*(6), 650–667.

Nisbet, M., & Fahy, D. (2013). Bioethics in popular science: Evaluating the media impact of *The Immortal Life of Henrietta Lacks* on the biobank debate. *BMC Medical Ethics, 14*(1), 1–10.

Nordentoft, H., & Kappel, N. (2011). Vulnerable participants in health research: Methodological and ethical challenges. *Journal of Social Work Practice, 25*(3), 365–376.

Odeh, P. (2013). The informed consent process. *AMT Events, 30*(1), 24–28.

Office of Laboratory Animal Welfare. (2002). *Public Health Services policy on humane care and use of laboratory animals.* Bethesda, MD: Author. Retrieved from http://grants.nih.gov/grants/olaw/references/phspolicylabanimals.pdf

Parascandola, M. (2004). Five years after the death of Jesse Gelsinger: Has anything changed? *Research Practitioner, 5*(6), 191.

U.S. Department of Health, Education, and Welfare (HEW). (1978). *The Belmont report: Ethical principles and guidelines for the protection of human subjects of research.* DHEW Publication Number (OS) 78-0012. Washington, DC: U.S. Government Printing Office.

U.S. Department of Health and Human Services. (2005, June 23). CFR 45, Public Health. Part 46, Protection of human subjects. Retrieved from http://www.hhs.gov/ohrp/regulations-and-policy/regulations/45-cfr-46/index.html#

Wasserman, R. (2013). Ethical issues and guidelines for conducting data analysis in psychological research. *Ethics & Behavior, 23*(1), 3–15.

Williams, S. (2012). The ethics of internet research. *Online Journal of Nursing Informatics, 16*(2). Retrieved from http://ojni.org/issues/?p=1708

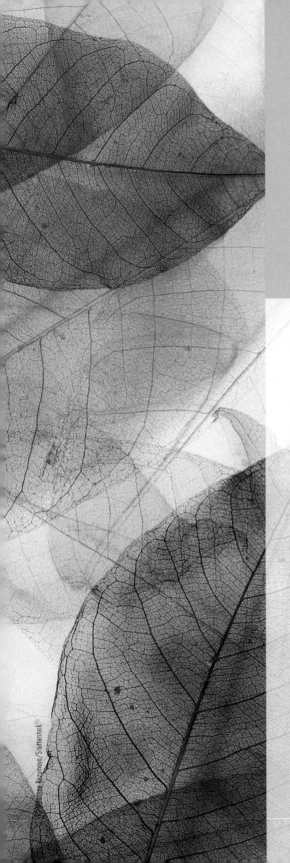

Part II

Planning for Research

© Oksana Razumova/Shutterstock

Chapter 4

Finding Problems and Writing Questions

CHAPTER OBJECTIVES

The study of this chapter will help the learner to

- Discuss strategies for identifying evidence-based practice problems.
- Describe the process for translating a practice problem into a researchable question.
- Define and contrast problem statements and purpose statements.
- Develop and articulate problem statements and purpose statements.
- Perform a critical analysis of the question, problem statement, and purpose statement from a research article.

KEY TERMS

Concepts	Inductive	Purpose statements
Deductive	Nondirectional hypothesis	Replication study
Directional hypothesis	Null hypothesis	Research question
Hypothesis	Problem statements	

Introduction

The best research starts with two words: "I wonder." A sense of curiosity is all that is needed to begin the research process. Observations about a practice problem become questions, and these questions lead to nursing research that provides evidence to solve the problem.

Finding and developing significant problems for nursing research is critical to improving outcomes for patients, nurses, organizations, and communities. The evolution of a research problem from a general topic of interest to the articulation of problem and purpose statements serves to narrow the focus to a researchable question. This progression moves the research problem from the conceptual (abstract concepts) to the operational (measurable concepts or variables). **FIGURE 4.1** depicts how the individual steps in translating a problem into a researchable question follow this path.

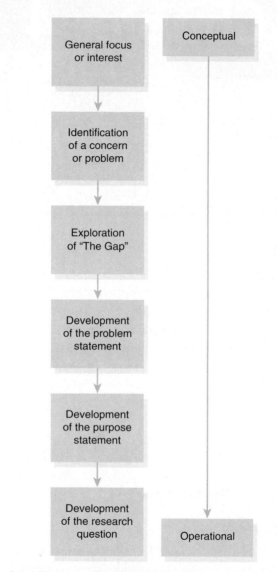

FIGURE 4.1 Traditional Evolution of the Research Process

VOICES FROM THE FIELD

The idea for this research study actually had its beginnings in a class on critically reading research that I took. I work on a medical–surgical unit, and my team decided that we would like to try to do a small project. We decided to do some observation and find a question to study, even though it is a really busy unit.

About that time, we had a physician who began doing more bariatric surgery. The standing orders for these patients were to have physical and occupational therapy personnel evaluate the patients and get them up and walking. We had always interpreted that order as being implemented on the next morning, because the therapists were generally not available in the evenings when these patients were in shape to start moving. We had patients who wanted to get up and start walking the first evening, though, so we would help them walk. We noticed that these patients seemed to get less nausea. Limiting nausea and retching is important in these patients because we cannot get their intravenous line (IV) out until they are not vomiting, and retching is very painful for them. They get their pain medications through the IV, and if they are vomiting we cannot switch to oral medications and pull their IV lines. If the patients had to wait until the second day to walk, it seemed they had more nausea and vomiting, and those reactions just backlogged everything. It usually meant that their discharge was delayed until the evening of the second day. We wondered if perhaps the earlier walking was helping with the nausea.

We started with a literature search. Originally, we planned to find a study and replicate it; we never thought we could do a study of our own. We just wanted to duplicate what someone else had done. But there were no studies to be found. We found lots of studies of the effects of ambulation in the postoperative period, but nothing dealing with this specific group of patients, and none of the studies measured nausea as the outcome measure. So we thought, "Maybe we need to do a study." We were going to do something very simple—not even go through the institutional review board (IRB), but instead undertake an investigation that was more like a quality study. We were nervous about having to go to the IRB; we thought that would be far too deep for us. We thought a little study would be a good way—a really simple way—for the staff to become involved in research, and we thought it was doable.

We had an opportunity to consult a researcher through our evidence-based practice council. The researcher told us, "This is a good study; this is publishable," and that was a turning point for us. We realized that this topic was as important as what other nurse researchers studied, and we recognized that we had an opportunity to make a contribution to practice.

What started as a simple little question—Does walking affect nausea?—has evolved into something more complicated. Our research question is now based on time—in other words, how soon does the patient have to walk to get a benefit? The process forced us to produce criteria for when a patient is ready to walk, which became a conversation in which the whole staff participated. We introduced another element after consulting with physical therapy personnel. We now have one group in which patients use a bedside pedaler and a second group in which patients walk, and we will see if one approach offers an advantage. That would be helpful to know, because when we have really chaotic days, we may not have a lot of time to stop and help someone walk. If we find that the pedaler does help the patient's gut "wake up" faster, then we can use this device instead of providing walking assistance, because it takes much less time.

When the people on the unit realized that our goal was publication, they got on board with our research. We have learned to appreciate the nurses with whom we work who have stayed in medical–surgical nursing. One of the driving forces behind this effort was our quest to gain some respect for the fact that we are a highly qualified group of nurses who care deeply about patient care and doing the right thing for patients. Taking our nursing practice to the next level through publication of original research could be a real source of pride for the staff—and we think that is why they are so solidly behind it.

Our study has encouraged us to look at our whole nursing practice and realize it is not insignificant—that our research is something someone would want to read. Now that we have finished the IRB process, we have realized, yeah, we really can do that.

Maureen Wenzel, FNP-BC

Deductive:
A process of reasoning from the general to the specific.

The traditional method for finding and developing research problems suggests a deductive, sequential process moving from a general interest to the development of a research question. **FIGURE 4.2** illustrates how the individual steps might look in the development of a specific researchable question.

In truth, the process of finding and developing research problems can be as chaotic as a busy parking lot. Some motorists drive their cars headfirst into the spaces, some motorists back their cars into the spaces, and still other motorists drive their cars into and out of the spaces until their cars are properly positioned. Research question development

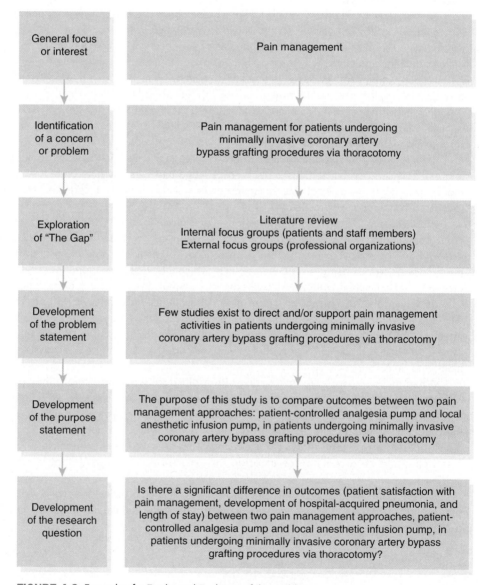

General focus or interest	Pain management
Identification of a concern or problem	Pain management for patients undergoing minimally invasive coronary artery bypass grafting procedures via thoracotomy
Exploration of "The Gap"	Literature review Internal focus groups (patients and staff members) External focus groups (professional organizations)
Development of the problem statement	Few studies exist to direct and/or support pain management activities in patients undergoing minimally invasive coronary artery bypass grafting procedures via thoracotomy
Development of the purpose statement	The purpose of this study is to compare outcomes between two pain management approaches: patient-controlled analgesia pump and local anesthetic infusion pump, in patients undergoing minimally invasive coronary artery bypass grafting procedures via thoracotomy
Development of the research question	Is there a significant difference in outcomes (patient satisfaction with pain management, development of hospital-acquired pneumonia, and length of stay) between two pain management approaches, patient-controlled analgesia pump and local anesthetic infusion pump, in patients undergoing minimally invasive coronary artery bypass grafting procedures via thoracotomy?

FIGURE 4.2 Example of a Traditional Evolution of the Problem

likewise is amenable to many different approaches. Some researchers do, indeed, use a sequential set of steps to arrive at a specific and well-articulated question. Many other nurse researchers use nontraditional methods for finding and developing research problems. These processes may be more **inductive**, in which specific observations serve as the starting points, leading to a general focus or interest. This approach is more common in evidence-based practice studies, as specific problems generally spark interest in finding an overall solution via research. **FIGURE 4.3** demonstrates a nontraditional example of finding and developing a research problem. Still other methods may begin somewhere in the middle of the traditional process by recognizing a gap, then proceed to identify the big picture as well as the specific research question.

Inductive:
A process of reasoning from specific observations to broader generalizations.

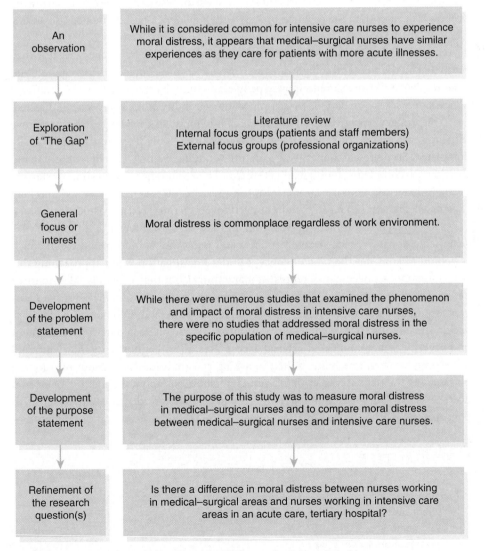

FIGURE 4.3 Nontraditional Example of the Evolution of a Research Problem

Concepts:
Abstract ideas or topics of interest that must be narrowed to researchable questions to be investigated.

Regardless of the approach—deductive, inductive, or somewhere in between—finding and developing research problems may be a process best characterized as a work in progress. The goal is always the same, though: to narrow the focus of the research problem so that a feasible research question emerges. The importance of narrowing the focus of the research cannot be overstressed. Research problems that have not been narrowed generate too many **concepts** and relationships to test.

The initial phase of implementing evidence-based practice is identifying the need for change that will improve patient care (Facchiano, Snyder, & Nunez, 2011). The need for change may become evident to nurses because of emerging problems or new knowledge (Boswell & Cannon, 2012). During this phase, the topic is selected and preliminary, problem-based questions are considered. Key words in problem-based questions drive the search and retrieval of literature and set the stage for research design. This narrowing process is used both in the research process and in evidence-based practice (Boswell & Cannon, 2012).

Subjects or topics that are overly broad are problematic for researchers because they mean that methodological complexities increase, expert methodologists are required, and resource demands (for example, money, people, and time) increase. With every additional concept or associated relationship examined, the feasibility of the study may be affected.

The primary objective of nursing research is to increase knowledge so as to improve nursing practice, but, of course, it can be accomplished only if the research is actually completed. Some researchers spend a lifetime studying a single concept; others spend their careers completing multiple, small studies. There is no shame in starting, or staying, small. Narrow questions are far easier for the novice researcher to address and may help the nurse learn skills that can then be applied to larger, more complex studies.

As the research problem moves from a broad topic of interest to a narrower, researchable question, measurable variables and outcomes should become evident. It is helpful to consider the type of concept under investigation when approaching this determination. Concepts may represent many things, but they generally fall into three categories: patient sensitive, staff member sensitive, or organizationally sensitive. Concepts studied by nurses, especially novice nurse researchers, should be limited to those within the nursing span of control. For example, a nurse interested in the development and severity of hematomas at arterial access sites after diagnostic or interventional arteriography would be better suited to asking research questions about positioning and turning the patient, rather than addressing questions about the method of arterial access used for the procedure. The first research question identifies nurse-sensitive concepts (repositioning and turning), whereas the second research question identifies

GRAY MATTER

Nursing research concepts can be organized into three categories:
- Patient sensitive
- Staff member sensitive
- Organizationally sensitive

medically sensitive concepts (arterial access methods). **Table 4.1** provides examples of each of these kinds of concepts.

Finding and Developing Research Problems

Often, research problems find the nurse, rather than the other way around. Frustrations with ineffective procedures, the search for a "better way," or the need to help a single patient may motivate the nurse to seek research-based evidence to improve patient care. The search for research problems is one of the easiest parts of the research process; researchable problems surround the contemporary nurse in practice.

Sources of Research Problems

Researchable problems can come from an almost unlimited number of sources (American Association of Colleges of Nursing [AACN], 2013; Boswell & Cannon, 2012; Schmidt & Brown, 2011). The following are some sources for researchable problems:

- Clinical practice observations
- Educational processes and experiences
- Consumer/customer feedback and personal experience
- Theoretical models and frameworks
- Professional literature
- Performance improvement studies
- Research reports and priorities
- Social issues

Clinical Practice

Research problems may be generated from active, passive, or other organizational activities. Active methods of problem discovery include experiences with direct patient care and discussion with other members of the healthcare team through formal or informal communications. Patient problems, ineffective clinical procedures, and changes in protocols all present opportunities for research. Passive methods for identifying problems include medical record review and observation. Data collection activities,

Table 4.1 Examples of Patient-, Nursing-, and Organizationally Sensitive Concepts		
Patient-Sensitive Concepts	**Nurse-Sensitive Concepts**	**Organizationally Sensitive Concepts**
Anxiety	Burnout	Cost
Skin integrity	Lower back injuries	Length of stay
Functional independence	Medication errors	Readmission
Blood glucose	Pain management	Resource utilization
Blood pressure	Patient falls	Satisfaction with nursing care
Quality of life	Restraint prevalence	
Satisfaction with nursing care		

such as those performed for quality improvement or risk management purposes, may also bring problems to light.

The need for confirmed evidence-based practice generates numerous research questions. Nurses are in a unique position to change and confirm clinical practices. Through structured decision-making processes, nurses, other members of the healthcare team, and patients and families together have the ability to improve healthcare-related processes, outcomes, safety, satisfaction, and costs (Boswell & Cannon, 2012). Nursing practice comprises a mixture of evidence and tradition. It is essential that nurses continually ask themselves and one another the crucial questions: What is the evidence for this approach to nursing care? Can I solve this problem with evidence?

Educational Processes and Experiences

Nursing students who are taking research courses are required to develop problem, purpose, and research statements from required and/or self-determined topics. Research-focused educational institutions may also support institution-driven research activities examining interests such as age-specific care, the effects of caring, or nursing shortage outcomes. Within the assignments and disciplined inquiry that occur during the educational experience, particularly graduate study, nursing students and their mentors may generate many researchable problems.

Consumer Feedback or Personal Experience

Research problems may be generated from consumer or personal experience. Such problems are distinguished from social issues; that is, consumers of health care have the opportunity to share ideas about and perceptions of care and treatment, and to suggest research questions that can potentially promote health throughout the continuum of care, improve patient outcomes and safety, and influence delivery models and cost-effectiveness (Centers for Medicare & Medicaid Services [CMS], 2013; Hospital Care Quality Information from the Consumer Perspective [HCAHPS], 2013; Patient-Centered Outcomes Research Institute [PCORI], 2013). Nurses may also have experiences as family members or as patients themselves. This unique perspective, in which nurses view nursing care from the other side of the bed, gives rise to opportunities to transform that care. Research problems generated from personal experience may expose clinical, consumer, social, and other opportunities for improvement and drive the research priorities of both individuals and organizations.

Research problems generated from the results of activities aimed at soliciting consumer and/or patient feedback may be generated from the following sources:

- Patients and customers of the institution, both external and internal
- Leaders who represent the interests of specific services (e.g., cardiac care)
- Departments (e.g., coronary care unit) and service lines (e.g., cardiac services) within an organizational structure
- Members of general or specialty professional organizations (e.g., American Nurses Association, American Association of Critical-Care Nurses)
- Advisory boards and other consumer/customer input organizations
- Accrediting, regulatory, and safety organizations

The feedback garnered from these groups may be used to generate problem statements, purpose statements, research questions, and testable hypotheses, as well as to set priorities for performance improvement or other research activities. Feedback may be solicited through surveys, during formal and informal meetings, and at conferences and workshops, or it may be received electronically.

Professional Literature

Research problems may be generated from the results of professional literature reviews. Sources of professional literature reviews include clinical and nonclinical works, databases, and letters and opinions. Clinical works include books and journals addressing nursing and medical topics, both general and specialty. Nonclinical works include books and journals presenting non-nursing and nonmedical topics from other fields of study that may be generalized into an appropriate, researchable problem to expand nursing knowledge. Many databases, both clinical and nonclinical, are capable of provoking inquiry. Examples of these databases include those that hold data from previous studies (clinical) and census data (nonclinical). Many research problems have been developed by using the data collected by other researchers and taking a unique approach to the analysis.

Published letters and opinions are another interesting source of research problems. Letters and opinions written by nurses and other medical professionals often express concern, as well as issue directives, about researchable problems, gaps in current knowledge, limitations of available research, and recommendations for future research.

Performance Improvement Activities

Performance improvement activities, also known as quality improvement activities, are used to improve processes and outcomes and to meet regulatory requirements. Tools and techniques specific to performance improvement activities do not meet the requirements of traditional research methods. In particular, performance improvement studies are often characterized by methodological limitations, a lack of control over extraneous variables, violation of assumptions for statistical testing, and small sample sizes in a single setting; all of these factors affect the generalizability of their findings. Nevertheless, the results of performance improvement activities may be used as a springboard to engage in formal research activities. Researchable problems may start as performance improvement activities and expand into formal research projects with alterations in methodological approach, sampling strategy, and informed consent procedures.

Research Reports and Priorities

Research problems may also be generated from the outcomes of other research studies and evidence-based practice reviews. Previous research may influence the generation of research problems either directly or indirectly. By convention, most research reports include a section on "suggestions for future research," which outlines ways to extend and expand on the currently available research. Researchers may directly influence the generation of subsequent research problems by explicitly stating remaining problems, gaps, and questions. One means of directly influencing subsequent studies is the type of research known as a **replication study**. Replication studies may be used to validate findings and knowledge, increase their generalizability (population and setting), or eliminate or minimize limitations (methodology). Replication studies are good exercises because they

Replication study:
A study generated from previous research studies in which the research is reproduced to validate findings, increase generalizability, or eliminate or minimize limitations.

Problem statements:
Statements of the
disparity between
what is known and
what needs to be
known and addressed
by the research.

increase the knowledge of inexperienced researchers. Research also may indirectly influence the generation of a problem when the reader identifies a problem with the written report (e.g., a discrepancy, gap, inconsistency, or unidentified limitation) or disagrees with the methodology and/or results of the original investigator.

The directives and recommendations of individuals and organizations may also serve as a source of research problems. In developing these directives and recommendations, individuals (educators and researchers) and organizations (clinical, educational, funding, and regulatory) apply their expertise to identify problems and gaps in current knowledge. Some of these experts may have developed problem statements and research questions to prioritize future research.

Social Issues

Research problems may be generated from social issues. Social issues include, but are not limited to, the effects of age, culture, education, gender, income, race, religion, and sexual preference. Social issues may be examined in the context of current events, the environment, and health policy. They may also be addressed in relation to local, state, national, or international populations. For example, obesity may be considered in terms of age, gender, race, and other social classifications. Notably, the "obesity epidemic" has given rise to equally epidemic rates of diabetes and heart disease. Additionally, obesity and its associated comorbidities affect national issues such as healthcare expenditures (percentage of the gross national product) and the ability of the government to maintain military readiness. Given this condition's widespread impacts, it should not be surprising that a large number of organizations are examining obesity-related research questions. Collaborative, multidisciplinary studies addressing research questions that are clinically and socially relevant and that could potentially improve outcomes in local, national, and international communities are more likely to receive support and to receive funding (White, 2012).

This list of sources for research problems is not exhaustive. Research problems are often the product of both internal and external driving forces; they are seldom generated from a single source. Any process or outcome associated with patient care, staff members' work environment, or organizational success may become the basis for study. The potential nurse researcher can scrutinize the current practices and ask the following questions:

- Why are we doing it this way?
- Is there a better way of doing it?
- Should we be doing it at all?

All of these questions may give rise to researchable problems, whose solutions may add valuable evidence to the effective practice of nursing.

Articulation of Research Problem Statements

Research **problem statements** are declarations of disparity: the difference (gap) between what is known and what needs to be known about a topic. They articulate a discrepancy that is to be addressed by the research process. The disparity, whether a small gap or a large chasm, defines the area(s) of concern and focuses the research methods (Boswell & Cannon, 2012; Schmidt & Brown, 2011). Most problem statements are explicitly stated; however, some problem statements may be inferred. The inferred research problem statement may describe the importance or potential consequences of the disparity as it pertains to clinical practice.

Problem statements, explicitly stated or inferred, are usually found at the beginning of a research report, in the introduction, or in the review of literature, and they may be repeated throughout the written report. The idea of a single problem statement is misleading; problem statements may resemble problem paragraphs and often can be several sentences long. Problem statements may be written as either questions or statements, and well-written ones contain clear, concise, and well-defined components.

Two examples of well-written problem statements from published articles follow:

- "The background research identified eight articles that looked at the gendered experience of being a nurse, six from the male perspective and two from the female, but none comparing these experiences" (Rowlinson, 2013, p. 218).
- "The majority of studies were quasi-experimental, and all examined disposable infant diapers under conditions of high humidity and/or radiant heat sources. One study found that no significant changes occurred after six hours; all others found that changes in diaper weights occurred. The question remained unanswered as to what changes might occur in diaper weights over time in open-air, open bed patient environments" (Carlisle et al., 2012, p. 224).

Development of Research Purpose Statements

Whereas research problem statements identify a gap in knowledge that requires disciplined study, research **purpose statements** are declarations of intent. Purpose statements indicate the general goal of the study and often describe the direction of inquiry (Boswell & Cannon, 2012; Schmidt & Brown, 2011). The purpose of the research should be clearly stated.

Purpose statements are written as objective statements. They are easily identified in reports by their inclusion of words such as *aim, goal, intent, objective,* or *purpose.* They contain clear, concise, and well-defined components including key variables to be studied, possible interrelationships, and the nature of the population of interest.

Two examples of well-written purpose statements from published articles follow:

- "The objective was to explore, analyze, and compare and contrast the gender differences with the existing literature" (Rowlinson, 2013, p. 219).
- "The purpose of this study was to examine changes in disposable infant diaper weights at selected intervals post-wetting" (Carlisle et al., 2012, p. 224).

Researcher bias is a limitation that may cause readers to question the validity of research processes and outcomes. When developing purpose statements, researchers should use unbiased verbs such as *compare, describe, develop, discover, explore, test,* and *understand* and avoid biased verbs such as *demonstrate, prove,* and *show.*

- *Example of using an unbiased verb:* The purpose of the study was to explore the effects of music therapy on speech recovery in adult stroke patients in a rehabilitation facility.
- *Example of using a biased verb:* The purpose of the study was to prove that music therapy improves speech recovery in adult stroke patients in a rehabilitation facility.

Purpose statements: Declarative and objective statements that indicate the general goal of the study and often describe the direction of the inquiry.

Table 4.2 lists some useful verbs for purpose statements. Carefully writing the purpose statement is the first step in demonstrating the research question's appropriateness for study. Although a purpose statement is relatively easy to compose, completing a study is a time-intensive, arduous process. It should be undertaken only when the researcher has a reasonable expectation of successfully achieving the purpose as stated.

Fit of the Purpose Statement

Research purpose statements indicate how variables will be studied within specific populations and settings. There should be a good fit between the design suggested in the purpose statement and the methods used in the research study (Boswell & Cannon, 2012; Schmidt & Brown, 2011). The following examples demonstrate potential purpose statements for a quantitative, correlation design:

- The purpose of the study was to determine the direction and strength of the relationship between depression and functional independence in patients at an urban rehabilitation center.
- The purpose of the study was to measure the effects of depression on functional independence in patients at an urban rehabilitation center.

The purpose statement in the first example exemplifies a good fit between the purpose statement and the study methods. Correlation methods measure the direction and strength of a relationship; they are not appropriate for assessing cause and effect. The purpose statement in the second example does not have a good fit with this method because it indicates the researchers intend to determine a causal relationship between the variables. This research focus would be better addressed with a quantitative, experimental design.

Table 4.2 Research Methods and Examples of Purpose Statement Verbs

Qualitative Methods	Quantitative Methods
Ethnographic	**Correlation**
Assess	Determine
Describe	Examine
Examine	Identify
Understand	Understand
Grounded Theory	**Descriptive**
Develop	Compare
Extend	Contrast
Identify	Describe
Validate	Identify
Phenomenological	**Experimental**
Describe	Determine
Develop	Examine
Generate	Investigate
Understand	Measure

Differentiating Research Problem Statements and Research Purpose Statements

Research problem statements are declarations of disparity (why); research purpose statements are declarations of intent (what). Although problem statements and purpose statements clarify and support each other, they represent different levels of the deductive process—that is, the process of moving from a general focus or interest to the development of a specific research question. As researchers identify problems, explore disparities or gaps, and develop problem and purpose statements, the focus of the research narrows, increasing the feasibility of carrying out the study as intended.

Problem and purpose statements are not limited to research based on empirical measurement—that is, to quantitative studies. Qualitative studies use subjective means to describe and examine concepts and their meanings, but will still have an identifiable problem focus and purpose statement. The problem and purpose statements of qualitative studies may be vaguer and less prescriptive than those for quantitative studies, primarily due to the emergent nature of research design in qualitative research. Although an overall problem is generally identified for a qualitative study, the purpose may be broader and less detailed than that of a quantitative study because the particulars of the study may become clear only after data collection has commenced. In other words, qualitative problem and purpose statements are more general and allow for the flexibility that is characteristic of an emergent design (Boswell & Cannon, 2012; Schmidt & Brown, 2011). Quantitative studies, by their very nature, are more prescriptive and use objective measures to describe and examine concepts and the relationships between concepts. Thus, quantitative problem and purpose statements are generally detailed, are based in previous literature, and outline the variables, populations, and settings to be studied.

It remains important for a clear problem to be identified and a purpose statement to be articulated before either type of research design begins. Table 4.3 and Table 4.4 provide examples of problem and purpose statements for selected qualitative and quantitative research designs.

Developing the Research Question

The problem statement is a general review of why a particular research study is necessary; the purpose statement gives an overview of the intent of the study. Neither of these is prescriptive enough to give specific guidance to the design and methodology of the study. Instead, a focused research question is necessary to fulfill this need. The research question is the final step prior to beginning research design, and it outlines the primary components that will be studied. In some cases, the research question is analogous to the purpose statement, but it is constructed as a question instead of a statement. Questions that are clear, simple, and straightforward provide direction for subsequent design decisions and enable the researcher to focus the research process.

Research question: A question that outlines the primary components to be studied and that guides the design and methodology of the study.

Table 4.3 Problem and Purpose Statements from Qualitative Research Studies

Design	Problem and Purpose Statements
Ethnography	**Title:** Parental involvement in neonatal pain management: Reflecting on the researcher-practitioner role (Skene, 2012)
	Problem statement: "I have been surprised to find that while the neonatal literature presents a description of what happens when parents in the neonatal unit are excluded from their babies' pain management, it does not provide a picture of what happens when they are involved" (p. 27).
	Purpose statement: "To fill this gap, I began a study to answer the following research question: 'How do parents interact with babies and nurses around the provision of comfort care in a neonatal intensive care unit where information and training in comfort care have been provided?'" (p. 27).
Grounded theory	**Title:** Patients' perspectives on timing of urinary catheter removal after surgery (Bhardwaj, Pickard, Carrick-Sen, & Brittain, 2012)
	Problem statement: "There is limited evidence to inform the patients' perspective of short-term urinary catheterization after surgical procedures" (p. S4).
	Purpose statement: "The aims of the study were to: Explore patients' beliefs and perceptions regarding perioperative urinary catheterization [and] Relate patients' beliefs to current and future practice" (p. S4).
Phenomenological	**Title:** Quality of life after ileo-anal pouch formation: Patient perceptions (Perrin, 2012)
	Problem statement: "Williams (2002), who studied preoperative pouch patients, highlighted that little attention is given to addressing their experiences of living with a pouch" (p. S11).
	Purpose statement: "This phenomenological research study explored whether having an ileo-anal pouch provides a good quality of life by asking six individuals who have undergone ileo-anal pouch formation about their own perception of their quality of life following ileo-anal pouch formation" (p. S12).

Examples of well-written research questions from published articles follow:

- "The research question explored was 'Is the lived experience of being a nurse different depending on your gender?'" (Rowlinson, 2013, p. 219)
- "The research question was: Does volume of urine, diaper configuration, and size of diaper lead to statistically significant changes over time in the weight of infant disposable diapers?" (Carlisle et al., 2012, p. 224)

As questions are refined, they should be critiqued continuously. The simple act of writing the question down and asking for input from colleagues may help to focus and refine the question. Does it make sense? Is it logical? Is this question important for clinical

Table 4.4 Problem and Purpose Statements from Quantitative Research Studies

Design	Problem and Purpose Statements
Correlation	**Title:** The relationship between clinical indicators, coping styles, perceived support and diabetes-related distress among adults with type 2 diabetes (Karlsen, Oftedal, & Bru, 2012) **Problem statement:** "To date, we have been unable to find any research that compares the relative contribution of (i) essential clinical indicators of diabetes regulation as listed in the introduction, (ii) coping styles, and (iii) perceived social support to the variation in diabetes-related distress among adults with type 2 diabetes" (p. 393). **Purpose statement:** "One aim of this study was to describe diabetes-related distress, coping styles, and perceptions of social support among adults with type 2 diabetes. The main aim was to investigate the extent to which (i) clinical indicators such as Hb_{A1c}, diabetes treatment, diabetes-related complications, disease duration and BMI, (ii) coping styles, and (iii) perceived support from healthcare professionals and family are related to diabetes-related distress" (p. 393).
Descriptive design	**Title:** Quality of life after percutaneous coronary intervention: Part 2 (Cassar & Baldacchino, 2012) **Problem statement:** "Quality of life (QoL) has been found to be affected by demographic factors and cardiac risk factors. Research that concentrates on physical health and functional ability after this coronary intervention gives only a partial picture of life quality (Groeneveld et al., 2007; Konstantina & Dokoutsidou, 2009; Moons et al., 2006; Seto et al., 2000; Szygula-Jurkiewicz et al., 2005)" (p. 1125). **Purpose statement:** "The study aimed to: Assess the holistic QoL of patients who have undergone a PCI [and] identify significant differences in QoL between subgroups of patients by demographic characteristics and perceived cardiac risk factors" (p. 1125).
Experimental	**Title:** Pain after lung transplant: High frequency chest wall oscillation (HFCWO) vs chest physiotherapy (CPT) (Esquerra-Gonzalez et al., 2013) **Problem statement:** "Two studies used a randomized design to compare HFCWO and CPT on outcome variables of comfort and preference . . . No published studies have investigated which treatment is less painful and preferred by lung transplant recipients" (p. 116). **Purpose statement:** "Given the lack of evidence supporting the effectiveness of HFCWO and CPT among lung transplant recipients, the purposes of this pilot, feasibility study were to (1) explore the effect of HFCWO versus CPT treatment on patients' pain patterns by measuring pain scores before and after treatment and (2) compare lung transplant recipients' preference for HFCWO versus CPT" (p. 117).

care? Could this research yield practical benefits? This kind of feedback can help the nurse researcher generate a strong research question that provides guidance for subsequent research design and methodology. The time invested in carefully constructing the final research question is well worth the effort; it provides a foundation for the remaining decisions that must be made about the research process.

The Elements of a Good Research Question

Two guides are helpful in developing a good research question. One of them is described by the acronym *PICO*, which outlines the elements of a good quantitative question. PICO stands for population, intervention, comparison, and outcome. Using preoperative education for short-stay patients undergoing prostatectomy as an example, a research question based on PICO might look like this:

- *Population:* In radical prostatectomy patients staying in the hospital one day after surgery . . .
- *Intervention:* Does customized preoperative teaching . . .
- *Comparison:* Compared to standard preoperative teaching . . .
- *Outcomes:* Lead to better pain control as measured by a visual analog scale?

A qualitative research question is the least prescriptive type of research question. It outlines, in a general way, the phenomenon to be studied and the people who can best inform the question. The researcher defines the general boundaries of the inquiry, but even these are subject to change. The study begins with the researcher having a general question in mind, but the researcher is flexible enough to change the particulars of the question if the information gathered suggests that step would be appropriate. Measurements, interventions, and comparison groups are irrelevant in qualitative research, so they are not parts of the qualitative question. Specification of outcomes may be incorporated into the qualitative question but are not necessary elements. Because qualitative questions may actually evolve over the course of the study, they are reported in detail only after the study is complete.

Clearly, the elements of the research question are very similar to those in the purpose statement. The primary distinction relates to format—a purpose statement is given as a statement, whereas a research question is stated as a question. In addition, the research question often spells out the outcome in a statement such as "as measured by the Wong Faces Pain Scale," and so gives more specificity to what is to be measured.

A Well-Done PICO Question

Among parents of children diagnosed with type 1 diabetes in a small Midwestern city, what are parents' self-reported self-efficacy scores related to diabetic care management pre- and post-implementation of a web-based social support platform? (Merkel & Wright, 2012)

A Well-Done PICOT Question

Will the implementation of a popup prompt in the health record increase adherence and decrease time to administration of aspirin from Emergency Department presentation of women who are having symptoms suspicious of acute cardiac syndrome? (Carman et al., 2013)

Box 4.1 PICO Versus PECO Versus PICOT

Any research question will be strengthened by a systematic approach to developing some fundamental elements.

- *Population:* In almost every study, the population addressed needs to be clearly identified. Begin by deciding how broad the population should be. Who are the specific people of interest? Can selecting a subset of this population as the sample make the study more focused and feasible? Are there specific conditions, risk factors, or characteristics that are of interest? By thinking through these elements, a clear population of interest may emerge. Describe the population as succinctly and specifically as possible.

- *Intervention:* Determine exactly what the "intervention" is for the study. What will the researcher introduce into the study or manipulate? Is the "cause" a naturally occurring characteristic? The former will be better represented in a PICO question; the latter in a PECO question (discussed later in this feature). Interventions may include process measures, specific treatment practices, or exposure to an event or substance. Describe the intervention or risk factor in a focused but clear way.

- *Comparison:* Without a comparison, all we can say about the intervention is that it was better than nothing. The object of comparison will likely be the standard practice, but it may also be a group without a risk factor. This issue does not usually require in-depth description in the statement of the research question.

- *Outcomes:* The outcome should reflect the nature, direction, and degree of results anticipated. This definition should be precise and, in most cases, will indicate the way the outcome will be measured.

In many cases, the "intervention" is not introduced, so much as it is "found." In these cases—where the effects of a naturally occurring event are of interest—some researchers prefer the PECO approach. PECO includes the following four elements:

- Population of interest
- Exposure to a factor of interest
- Control or comparison group
- Outcome of interest

It is clear that the PECO approach mirrors the PICO method closely, except that the "intervention" is not manipulated or artificially introduced into the experiment. PECO research questions are commonly encountered in population health or epidemiology studies (McKeon & McKeon, 2015).

Some researchers recommend adding elements to the model. The most common extension is found in the PICOT model. The final "T" in this acronym stands for time, referring to the duration of data collection or the expected time to observe an effect (Carman et al., 2013).

The PICO model is not appropriate for every research problem. This format must be modified for descriptive studies—in which no intervention is applied—and for studies describing relationships. In these cases, the research question should include at a minimum a clear identification of the population and the variables being studied.

Another acronym—FINER—gives guidance in the appraisal of a research question. This model gives the nurse researcher a framework for evaluating the desirable characteristics of a good question:

- *Feasible:* Adequate subjects, technical expertise, time, and money are available; the scope is narrow enough for study.
- *Interesting:* The question is interesting to the investigator.

- *Novel:* The study confirms or refutes previous findings, or provides new findings.
- *Ethical:* The study cannot cause unacceptable risk to participants and does not invade privacy.
- *Relevant:* The question is relevant to scientific knowledge, clinical and health policy, or future research directions.

Once the question is carefully defined, then the link to design elements often becomes obvious. If not, then the researcher may need to provide more specificity about the population, intervention, or outcomes in the research question. These three elements of the question will later provide guidance in the selection of a sample, the procedures, and the measurements.

The Link Between Questions and Design

Focusing the research question guides how that question will be answered. The question will lead to a sampling strategy (Who is the patient population?), an intervention protocol (Which treatment is being tested?), and the outcomes measured (How will the effect be demonstrated?). There are also direct links between the kind of words used in the question and the design that is used to answer it.

Descriptive questions ask simple questions about what is happening in a defined population or situation. For example, a descriptive question is "What are the characteristics of surgical patients reporting high satisfaction with pain management during their hospitalization?" Three general types of research questions are best answered with descriptive studies:

- Resource allocation questions
- Questions about areas for further research
- Questions about informal diagnostic information

Most qualitative questions are answered with descriptive studies, because a qualitative study is generally descriptive of a single sample. The broad nature of a qualitative research question lends itself to a variety of methods, ranging from interviews to focus groups to observation. The specific verbiage used in the qualitative question may guide the study's design, but in general the design emerges from the nature of the phenomenon under study, not from the particular way in which the research question is written.

Analytic studies compare one or more interventions to specific outcomes. For example, the questions "What is the effectiveness of individual or group educational sessions for hip surgery patients?" and "Is breast cancer associated with high fat intake?" may be answered with quantitative analysis. The objective of an analytic study is to determine whether there is a causal relationship between variables, so the research question reflects study of the effect of an intervention on one or more outcomes. Statistical procedures are used to determine whether a relationship would likely have occurred by chance alone. Analytic studies usually compare two or more groups.

Analytic studies are logical means to address questions that will be answered with numbers or with measurements. In this kind of quantitative study, the researcher performs tests related to the research question using statistical analysis. Although research questions are not directly testable with numbers, their transformed version—the hypothesis—is subject to numerical analysis. It is important, then, to translate quantitative research questions into hypothesis statements that lend themselves to statistical analysis.

From Question to Hypothesis

Just as the research question guides the design of a study, so a hypothesis guides the statistical analysis. A research hypothesis is a specific statement that predicts the direction and nature of the results of a study. It can be complex or simple, directional or nondirectional, and stated in statistical symbols or narrative form (Connelly, 2015). The way a hypothesis is written determines which tests are run, which outcome is expected, and how conservative the results are. A hypothesis is a restatement of the research question in a form that can be analyzed statistically for significance. It is specifically used in causal tests, such as experimental designs and quasi-experimental designs. For example, the research question "What is the association of environmental factors and reactive airway disease in otherwise healthy adults?" can be rewritten as the hypothesis "There is no association between environmental factors and reactive airway disease in otherwise healthy adults." Although stating that no relationship exists might seem a counterintuitive way to start a research analysis, it is, in fact, the only way that statistical significance can be measured. Although we can never be sure that a relationship exists, we can calculate the probability that it does not. Testing a null hypothesis in effect tells us how much uncertainty is present in the statistical conclusions, so the researcher can judge if it is within an acceptable range.

Two characteristics make a good hypothesis: the statement of an expected relationship (or the lack of a relationship) and an identified direction of interest. A **null hypothesis** states there is no difference between groups as a result of receiving the treatment or not receiving the treatment, whereas an alternative hypothesis specifies an expected difference between treatment groups. In either case, the relationship between variables is defined.

With respect to directionality, a **nondirectional hypothesis** is one for which the researcher is interested in a change in any direction, good or bad. In other words, a positive or negative association would be of interest. If we were testing a drug for hypertension, for example, a nondirectional hypothesis would indicate we are interested in reductions in blood pressure, but we would also be interested in rises in blood pressure. Sometimes called two-sided hypotheses, nondirectional hypotheses are appropriate for exploratory research questions or randomized trials of interventions. They require more rigorous tests than directional hypotheses. Research questions are often used alone, rather than being paired with hypotheses, when no direction of influence is predicted (Connelly, 2015); thus, studies with nondirectional hypotheses may not state them explicitly.

Directional hypotheses, or one-sided tests, are interested in only one direction of change. They are appropriate for research questions in which a great deal of literature or empirical support for an existing relationship can be found. Directional hypothesis tests are more liberal than nondirectional ones.

A good hypothesis statement includes the population, variables (dependent and independent), and the comparison (Boswell & Cannon, 2012). Using preoperative

Hypothesis:
A restatement of the research question in a form that can be analyzed statistically for significance.

Null hypothesis:
A statement of the research question that declares there is no difference between groups as a result of receiving the intervention or not receiving the intervention.

Nondirectional hypothesis:
A two-sided statement of the research question that is interested in change in any direction.

Directional hypothesis:
A one-sided statement of the research question that is interested in only one direction of change.

education for short-stay patients undergoing prostatectomy as an example, a research hypothesis might look like this:

- *Population:* In patients who undergo radical prostatectomy and stay in the hospital one day after surgery . . .
- *Comparison:* There will be no difference in . . .
- *Dependent variable:* Pain control as measured by a visual analog scale . . .
- *Independent variables:* Between patients receiving customized preoperative teaching and standard preoperative teaching.

It is easy to see the analogy between a PICO question and a hypothesis. In this example, the "I" of the PICO question is the independent variable, and the "O", or outcome, is the dependent variable. Note, however, that hypotheses are sequenced slightly differently than PICO questions. Hypotheses are best used for experimental designs, but they can serve as a PICO statement when the results will be statistically driven.

Examples of null, alternative, directional, and nondirectional research hypotheses appear in Table 4.5.

GRAY MATTER

Two essential aspects of a good hypothesis are
- A statement of an expected relationship (or lack of one)
- An identification of a direction of interest

Reading Research for Evidence-Based Practice

The primary reason for critically reading problem statements is to identify concerns or problems and to understand the disparities or gaps between what is known and what still needs to be known about concepts. A secondary reason is to determine the significance of the concerns or problems. The primary reason for critically reading purpose statements is to identify the variables and study design within the context and scope of specific populations and settings. A secondary reason is to determine feasibility and fit.

When reading research as evidence for practice, many novice researchers are tempted to search by key words, retrieve by titles, and scan conclusion sections of abstracts and articles. In fact, novice researchers should avoid such practices. Instead, the problem and purpose statements must be reviewed to ensure fit between the nurse's problem and purpose and the researcher's problem and purpose. Does the problem statement address the same or similar concepts and gaps in knowledge? Does the purpose statement address the same or similar variables, populations, and settings? Often these elements are defined and explained in the introduction, literature review, and study design sections of a research report.

Problem and purpose statements, as well as research questions, should be stated early in the research report. The problem statement may be inferred and incorporated into the introduction and review of the need for the study. Often the context of the problem

Table 4.5 Examples of Hypotheses

Research Question	Null Hypotheses	Alternative, Nondirectional Hypotheses	Alternative, Directional Hypotheses
Do collaborative interdisciplinary rounds change the nurse's perception of collaboration on a patient care unit?	There will be *no difference* in nurses' perception of collaboration when interdisciplinary rounds are implemented on a patient care unit.	Nurses' perception of collaboration will be *different* when interdisciplinary rounds are implemented on a patient care unit.	Nurses' perceptions of collaboration will be *improved* when interdisciplinary rounds are implemented on a patient care unit.
Does a school-nurse educational campaign on the importance of sleep change the average amount of school-night sleep of middle school students?	There will be *no difference* in the average amount of school-night sleep among middle school students as a result of a school-nurse educational campaign.	Middle school students will have a *different* average amount of school-night sleep as a result of a school-nurse educational campaign.	Middle school students will have a *greater* average amount of school-night sleep as a result of a school-nurse educational campaign.

appears in the literature review. The purpose statement should be explicit and found near the beginning of the study; it might also be called "objectives," "aims," or "goals." The research question itself should be specific and made clear early in the study. The study may or may not report hypotheses, even if it is clearly quantitative and experimental in design. If they are reported, hypotheses often appear in the results section with their associated statistical conclusions.

Using Research in Evidence-Based Practice

By understanding problems, their related concepts or variables, the definition of the population, and the context for a research study, the nurse may be able to generalize the findings from that study to his or her specific nursing practice. The best evidence may then be used to design changes to improve processes and outcomes.

Literature searches may produce hundreds or even thousands of applicable and nonapplicable results. To easily and quickly identify applicable studies, look for the problem statements and the purpose statements in research reports. Problem statements and purpose statements provide readers with the focused context and scope required to generalize research findings to their own nursing practice and establish and support evidenced-based practice within their organizations. Efficient literature searches include not only key words related to research problems, but also key words related to the level of evidence. For example, key words such as *meta-analysis, randomized,* or *controlled* may yield higher levels of evidence for critiquing, weighting, and synthesizing activities (Facchiano et al., 2011).

Creating Evidence for Practice

Finding and developing research problems begins with a general concern or focus related to a subject or topic. Subjects and topics consist of broad categories and may include examples such as hospital-acquired infections, pain management, patient falls, physiological monitoring, and pressure ulcer prevention. As the process evolves, a problem is identified. Research problems consist of narrower topics and may include examples such as ventilator-associated pneumonia, patient-controlled analgesia, blood pressure monitoring, and use of specialty beds to prevent skin breakdown.

Once a problem is identified, the gap between what is known about the problem and what remains to be known about the problem is examined. Special consideration should be given to exploring the gap within the context and scope (population and setting) of the problem. This gap examination occurs primarily through a literature review. Research activities should focus on narrowing or filling in the gaps.

After the gap has been identified, the problem statement(s), purpose statement(s), and research question(s) are developed. The problem statement indicates the focus or interest of the study and raises concerns and questions (disparities and gaps) about general concepts. The purpose statement indicates why the study is being conducted and suggests methods for examining the concepts or variables, and the relationships among them, within a specific population and setting. The research question is a rewording of the purpose statement into a question that suggests methods for examining the concepts or variables and the relationships between them.

CHECKLIST FOR CRITICALLY READING PROBLEM STATEMENTS

Development

❑ Deductive narrowing from the general to the specific

Articulation

❑ The problem is stated or inferred
❑ The statement is provided early in the article and is easy to find
❑ The concern, disparity, or gap is clear

Significance

❑ Develops, expands, or validates nursing knowledge
❑ Develops, expands, or validates conceptual models or theoretical frameworks
❑ Improves patient care, staff member, and/or organizational processes and/or outcomes

---

CHECKLIST FOR CRITICALLY READING PURPOSE STATEMENTS

Development

❑ Deductive narrowing from problem statement

Articulation

❑ The purpose is stated or inferred but can be described
❑ The statement is provided early in the article and is easy to find
❑ The purpose is written as a statement
❑ The statement uses an unbiased verb
❑ The design is described
❑ The variables are described

❑ The population is defined
❑ The setting is specified

Feasibility

❑ Required resources (people, time, money, equipment, materials, and facilities) are accessible
❑ Ethical issues have been considered

Fit

❑ There is obvious alignment between purpose statement and design

You should look for information about the research question or hypothesis in the following places:

- The research question may be explicitly stated in the research abstract, but is often simply implied by the title of the article, purpose statement, or objectives for the study.
- Ideally, the question is discussed at the beginning of the article, often at the end of the introduction. When it is stated early, it is followed by evidence from the literature review to support the researcher's contention that this question is important to investigate further. It may be written as a statement instead of a question. If it is not found at the beginning of the research report, look for the question at the end of the literature review.
- The null and alternate hypotheses are often found in the methods section where statistical methods are discussed, along with the rationale for the statistical tests used to test the hypotheses. Hypotheses are typically easy to find and are explicitly identified as such.
- Sometimes a separate section is created for a formal statement of the problem, the purpose of the study, and the research question. It may be labeled "Purpose," "Aims," or "Objectives." The research question may similarly have its own heading.
- If the researcher used any inferential statistical tests, which most quantitative studies do, then there were hypotheses, whether they are stated or not. Sometimes the reader needs to guess what the hypotheses were, based on the tests that were reported. Most studies do not report a hypothesis. This is not a weakness; except for the most scientific of journals, formal explication of hypotheses is not a standard part of a write-up.

That said, there may be no properly constructed research question explicitly stated in the report. Three researchers in rehabilitation medicine reviewed more than 250 research articles to identify what proportion of them described appropriate research questions. More than 30% of the articles reviewed had questions that required reworking to match the work undertaken (Mayo, Asano, & Barbic, 2013). When the research question is not specifically identified, the reader may need to infer the elements of the research question from the descriptions of the study's design, methods, and sampling.

SKILL BUILDER   Write Stronger Research Questions

The most important part of the research process is getting the question right. How the problem is stated determines which measures will be used, which data will be collected, which kind of analysis will be used, and which conclusions can be drawn. It is worth the time, then, to carefully consider how this element of the research study is developed. A thoughtful process does not necessarily mean a complicated process, however. Here are some simple suggestions for creating strong research questions:

- Answer the "why" question first. With a solid understanding of the reason for the study, the specifics of the research question become easier to identify.
- Review the literature before finalizing the question. Do not hesitate to replicate the question of a research study that accomplishes similar goals. It is flattering to researchers—even established, well-known ones—to have their work replicated. Be sure to give credit where credit is due.

- Focus, focus, focus. Refine the research question, mull it over for a bit, and then refine it again. The effort spent to get the question just right will be worth it, because less confusion will arise later about how to answer the question.
- That said, do not wait until the question is perfect to begin the design of the study. The question is, to some extent, a work in progress as the specifics of the research unfold. The question can,

and likely will, be revised as new information, resources, and constraints come to light.
- Keep the research questions focused; do not include more than one major concept per question. Compound questions are challenging to study and make it more difficult to isolate the effects of a single independent variable. Multiple research questions should be used instead of multiple parts of a single question.

Summary of Key Concepts

- Finding and developing significant problems for research are critical for improving processes and outcomes for patients, staff members, and organizations. For both the researcher and the reader, problem statements, purpose statements, and research questions serve to guide and direct research activities.
- The evolution of a research problem from a general topic of interest to the articulation of a problem statement and a purpose statement serves to narrow the focus of the research to a researchable question. Subjects or topics that are too broad are problematic for researchers—because methodological complexities increase, experienced researchers or consultants are required, and resource demands (for example, money, people, and time) increase.
- Sources for researchable problems include clinical practice, educational institutions, consumer/customer feedback, personal experience, frameworks and models, professional literature, performance improvement activities, research reports and priorities, and social issues.
- Research problem statements are declarations of disparity: the difference (gap) between what is known and what needs to be known about a topic. They are written as questions or statements and contain clear, concise, and well-defined components (disparities or gaps and concepts).
- Research purpose statements are declarations of intent: what will be studied, how it will be studied, who will be studied, and what the context for the study is. They are written as declarative, objective statements and contain clear, concise, and well-defined components (design, variables, population, and setting).
- There should be a good fit between the design suggested in the purpose statement and the methods used in the research study. There should also be a good fit between the research question and the specifics of the research design, sampling strategy, and measurement.
- Qualitative problem and purpose statements, as well as research questions, are generally broader, vaguer, and less prescriptive than those created for quantitative studies. Qualitative designs are emergent and may be revised frequently as the study unfolds.
- Research questions for quantitative studies can be developed using the PICO guide by specifying population, intervention, comparison, and outcome. Some researchers add a "T" to the PICO acronym (PICOT) to identify the time period of interest.

- Epidemiology studies often use questions constructed in the "PECO" format, in which an exposure of interest is substituted for an intervention.
- All elements will not necessarily be in every question, because PICO guidelines are most appropriate for experimental designs.
- The FINER criteria—feasible, interesting, novel, ethical, and relevant—serve as a good basis for analysis of the quality of a researchable question. The research question should have an identifiable link to the research design.

For More Depth and Detail

For a more in-depth look at the concepts in this chapter, try these references:

Chang, S., Carey, T., Kato, E., Guise, J., & Sanders, G. (2012). Identifying research needs for improving health care. *Annals of Internal Medicine, 157*(6), 439–445.

Curley, M. (2012). Clinical research: Together, stronger, bolder. *American Journal of Critical Care, 21*(4), 234–241.

Houghton, C., Hunter, A., & Meske, U. (2012). Linking aims, paradigm and method in nursing research. *Nurse Researcher, 20*(2), 34–39.

Krill, C., Raven, C., & Staffileno, B. (2012). Moving from a clinical question to research: The implementation of a safe patient handling program. *Medsurg Nursing, 21*(2), 104–116.

O'Brien, M., & DeSisto, M. (2013). Every study begins with a query: How to present a clear research question. *NASN School Nurse.* doi: 10.1177/1942602X12475094

Toledo, A., Flikkema, M., & Toledo-Pereyra, L. (2011). Developing the research hypothesis. *Journal of Investigative Surgery, 24*(5), 191–194.

Welford, C., Murphy, K., & Casey, D. (2011). Demystifying nursing research terminology: Part 1. *Nurse Researcher, 18*(4), 38–43.

Welford, C., Murphy, K., & Casey, D. (2012). Demystifying nursing research terminology: Part 2. *Nurse Researcher, 19*(2), 29–35.

CRITICAL APPRAISAL EXERCISE

Retrieve the following full-text article from the Cumulative Index to Nursing and Allied Health Literature or similar search database:

Baker, N., Taggart, H., Nivens, A., & Tillman, P. (2015). Delirium: Why are nurses confused? *MedSurg Nursing, 24*(1), 15–22.

Review the article, looking for information about the problem and purpose statements and the research questions and hypotheses. Consider the following appraisal questions in your critical review of these elements of the research article:

1. These authors do not specify a problem statement, or a statement about the gap between what is and what is not known about the problem. From the authors' introduction and review of the literature, what can you infer is the problem they want to address?
2. Are the research questions appropriate to achieve the given purpose of the study?
3. Does the research question meet the FINER criteria? Why or why not?
4. Which elements of the PICO question are evident here? How could these questions be strengthened using a PICO approach?
5. Are these hypotheses directional or nondirectional?
6. Discuss whether and how this study will contribute to nursing practice.

References

American Association of Colleges of Nursing (AACN). (2013). Nursing research. Retrieved from http://www.aacn.nche.edu/publications/position/nursing-research

Bhardwaj, R., Pickard, R., Carrick-Sen, D., & Brittain, K. (2012). Patients' perspectives on timing of urinary catheter removal after surgery. *British Journal of Nursing, 21*r(18), Urology Supplement, S4–S9.

Boswell, C., & Cannon, S. (2012). *Introduction to nursing research: Incorporating evidence-based practice* (3rd ed.). Burlington, MA: Jones & Bartlett Learning.

Carlisle, J., Moore, A., Cooper, A., Henderson, T., Mayfield, D., Taylor, R., . . . Sun, Y. (2012). Changes in infant disposable diaper weights at selected intervals post-wetting. *Pediatric Nursing, 38*(4), 223–226.

Carman, M., Wolf, L., Henderson, D., Kamienski, M., Koziol-McLain, J., Manton, A., & Moon, M. (2013). Developing your clinical question: the key to successful research. *Journal of Emergency Nursing, 39*(3), 299–302.

Cassar, S., & Baldacchino, D. (2012). Quality of life after percutaneous coronary intervention: Part 2. *British Journal of Nursing, 21*(19), 1125–1130.

Centers for Medicare & Medicaid Services Partnership for Patients (CMS). (2013). Retrieved from http://partnershipforpatients.cms.gov/

Connelly, L. (2015). Research questions and hypotheses. *MedSurg Nursing, 24*(6), 435–436.

Esquerra-Gonzalez, A., Ilagan-Honorio, M., Fraschilla, S., Kehoe, P., Lee, A., Marcarian, T., . . . Rodman, B. (2013). Pain after lung transplant: High frequency chest wall oscillation vs chest physiotherapy. *American Journal of Critical Care, 22*(2), 115–125.

Facchiano, L., Snyder, C., & Nunez, D. (2011). A literature review on breathing retraining as a self-management strategy operationalized through Rosswurm and Larrabee's evidence-based practice model. *Journal of the American Academy of Nurse Practitioners, 23*(8), 421–426.

Hospital Care Quality Information from the Consumer Perspective (HCAHPS). (2013). Retrieved from http://www.hcahpsonline.org/home.aspx

Karlsen, B., Oftedal, B., & Bru, E. (2012). The relationship between clinical indicators, coping styles, perceived support and diabetes-related distress among adults with type 2 diabetes. *Journal of Advanced Nursing, 68*(2), 391–401.

Mayo, N., Asano, M., & Barbic, S. (2013). When is a research question not a research question? *Journal of Rehabilitation Medicine, 45,* 513–518.

McKeon, J., & McKeon, P. (2015). PICO: A hot topic in evidence-based practice. *International Journal of Athletic Therapy & Training, 20*(1), 1–3.

Merkel, R., & Wright, T. (2012). Parental self-efficacy and online support among parents of children diagnosed with type 1 diabetes mellitus. *Pediatric Nursing, 38*(6), 303–308.

Patient-Centered Outcomes Research Institute (PCORI). (2013). Retrieved from http://www.pcori.org/

Perrin, A. (2012). Quality of life after ileo-anal pouch formation: Patient perceptions. *British Journal of Nursing, 21*(16), Stoma Care Supplement, S11–S19.

Rowlinson, L. (2013). Lived experience of being a nurse. *British Journal of Nursing, 22*(4), 218–222.

Schmidt, N., & Brown, J. (2011). *Evidence-based practice for nurses: Appraisal and application research.* Burlington, MA: Jones & Bartlett Learning.

Skene, C. (2012). Parental involvement in neonatal pain management: Reflecting on the researcher-practitioner role. *Nurse Researcher, 19*(4), 27–30.

White, E. (2012). Challenges that may arise when conducting real-life nursing research. *Nurse Researcher, 19*(4), 15–20.

Williams, J. (2002). The Essentials of Pouch Care Nursing. London, England: Whurr Publishing Ltd.

Chapter 5

The Successful Literature Review

CHAPTER OBJECTIVES

The study of this chapter will help the learner to

- Discuss the rationale for conducting a thorough search of the literature.
- Discuss tools that measure the impact of studies.
- Review the concept of "open access" and describe how it is making research information more accessible.
- Describe the types of literature used to support a research study, including studies that constitute the "evidence pyramid."
- Understand the steps of a well-thought-out search strategy to find evidence-based information.
- Compare a literature search for research to a literature search for a practice guideline.
- Critically appraise the literature review section of a research article.
- Reflect on the ways that research literature can be used as evidence for nursing practice.

KEY TERMS

Altmetrics	Journal impact factor	Search strategy
Bibliometrics	Levels of evidence	Search terms
Boolean operators	Literature review	Secondary sources
Cited reference search	Open access	Seminal work
Empirical literature	Peer review	Subject headings
Evidence pyramid	Primary sources	Systematic review
h-Index	Scholarly	Theoretical literature
Information literacy	Search concepts	

Literature review:
A critical component of the research process that provides an in-depth analysis of recently published research findings in specifically identified areas of interest. The review informs the research question and guides development of the research plan.

An Introduction to the Literature Review

The literature review is a critical component of the research process. It provides an in-depth analysis of what is known and what is missing related to a specific subject. This forms the foundation for research and ultimately patient care. Through online access to health information, today's students and professionals can tap into a wide variety of complex

VOICES FROM THE FIELD

I was on the Evidence-Based Practice (EBP) Council for my hospital, and one of the questions we wanted to study was whether hourly rounding—a nurse checking every patient, every hour, and documenting it—was worth the amount of time it required of the nurse. The policy had come down from administration, and the rank and file who were expected to carry it out were not sure it would achieve the expected outcomes of decreasing the number of adverse events and enhancing patient satisfaction.

We talked about designing our own little study, but concluded we would see if there was already enough literature to show its effectiveness. We started with the question, "What are the outcomes associated with hourly rounding?" and identified search terms. We found quite a bit of literature through our initial search, but much of it focused on physicians' rounds, not nurses'. We asked the health sciences librarian for help, and she combined our terms in novel ways that brought us more focused literature. She also helped us search dissertations and conference proceedings. This turned up a few dozen applicable abstracts. After applying our criteria to the list, we ended up with six articles that measured some aspect of hourly rounding. One of them was a review of other articles, so that was like hitting the evidence jackpot.

We started the study expecting to prove that hourly rounding did not really improve things. What we found—when we used objective criteria for including studies—was that evidence supported the effectiveness of this policy. Adverse events were decreased in two of the studies; patient satisfaction improved in almost all of them. So we were both surprised and a bit dismayed by the findings: We found something we did not expect that supported continuing a time-consuming policy.

When we looked closer, however, it became clear that it was the nurse contact that made the difference. That did not surprise us when we thought about it. There really was no evidence that we needed in-depth documentation of the rounding for it to be effective. So we suggested to our nurse administrator, "We recognize the evidence for hourly rounds, but can we find a faster way to show it was done?" We brainstormed for some time and decided the rounds could just be marked off on a small whiteboard in the room. Check the patient, check the whiteboard.

This was a case when the literature showed us something we did not expect but helped us pose alternative solutions. I think it convinced most of the team of the value of going to the literature first—you do not have to reinvent the wheel—and doing so in an objective, deliberate way.

Eunice Nolan, RN, DNP

resources that provide an unending source of data. Moreover, this information is so dynamic that the nurse researcher or clinician can no longer rely on a handful of familiar resources, but rather must constantly remain alert to new findings from a multitude of sources. In turn, nurses must develop the skills needed to search health sciences databases efficiently and to assess the authority, objectivity, and validity of the information they retrieve.

While this chapter can serve as a guide for nurses to help them find evidence-based information, both students and professionals should not hesitate to contact a health sciences librarian for further assistance. Whether they work at a major academic center or in a one-room hospital library, such librarians are skilled at searching the relevant resources and are experts in the science of comprehensive literature retrieval.

Purpose, Importance, and Scope of the Literature Review

Literature reviews add credence to the researcher's assertions of the importance of the topic proposed for investigation. It is the researcher's responsibility to determine what others have discovered on the same topic. A thorough literature review may turn up studies that can be replicated, instruments that have been standardized and tested for use, or procedures that can be adapted to the proposed study. In addition, the literature often reveals an appropriate theoretical framework.

The literature review may enhance the body of knowledge on a particular issue, or it may establish that there is a paucity of knowledge on the subject in question. Although many researchers are discouraged by a lack of published findings on a specific topic, this may actually be a benefit. A gap in the knowledge of a healthcare issue creates an area that is ripe for exploratory or interventional study and signals that the researcher is pioneering a new issue for investigation. It also increases the likelihood of publication and can serve as the basis for advanced academic study. Either way, the literature review is the first step in evaluating the importance of a research question and potential methods for its study.

Although the researcher needs to provide substantial literature support that directly relates to the problem, it is important to resist the temptation to include everything. A researcher must decide when to stop searching—perhaps an obvious point in theory, but one that is sometimes difficult to put into practice. A researcher may want to consciously note that nothing new is being revealed or that literature resources are exhausted. The scope of a scholarly literature review will obviously go into greater depth than a literature review for a small bedside science project. Likewise, a study directed toward a journal focused on practice may have fewer references than one intended for publication in a research journal. The type of study, the expectations of the readers, and the level of scholarly sophistication required will drive the scope of the literature review.

Scholarly:
Concerned with or relating to academic study or research.

Theoretical literature:
Published conceptual models, frameworks, and theories that provide a basis for the researcher's belief system and for ways of thinking about the problem studied.

GRAY MATTER

A literature review will
- Add credence to the importance of the topic proposed for investigation
- Identify studies that can be replicated, instruments that have been standardized and tested, or procedures that can be adapted
- Reveal appropriate theoretical frameworks
- Contribute to the body of knowledge or establish the lack of published research on a subject

Types of Literature Used in the Review

Multiple types of information are used to enhance the scope and depth of the review, and one way to consider them is to recognize theoretical versus empirical literature. **Theoretical literature** includes published conceptual models, frameworks, and theories. It provides a basis for the researcher's belief system and a road map for ways to think

Empirical literature:
Published works that demonstrate how theories apply to individual behavior or observed events.

Seminal work:
A classic work of research literature that is more than 5 years old and is marked by its uniqueness and contribution to professional knowledge.

Primary sources:
Reports of original research authored by the researcher and published in a scholarly source such as a peer-reviewed research journal or scholarly book.

Secondary sources:
Comments and summaries of multiple research studies on one topic, such as systematic reviews, meta-analyses, and meta-syntheses, which are based on the secondary author's interpretation of the primary work.

about the problem under study. **Empirical literature**, by comparison, includes works that demonstrate how theories apply to individual behavior or observed events. Both types of literature may take the form of research journals, books, theses and dissertations, conference proceedings, government reports, and practice guidelines.

GRAY MATTER

Scholarly literature includes the following types of sources:
- Journals
- Books
- Conference proceedings
- Practice guidelines
- Theses and dissertations
- Government reports

Comprehensiveness in terms of both the time period reviewed and appropriate coverage of the subject matter is important. The delay between completion of a research study and the publication of its results can be significant; thus articles that are more than a few years old may refer to findings that are, in reality, much older. Researchers continually discover new facts, methods, and outcomes, which in turn change what is known about a subject. Consequently, the healthcare literature is highly dynamic. Failure to keep up with the latest findings or recommendations can potentially affect patient care, so it is essential for healthcare providers to keep abreast of the evolving literature.

There are exceptions to every rule, of course. A **seminal work**—one that is a classic in its field—may go back many more years than is common in the healthcare literature and is not bound by time. For example, the important contributions to the literature made by Florence Nightingale, Dorothea Orem, and Jean Watson—all trailblazers in the field of nursing theory—are considered seminal works. Likewise, research supporting statistical treatments or measurement instruments may be from less recent literature, if one can show that they are still relevant and their properties are still applicable to today's practice.

Research literature may be further defined in terms of its sources. **Primary sources** are reports of original work that are published in a peer-reviewed journal, government report, manuscript, or other scholarly work. **Secondary sources** include comments on and summaries of multiple research studies on one topic. For example, reviews of studies that provide synopses of clinical studies are secondary sources. If the conclusions drawn in the secondary source are based on that author's interpretation of the primary work, it is necessary, then, to review primary sources whenever possible to ensure accuracy. **Table 5.1** defines primary and secondary sources and gives examples for each.

Searching for the Evidence in a Research Problem

Selecting the appropriate resource, often an online database, is among the most important initial steps in the literature search. Electronic databases vary in subject (e.g., biomedical versus nursing), search interface (the search engine and appearance), content type

Table 5.1 Primary and Secondary Sources of Information	
Primary Source Definition	Resources that publish the findings of original research and other types of studies in their first and original form
Examples of resources with primary source information	Clinical trials Dissertations/theses
Potential search tools and sources	CINAHL MEDLINE/PubMed PsycINFO Cochrane Central Register of Controlled Trials
Secondary Source Definition	Resources that synthesize, summarize, or comment on original research
Examples of resources with secondary source information	Systematic reviews Meta-analyses Qualitative synthesis Reviews of individual articles Clinical practice guidelines
Potential search tools and sources	CINAHL MEDLINE/PubMed PsycINFO Cochrane Database of Systematic Reviews National Guidelines Clearinghouse (AHRQ) Professional association databases of practice guidelines Clinical point-of-care tools (e.g., UpToDate)

(e.g., bibliographic records versus full text), and indexing (e.g., subject headings versus searching for key words), among other characteristics. A researcher can spend an inordinate amount of time searching in a broad science database when, in fact, the question is more appropriately addressed in a specialized database. Additionally, books, dissertations, websites, and individual journals will yield relevant and authoritative information not included in major databases.

A well-planned search strategy is helpful in ensuring that the literature search is comprehensive and unbiased. The PICO statement (population, intervention, comparison, outcome) is a useful tool that aids in identification of major concepts for the search (Carman et al., 2013).

Open Access

Many databases and sources of literature are proprietary; in such a case, individual researchers or an organization must be a subscriber to gain access to them. In recent years, digital technology has dramatically increased the ease of dissemination and access to research results, building an expectation that everyone—not just subscribers—should have access to articles published in scholarly journals, especially publications resulting from government-funded (i.e., taxpayer-funded) research. The open access movement has gained prominence in response to readers and authors alike demanding that research information be readily available. The most frequently quoted definition of **open access** (OA) literature, attributed to Peter Suber, Director of the Harvard Open Access Project, is "digital, online, free of charge, and free of most copyright and licensing restrictions" (Suber, 2004).

Researchers, healthcare professionals, patients, and funding agencies have been urging scholarly publishers to provide research information freely and to permit unlimited downloading, copying, distributing, and printing of the articles, or data-mining for analysis. In the United States, the National Institutes of Health's (NIH) Public Access Policy requires that authors of articles that result from research funded by NIH submit their work to PubMed Central, a free digital repository of peer-reviewed articles, within 12 months of publication (Consolidated Appropriations Act, 2007). In early 2013 and again in 2015, Congress introduced and reauthorized the Fair Access to Science and Technology Research Act (FASTR) (2015a, 2015b), which takes the NIH policy a step further, by requiring open access within 6 months of publication in a peer-reviewed journal.

With the growing strength of the open access movement, it is increasingly feasible for nurses, whether affiliated with an academic institution or not, to readily access evidence-based information.

Assessing Study Quality and Its Influence

How can readers of research publications be assured of the quality of the information? One of the hallmarks of high-quality research is **peer review** of the study's rationale, design, methodology, results, and conclusions. Peer-reviewed publications have been subjected to critical assessment provided by "blinded" reviewers who are unaware of the author's name, credentials, or professional status. This practice ensures a thorough evaluation of the paper using the same standard applied to other, similar works, without being influenced by the status of the author. When a researcher submits his or her manuscript to a peer-reviewed (sometimes called refereed) professional journal, it is understood that it will be evaluated by a team of experts who are experienced in the content and methodology reflected in the manuscript. This rigorous review process adds legitimacy to the findings reported in the study.

The peer review process itself, however, may vary. Quantitative research studies are generally subjected to a thorough analysis that focuses on potential sources of bias and error and then applies strict standards to the evaluation of methodology and design. Qualitative research, in contrast, lends itself more appropriately to peer review that focuses on the efforts the author has made to ensure credibility and trustworthiness.

Readers and authors alike may obtain further evidence of a study's quality by examining the subsequent references to its publication. Authors must always attribute an idea or finding first reported in another publication by citing the source. In turn, the number of times an article is cited in other articles is an indication of the visibility and credibility of the work. With the help of online tools and applications, the discipline of **bibliometrics** (a term coined by Alan Pritchard in 1969) collects data on the impact of a publication. Pritchard (1969) defined bibliometrics as "the application of mathematics and statistical methods to books and other media of communication." With the rise of digital information, the ability to track a scholarly publication's impact and reach has greatly expanded.

Many methods exist that try to quantify this reach. The **journal impact factor** is a measure of the influence and ranking of a journal within a discipline (Thomson Reuters, 2015). The **h-index** is a calculation that provides a measure of a particular individual researcher's output (Hirsch, 2005). A newer tool that looks at the extent of a publication's influence is **altmetrics**, a method developed by Jason Priem. On his website (www.altmetrics.org), Priem and his colleagues (2010) define altmetrics as "the creation and study of new metrics based on the Social Web for analyzing and informing scholarship." In their own literature searches, nurses will notice that publishers use various tools to discern an article's impact.

Competencies for Information Literacy

It is clearly important that clinicians and researchers alike possess the competencies necessary to access, retrieve, and analyze research evidence for their practice throughout their career. **Information literacy** is important for nurses to acquire because they must decipher the vast expanse of knowledge generated through healthcare research. Nurses are required to make patient care decisions on a daily basis, so they must be able to incorporate evidence-based research into their clinical nursing practice. These skills can be mastered through repeated practice and application throughout the nursing curriculum, with feedback and instruction from the faculty in partnership with the health sciences librarian (Schardt, 2011). When students graduate, they then bring their information literacy skills to their employing organizations.

Today, competent nurses must possess lifelong learning and information literacy skills that include the following abilities:

- Identifying and succinctly stating the question or problem to be researched
- Using the appropriate online databases, websites of professional and government organizations, and other reliable resources for the retrieval of scholarly research and the best evidence
- Creating effective search strategies that yield relevant, current, research-based results
- Thinking critically to analyze problems and issues, and to appraise evidence
- Integrating evidence into practice
- Working with computers, the Internet, word processing, spreadsheet analysis, databases, and new applications that are relevant to the job

The process of searching the literature for evidence-based nursing resources begins with a focused clinical question that is limited in its time frame so that the evidence is current and directly applicable to nursing practice. **Table 5.2** highlights some of the differences between a literature review for a research study and a literature review for the development of practice guidelines.

Journal impact factor:
A way to measure the visibility of research by calculating a ratio of current citations of the journal to all citations in the same time period.

h-Index:
An indicator of a researcher's lifetime impact in his or her field.

Altmetrics:
The creation and study of new metrics based on the Social Web for analyzing and informing scholarship.

Information literacy:
The competencies necessary to access, retrieve, and analyze research evidence for application to nursing practice.

Table 5.2 Contrast of Literature Review for Research and for Practice Guideline Development

	For a Research Study	For Practice Guidelines
Conceptual basis	Provides background and context for the particular study that is planned Incorporates a theoretical framework Specific to the research question	Provides evidence that can be applied to a clinical problem Focuses on application of research to practice Specific to the clinical question
Type of evidence appraised	Scholarly works that are published in peer-reviewed journals Research reported in other peer-reviewed venues such as symposia, dissertations, and monographs	Scientific works that are published in peer-reviewed journals Systematic reviews, meta-analyses, and integrative reviews published in journals, by professional associations, or by other organizations Opinions presented by expert panels or task forces
Critical appraisal skills used	Critical appraisal of single focused research reports	Critical appraisal of single studies and aggregate research report

GRAY MATTER

A literature search for evidence-based nursing practice should meet the following criteria:
- Be focused on a clinical question
- Be limited in its time frame so that the evidence is current
- Be applicable directly to nursing practice

Reading the Literature Review Section

The literature review section of a research study provides rich information about the context of the study in the field and its potential for use in direct practice. Studies based on thoroughly searched and synthesized literature produce evidence that is more standard, easily aggregated, and likely to be valid. A well-done literature review section will support the authors' contention that the research question is important and has significant implications for practice. It may also provide a link to the theoretical basis of the question and offer support for the methods and procedures used. The literature review should present a logical argument, in essence, that builds a case for the significance of the study and its particular design.

The literature review should include a variety of sources of data; these sources should be sorted and analyzed for their usefulness to the study. The literature review can be arranged in chronological order or by subject matter. The review should also be unbiased; that is, there should be a mix of previous studies related to the research question—some

WHERE TO LOOK

A review of literature can appear throughout a published research article, but typically will be concentrated in a special section that follows the introduction, purpose statement, and research question. Citations to literature that support and discuss the scope of the research problem generally first appear in the literature review section, which may be labeled straightforwardly as "Literature Review"; alternatively, it may be called "Background" or "Context of the Problem." On occasion, this information might not be presented in a separate section, but rather will be embedded into the introductory paragraphs.

Literature may also be cited to support the measurements that were used, the intervention protocol, or the data analysis procedures. The literature is often referred to during discussion and conclusions; it is here that the authors compare their findings to the findings of previous studies. In discussing the findings of their own study, the researcher should identify results that confirm previous studies, clear up contradictions, or highlight inconsistencies with the findings of other studies. Each citation in the text should be linked to an entry in the references list.

The use and placement of the literature review is standardized in most quantitative studies. Qualitative studies, however, may refer to and cite the literature in various ways. Some qualitative researchers believe the researcher should not have preconceived notions about a study and so should complete the literature search only after completing the study. Others use a fairly traditional approach. The literature review for qualitative studies often appears sprinkled throughout the sections noted earlier but may also appear in the results section, supporting the themes recorded and the words of informants.

CHECKLIST FOR EVALUATING AN EVIDENCE-BASED LITERATURE REVIEW

- ❏ The literature review relies primarily on studies conducted in the last 5 years.
- ❏ The relationship of the research problem to the previous research is made clear.
- ❏ All or most of the major studies related to the topic of interest are included.
- ❏ The review can be linked both directly and indirectly to the research question.
- ❏ The theoretical or conceptual framework is described.
- ❏ The review provides support for the importance of the study.
- ❏ The authors have used primary, rather than secondary, sources.
- ❏ Studies are critically examined and reported objectively.
- ❏ The review is unbiased and includes findings that are conclusive and those that have inconsistencies.
- ❏ The author's opinion is largely undetectable.
- ❏ The review is logically organized to support the need for the research.
- ❏ The review ends with a summary of the most important knowledge on the topic.

that support the author's viewpoint and some that do not. Contradictory results from the literature should be reported, because one goal of nursing research is to clarify previous confusing results. Ideally, the studies should be dated within the past 5 years, unless the work is a seminal one or a theoretical selection.

Using Evidence-Based Literature in Nursing Practice

Nurses use literature reviews for a variety of reasons. Students will use them to compose scholarly papers and to design research studies. Practicing nurses may rely on literature reviews to make decisions supported by evidence when dealing with specific patient care problems. For the use of the profession as a whole, articles may be combined to develop evidence-based practice guidelines. All of these applications require competency in retrieving and using the literature appropriately. Table 5.3 highlights how nurses are expected to use the literature in education and in practice, while Table 5.4 reviews some of the ways that research literature is integrated into clinical practice.

When thinking about evidence-based literature, it may be helpful to visualize the various levels of information as a pyramid. Although many versions of this pyramid exist, one that has been widely cited and adapted for nursing research was produced through the efforts of librarians at Yale University and Dartmouth College (Glover, Izzo, Odato, & Wang, 2006). The **evidence pyramid** (**FIGURE 5.1**) illustrates the hierarchy of literature related to the strength of the evidence presented. This literature may be associated with a **level of evidence** tool—that is, a ranking system that allows a clinician to quickly assess the quality of the evidence supporting a claim.

Table 5.3 Expectations for Use of Literature in Education and Practice

Baccalaureate (BSN)

Conduct literature reviews on a clinical subject
Critically appraise the data retrieved
Synthesize summaries of literature
Apply research findings to clinical practice
Write academic papers
Prepare academic presentations

Graduate

The BSN skills plus the following:
- Test the efficacy of nursing interventions yielding evidence for "best practices"
- Develop research and/or evidence-based proposals
- Develop research and/or evidence-based scholarly projects

Postgraduate

The BSN and graduate skills plus the following:
- Conduct research on proposals
- Publish research and/or evidence-based findings from own research
- Develop systematic reviews
- Collaborate with other nursing colleagues to develop future studies

Clinical

Conduct literature reviews on a clinical subject being studied
Critically appraise the data retrieved
Synthesize summaries of the literature reviewed
Apply research findings to clinical practice
Develop research and/or evidence-based proposals
Develop research and/or evidence-based scholarly projects

Table 5.4 Integration of Literature Review into Clinical Practice		
	Definition	**Application to Clinical Practice**
Independent reading	Personal reading for enrichment and professional knowledge	Improvement of patient care Improvement of professional self
Journal clubs	Group discussions regarding clinical issues and the scientific evidence that addresses them via critical appraisal of selected journal articles	Improvement of patient care Improvement of professional self Increase in new knowledge of clinical issues with associated evidence Learning research methodologies Learning new clinical practice techniques Discussing professional nursing issues
Research conferences	Professional meetings focusing on research findings	Improvement of patient care Improvement of professional self Increase in new knowledge of clinical issues with associated evidence Learning research methodologies Learning new clinical practice techniques Discussing professional nursing issues
Nursing practice councils/ committees	A forum to research, craft, and revise nursing practice standards	Learning about evidence-based practice Development of professional practice guidelines: standards of care, procedures, protocols, and practice changes Identification of "best practices"
Performance improvement councils/ committees	A forum that focuses on analysis and improvement of care	Evidence-based measurement outcomes: nursing-sensitive indicators Use of the plan–do–check–act (PDCA) or PICO assessment form for quality management
Peer reviews	Processes wherein nurses review the practice of other nurses and compare actual practice to evidence-based professional standards	Promoting excellence in professional practice Identification of the need for safety and quality interventions

Data from Levin, R. F., & Feldman, H. R. (2006). *Teaching evidence-based nursing*. New York, NY: Springer.

The evidence pyramid model shows both filtered and unfiltered resources. Filtered resources are those that are reviewed by experts in the subject area and distilled into a publication such as a review, guideline, or evidence-based synopsis of a problem. The bottom section of the pyramid includes unfiltered works such as clinical trials, qualitative studies, and opinion pieces published by authors but not reviewed or appraised by others.

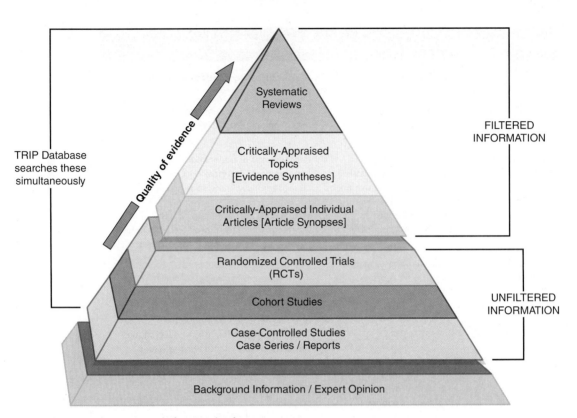

FIGURE 5.1 Evidence Pyramid of Research Information

Reproduced from EBM Pyramid and EBM Page Generator, copyright 2008 Trustees of Dartmouth College and Yale University. All Rights Reserved. Produced by Jan Glover, David Izzo, Karen Odato and Lei Wang. Retrieved from http://www.dartmouth.edu/~biomed/resources.htmld/guides/ebm_resources.shtml

Systematic review:
A highly structured and controlled search of the available literature that minimizes the potential for bias and produces a practice recommendation as an outcome.

Systematic reviews are positioned at the top of this pyramid example. This type of literature is typically considered the highest level of evidence because multiple studies are judged related to a specific research question and reviewed to reveal the best practices or results pertaining to that question. As the pyramid indicates, there is generally less literature available at this level. The Cochrane Collaboration—a global partnership whose members have been developing systematic reviews since the early 1990s—creates such reviews, which are found in the *Cochrane Database of Systematic Reviews (CDSR),* part of the Cochrane Library. These systematic reviews are considered to be the gold standard of evidence. The Preferred Reporting Items for Systematic reviews and Meta-Analyses Guidelines describe steps for developing systematic reviews and provide specific guidance on the literature search involved in creating the review (Liberati et al., 2009).

Critically appraised topics and articles are the next level in the evidence. These sources include guidelines developed on a specific health problem or articles reviewed for a journal club exercise.

Randomized controlled trials (RCTs) fall in the middle of the evidence pyramid. They include original research published in scholarly journals and indexed in bibliographic databases such as CINAHL and MEDLINE. The quantity of information here is vast, so a specialized topic is more likely studied. The most relevant information may be hidden in this abundance, however, and only someone with well-practiced search skills may be able to effectively locate it. Furthermore, these studies are not preappraised or filtered, so it is up to the researcher to assess the quality of the studies. Cohort and case-controlled studies are single studies that are also indexed in the bibliographic databases. The have less rigorous study designs than RCTs and, therefore, represent a lower level of evidence.

Expert opinion and background publications, such as encyclopedias and textbooks, fall at the lowest level of the pyramid. While important, these sources simply present the authors' viewpoint based on their experience and knowledge or general information about a topic and may not be supported by research.

Creating a Strong Literature Review

To successfully conduct a literature review, an organized approach must be used to address the clinical problem and research question. The most important steps are described here.

Identify the Research Problem and Question

Clinicians and researchers are often inundated by information and data coming from many sources: the medical record, a physical examination, the patient's story, practice guidelines, expert opinion, and the research literature. In the face of this wealth of data, it is easy to become overwhelmed. The key to finding evidence-based information is to boil it down to a handful of—and perhaps even one—*searchable* and ultimately *answerable* questions. The identification of these questions, in turn, presents the basic terms that are used for the literature search process. The study population, health problem, treatment options, differential diagnoses, prognosis, and expected outcomes are common considerations when formulating the research question. The PICO mnemonic takes many of these factors into account to help the searcher identify major concepts in the research problem.

Select the Resources

Table 5.5 includes many resources for clinical and research information. Increasingly, clinical resources are available as mobile applications, which are also noted here. Professional journals that commonly focus on nursing research and evidence-based practice are listed in Table 5.6.

Early in the literature review process, the researcher selects appropriate resources to locate prior studies that address the topic. The resource could be a review article with a lengthy bibliography, but it is often more fruitful to search an electronic resource that contains millions of records. This type of bibliographic database—that is, an electronic index of journal article citations—is searchable by key words, subject, author names, journal names, and other relevant categories.

Among the most important databases for nursing research is CINAHL (Cumulative Index to Nursing and Allied Health Literature), a collection of bibliographic records of articles, books, dissertations, and conference proceedings in nursing, biomedicine, and allied health. A subscription-based service, it is currently offered through EBSCO, a scholarly publisher.

Table 5.5 Databases and Websites Used for Nursing Literature Searches

Databases	Proprietary or Free	Comments
Academic Search Premier (EBSCO; http://www.ebscohost.com/academic/academic-search-premier)	Proprietary	General science, social science bibliographic database.
ACP PIER (American College of Physicians; http://pier.acponline.org/index.html)	Proprietary	Point-of-care database available online and as a mobile app.
CINAHL: Cumulative Index to Nursing and Allied Health Literature (EBSCO; https://health.ebsco.com/subjects/allied-health-nursing)	Proprietary	Nursing and allied health bibliographic database. Mobile app available.
Cochrane Library (Wiley; http://www.thecochranelibrary.com/)	Proprietary	Includes the Cochrane Database of Systematic Reviews (CDSR), Cochrane Register of Controlled Trials (CENTRAL), Database of Abstracts of Reviews of Effects (DARE), and other evidence-based databases.
Epocrates Rx (http://www.epocrates.com/)	Free	Point-of care drug database available as a mobile app and online.
ERIC: Educational Resources Information Center (U.S. Department of Education; http://eric.ed.gov)	Free	Education bibliographic database.
EMBASE: Excerpta Medica Online (Elsevier; https://www.elsevier.com/solutions/embase-biomedical-research)	Proprietary	Biomedical bibliographic database having considerable overlap with PubMed. Strength is in drug information; focus is somewhat more European than PubMed.
Google Scholar (http://scholar.google.com)	Free	Conducts citing-articles searches.
Grey Literature Reports (http://www.greylit.org)	Free	Gray (unpublished) literature such as government reports and white papers focusing on the health sciences.
Joanna Briggs Institute (http://www.joannabriggs.org)	Proprietary	Based at the University of Adelaide in Australia, the Joanna Briggs Institute develops systematic reviews and other resources with evidence-based information, particularly for nursing.

Databases	Proprietary or Free	Comments
Micromedex (Truven Health Analytics; http://www.micromedex.com/)	Proprietary	Drug database used by pharmacists as well as other clinicians. Available online and as a mobile app.
National Guidelines Clearinghouse (AHRQ; http://www.guideline.gov)	Free	Practice guidelines.
Natural Medicines Comprehensive Database (Therapeutic Research Faculty; http://naturaldatabase.therapeuticresearch.com/)	Proprietary	Database of natural products searchable with brand names. Includes herbals and other supplements. Online and via mobile app.
Networked Digital Library of Theses and Dissertations (http://www.ndltd.org/)	Free	Bibliographic database of dissertations and theses.
Nursing Best Practice Guidelines (http://rnao.ca/bpg)	Free	Guidelines developed by the Registered Nurses Association of Ontario (Canada).
PubMed (U.S. National Library of Medicine; http://www.pubmed.gov)	Free	Biomedical bibliographic database with wide global reach. Mobile app available.
PsycINFO (American Psychological Association; http://www.apa.org/)	Proprietary	Behavioral health, psychology, and psychiatry bibliographic database.
SCOPUS (Elsevier; https://www.elsevier.com/solutions/scopus)	Proprietary	General science bibliographic database. Conducts citing-articles searches.
Web of Science (Thomson Reuters; http://wokinfo.com/)	Proprietary	General science and social science bibliographic database. Conducts citing-articles searches.

Another key resource is MEDLINE, a large biomedical database that is freely available through the National Library of Medicine's PubMed portal as well as via other search interfaces such as Ovid and EBSCO. Additional relevant databases include the Cochrane Library—in particular, the CDSR and the Cochrane Register of Controlled Trials (CENTRAL). Health and Psychosocial Instruments (HaPI) is a unique bibliographic database of behavioral instruments and scales, while PsycINFO includes citations on behavioral medicine and mental health. Google Scholar is the academic database offered by Google.com and an increasingly important source of scholarly information.

Table 5.6 Professional Nursing Research and Evidence-Based Practice Journals

Advances in Nursing Science

Applied Nursing Research

Biological Research for Nursing

Canadian Journal of Nursing Research

Clinical Nursing Research

Evidence-Based Nursing

Journal of Nursing Measurement

Journal of Nursing Scholarship

Journal of Research in Nursing

Nurse Researcher

Nursing Research

Nursing Science Quarterly

Oncology Nursing Forum

Research in Nursing and Health

Research and Theory for Nursing Practice

Western Journal of Nursing Research

Worldviews on Evidence-Based Nursing

Information from websites must be used with caution. Not every site, database, or other Internet resource is supported by a reputable provider. The reader in general has little assurance that information on Internet sources is authoritative and objective and must do his or her homework to confirm that a source is reputable.

Researchers must secure information from bona fide, established, and credible sources. Nursing associations, healthcare organizations, major hospital systems, and government agencies are often reliable and objective hosts for evidence-based information. To aid researchers and users, the Medical Library Association (2015) has developed guidelines for evaluating websites.

Identify Inclusion and Exclusion Criteria

When beginning the literature review, it is important to determine which types of studies will be included and which will be excluded. Common questions to address when identifying appropriate criteria relate to the study design, publication year, population of interest, intervention, and outcomes of significance. If the researcher is interested in just the effectiveness of an intervention, for example, then citations may be retained only if the studies used experimental or quasi-experimental designs. If the evidence that is needed relates to patient preferences, however, then the researcher may choose to focus on qualitative studies. Using criteria related to the topic and type of studies ensures that the researcher remains focused on the most relevant studies without getting bogged down by literature that is only indirectly related to the topic.

Build the Search Strategy and Conduct the Search

The **search strategy** starts with identification of major **search concepts**—that is, ideas and themes in the research question—that will serve as the foundation for the search strategy. These concepts may be the exact words and phrases included in the problem statement.

The researcher next determines which **search terms** most closely describe each of the concepts and utilizes **Boolean operators** (AND, OR, NOT) to connect the terms and create the search strategy. Finding many similar terms or synonyms to describe the concepts ensures that the search strategy is extensive, helping the researcher avoid the problem of overlooking a key study that happens to use slightly different terminology.

An example of basic search strategy development can be found in **Table 5.7**. While the approach illustrated is applicable across databases, the specific syntax used for each strategy will vary from one resource to another, especially in databases that utilize **subject headings**, meaning fixed key words assigned by the publishers and authors that describe many concepts in the database's subject field. Furthermore, many search interfaces include filtering tools to limit the retrieved records by publication date, language of the article, and evidence-based criteria. PubMed, for example, supports Clinical Queries (http://www.ncbi.nlm.nih.gov/pubmed/clinical), a tool with built-in search strategies that provides a quick way to retrieve controlled trials or systematic reviews on a particular topic.

Database searching usually involves the location of specific words or phrases in the content of the resource within one or more of the bibliographic fields (e.g., article title field, abstract field, author field). Another, quite different way of searching is the process of finding citing articles. Unlike the usual approach of locating words in the text, a **cited reference search** finds works included in the list of references. It is based specifically on the bibliography. The results turned by a cited reference search may be often quite different from the results retrieved using conventional searching for key words, sometimes reflecting more closely the authors' deliberations on what they regard as important (see Table 5.5 for a list of databases that conduct a cited reference search).

Screen the Initial List of Citations and Organize Them

The initial literature search will almost certainly return a list that includes both relevant and irrelevant citations. Rather than expending time reading articles that are not appropriate, the researcher should start by screening the citations list for relevance using the preestablished set of inclusion and exclusion criteria, as discussed earlier.

Organizing citations using a bibliographic management application is a valuable time-saving step. The initial exploratory search of a broad topic may result literally in thousands of citations, but using applications such as Endnote (http://endnote.com/) or RefWorks (http://www.refworks.com/) to store and organize them can save time and help

Search strategy: The identification of search concepts and terms and the way they are combined that will be used to search for resources for the literature review.

Search concepts: Major ideas or themes in a research question.

Search terms: Words or phrases that describe each search concept used to conduct the literature search. They may include variables in the research question, characteristics of the population of interest, or the theoretical framework of the research problem.

Boolean operators: The words AND, OR, and NOT, which are used to join or exclude search terms.

Subject headings: Fixed "official" key words used by many databases to describe major concepts and assigned by indexers to bibliographic records.

Cited reference search: A search that finds articles that are cited by another article.

Table 5.7 Developing the Search Strategy

a. Planning Table. Included are the research question, major concepts, and the terms that describe the concepts.

Question

What are the metabolic consequences of traumatic brain injury in pediatric patients?

Concepts

pediatric patients	traumatic brain injury	metabolic consequences

Terms

children	traumatic brain injury TBI	metabolic consequences
child		metabolic response
pediatric		hypothermia

b. Search Strategy Using Sets

Sets	Search Terms and Combinations
1	children
2	child
3	pediatric
4	1 OR 2 OR 3
5	traumatic brain injury
6	TBI
7	5 OR 6
8	metabolic consequences
9	metabolic responses
10	hypothermia
11	8 OR 9 OR 10
12	4 AND 7 AND 11

c. All-at-Once Search Strategy

(children OR child OR pediatric) AND (traumatic brain injury OR TBI) AND (metabolic consequences OR metabolic response OR hypothermia)

the researcher keep track of the citations. While many applications that perform this function require the purchase of software or an institutional license, there are also several free online resources, such as Zotero (http://www.zotero.org/), CiteULike (http://www.citeulike.org/), and Mendeley (http://www.mendeley.com/). Notably, Mendeley serves as a social-networking site where researchers can exchange information or discover new studies shared by other members.

Retrieve the Full Text and Summarize Relevant Articles

Although full-text versions of many articles will be available electronically through a library's subscription, others may be available only through interlibrary loan—a nationwide borrowing and lending service available at most libraries. The librarian's assistance can be very helpful in this process.

Most researchers will find they need to organize the review of the full-text articles so the summary of their content is both complete and efficient. The research question, methods, findings, and conclusions of each study should be summarized. The review should focus on relevant results and the quality of the evidence. At this point, it is helpful to record any quotes the researcher may want to include in the write-up, along with page numbers so the quote can be attributed appropriately. All of these elements can be recorded in bibliographic management software. In general, it is helpful to record the following items for any study that may end up in the literature review:

- Full article citation
- Purpose of study
- Research design
- Sample size
- Methodology and measurements
- Treatment(s)
- Results
- Findings
- Implications for the current research question
- Implications for nursing practice

Critically Appraise the Study Quality and Findings

Once the researcher has a final stack of relevant articles, the next step is to appraise the studies for quality of design and methodology. Many useful articles and books can serve as guides to critical appraisal; while their details may differ, they tend to ask some of the same fundamental questions (Greenhalgh, 2010; Scottish Intercollegiate Guidelines Network, 2013; Young & Solomon, 2009):

- Is the study question relevant, and how do the findings add to the body of knowledge?
- Was the study design appropriate for the question?
- Are there potential sources of bias?
- Does the conclusion match the data results?
- How does this study contribute to patient care?

CASP (Critical Appraisal Skills Programme), a nonprofit organization based in the United Kingdom, has created tools and checklists to assist in the appraisal process (http://www.casp-uk.net/).

Summarize and Synthesize the Findings

The final step of any literature review is to compose a synthesis of the key findings of the studies that organizes them into a coherent summary. This summary should not be a simple reiteration of the studies that were reviewed, but rather a logical unfolding of the relationships discovered in the research studies. It should emphasize the significance of the research that was reviewed and link it to the current research question.

SKILL BUILDER   Develop a Strong Literature Review

It is easy to see the literature search as a task that must be done to get at the "real" work of research. In fact, if it is done well, a thorough review of previous work can actually save the researcher time in the long run. The literature search can help focus the research question, develop the details of a study design, and put the study in a larger context. Doing a literature search requires time and a bit of frustration tolerance—but there are ways to get the most from this critical step.

- Involve a health sciences librarian in the literature search early in the process. Searching the literature is a methodical science, and the expertise a librarian brings can prove invaluable. A health sciences librarian can help locate databases and assist in developing a search strategy, both of which can improve the chances of a successful search.
- Go from general to specific in the search strategy. Look for studies on the overall topic first, and then search for research that is more specific to the unique question.
- Select references to review from the lists of the most relevant studies.
- Resist the urge to look only at full-text databases. Valuable studies may be missed, and the research

may end up with an incomplete literature review if the focus is exclusively on easily accessible articles.
- Use a broad range of sources, including "gray literature" such as conference proceedings, dissertation abstracts, and government reports. Though time consuming, manual searches of the tables of contents of the most relevant journals may reveal studies that were missed in the electronic search.
- Rely on primary sources—in other words, the original studies—instead of quotes or summaries from other articles. Studies may be misquoted and findings reported incorrectly, so the primary source must be evaluated to ensure the findings are reported correctly.

A strong literature review will include studies that both support and refute the researcher's ideas. Any gaps, particular strengths, or evident weaknesses in the current evidence should be revealed. The goal of a literature review is to explore the support for a research project, not to prove a point. The best literature reviews provide direction while reinforcing the need for specialized inquiry.

Summary of Key Concepts

- The literature review provides an in-depth analysis of recently published research findings.
- Health information is dynamic and vast in quantity. Nurses must learn to search effectively for evidence-based information.
- Peer review is critical for ensuring the credibility of research publications.
- Bibliometrics includes various measures that try to quantify the influence of journals, articles, and researchers.
- The open access movement is making research information more readily accessible.
- Information literacy is a key competency for students and practicing nurses to ensure nursing practice is based on appropriate evidence.

- Evidence-based information can be represented in the form of an evidence pyramid that depicts the potential quality of information, the amount of information, and the amount of work required to find evidence.
- To find evidence, it is important to formulate a handful of searchable and answerable questions.
- Numerous health databases exist. Some are accessed only via a library subscription, some are open and freely accessible, and some are available as mobile applications.
- Plan a search strategy by identifying major search concepts and in turn search terms. Combine the terms using appropriate Boolean operators.
- Critically appraise studies by examining their designs and assessing the importance of the research question and the findings.
- Take advantage of librarians. They have the experience and skills to search many healthcare resources.

For More Depth and Detail

For a more in-depth look at the concepts in this chapter, try these references:

Facchiano, L., & Snyder, C. (2012). Evidence-based practice for the busy nurse practitioner: Part two: Searching for the best evidence to clinical inquiries. *Journal of the American Academy of Nurse Practitioners, 24,* 640–648.

Greenhalgh, T. (2010). *How to read a paper: The basics of evidence-based medicine.* New York, NY: John Wiley & Sons.

Lefebvre, C., Manheimer, E., & Glanville, J. (2011). Searching for studies. In J. P. T. Higgins & S. Green (Eds.), *Cochrane handbook for systematic reviews of interventions.* Version 5.1.0 (updated March 2011). The Cochrane Collaboration. Retrieved from http://handbook.cochrane.org/

Winsett, R., & Moutseous, M. (2012). Collaborating with hospital librarians to engage nurses in evidence-based practice education. *Journal of Hospital Librarianship, 12*(4), 309–316.

CRITICAL APPRAISAL EXERCISE

Retrieve the following full-text article from the Cumulative Index to Nursing and Allied Health Literature or similar search database:

Assante, J., Collins, S., & Hewer, I. (2015). Infection associated with single-dose dexamethasone for prevention of postoperative nausea and vomiting: A literature review. *AANA Journal, 83*(4), 281–288. Retrieved from http://dml.regis.edu/login?url=http://search.ebscohost.com/login.aspx?direct=true&db=ccm&AN=109825547&site=ehost-live&scope=site

Refer to the authors' procedures for searching and reporting the literature to address the following questions:

1. What is the goal of this literature review? How is it related to nursing practice?
2. What do the authors of this literature review do to ensure they retrieved the largest number of relevant articles? How could they have expanded their search?

3. Which actions are taken by these authors to reduce bias in selection and review of articles?
4. Which level of evidence is provided by this article, on the evidence pyramid?
5. How do these authors link the review to practice?

References

Carman, M., Wolf, L., Henderson, D., Kamienski, M., Koziol-McLain, J., Manton, A., & Moon, M. (2013). Developing your clinical question: The key to successful research. *Journal of Emergency Nursing, 39*(3), 299–302.

Consolidated Appropriations Act, 2008, Pub. L. No. 110-161 § Div G, Title II, Sec 218. (2007).

Fair Access to Science and Technology Research Act of 2015, H.R. 1477, U.S. House of Representatives. (2015a).

Fair Access to Science and Technology Research Act of 2015, S.779, U.S. Senate. (2015b).

Glover, J., Izzo, D., Odato, K., & Wang, L. (2006). EBM pyramid. Dartmouth University/Yale University. Retrieved from http://www.dartmouth.edu/~biomed/resources.htmld/guides/ebm_resources.shtml

Greenhalgh, T. (2010). *How to read a paper: The basics of evidence-based medicine.* New York, NY: John Wiley & Sons.

Hirsch, J. E. (2005). An index to quantify an individual's scientific research output. *Proceedings of the National Academy of Science U.S.A., 102*(46), 16569–16572.

Liberati, A., Altman, D. G., Tetzlaff, J., Mulrow, C., Gotzsche, P. C., Ioannidis, J. P., . . . Moher, D. (2009). The PRISMA statement for reporting systematic reviews and meta-analyses of studies that evaluate health care interventions: Explanation and elaboration. *Journal of Clinical Epidemiology, 62*(10), e1–e34. doi: 10.1016/j.jclinepi.2009.06.006

Medical Library Association. (2015). Find good health information. Retrieved from http://www.mlanet.org/resources/userguide.html

Priem, J., Taraborelli, D., Groth, P., & Neylon, C. (2010). Altmetrics: A manifesto. Retrieved from http://altmetrics.org/manifesto

Pritchard, A. (1969). Statistical bibliography or bibliometrics? *Journal of Documentation, 25*(4), 348–349.

Schardt, C. (2011). Health information literacy meets evidence-based practice. *Journal of the Medical Library Association, 99*(1), 1–2. doi: 10.3163/1536-5050.99.1.001

Scottish Intercollegiate Guidelines Network. (2013). Critical appraisal: Notes and checklists. Retrieved from http://www.sign.ac.uk/methodology/checklists.html

Suber, P. (2004). Open access overview. Retrieved from http://legacy.earlham.edu/~peters/fos/overview.htm

Thomson Reuters. (2015). The Thomson Reuters impact factor. Retrieved from http://thomsonreuters.com/products_services/science/free/essays/impact_factor/#ref.4

U.S. National Library of Medicine. (2015). Fact sheet. MEDLINE, PubMed, and PMC (PubMed Central): How are they different? Retrieved from http://www.nlm.nih.gov/pubs/factsheets/dif_med_pub.html

Young, J. M., & Solomon, M. J. (2009). How to critically appraise an article. *Nature Clinical Practice Gastroenterology & Hepatology, 6*(2), 82–91. doi: 10.1038/ncpgasthep1331

Chapter 6

Selecting an Appropriate Research Design

CHAPTER OBJECTIVES

The study of this chapter will help the learner to

- Establish the link between the research question and the study design.
- Evaluate the characteristics that are the basis for design decisions.
- Differentiate the kinds of questions that require quantitative, qualitative, and mixed method designs.
- Identify the types of variables that reflect the concepts in a research question.
- Review designs that describe populations, test relationships, or examine causality.
- Relate the type of design to the strength of evidence it can support.

KEY TERMS

Confirmatory studies	Descriptive variables	Predictive research
Correlation research	Exploratory studies	Research design
Dependent variable	Extraneous variables	Variable
Descriptive studies	Independent variable	

Introduction

In the best of all possible worlds, evidence would be the result of well-controlled, perfectly designed studies. Of course, most nurses do not practice in the best of all possible worlds; nursing research is planned by making a series of decisions, each of which involves weighing alternatives and options in the search for knowledge. It is important, then, to understand each of the predominant research designs so a study can be planned that best answers the research question and therefore is the strongest evidence for practice.

To call this process "design" may give the wrong impression. This singular word implies that design is an event that happens and then is complete. In reality, design may be a circuitous process, with each decision having a variety of implications that require consideration and that may even compel the researcher to revisit earlier decisions. The ultimate result of this process is a detailed plan for the ensuing research project, which addresses the research question with a minimum of bias. Bias may come from several sources in a research study—the researcher, the subjects, the measurements, the sampling procedures—and solid design is the best way to control the threat that bias presents to the overall credibility of the results.

VOICES FROM THE FIELD

I used to just accept that the way things were done on my surgical unit was the way they should be done, until I went back to school to get my BSN and took a course in evidence-based practice. My instructors taught me to be curious and to question the status quo if I suspected I could find a better way to care for patients.

One day, I was pulling up pressure hosiery on one of my postoperative patients and cursing under my breath. It was the third time that day I had found the hosiery either wadded up around her ankles or rolled down at the top into something that looked disturbingly like a tourniquet. She was 78 years old and had experienced abdominal surgery, but was otherwise quite healthy. For the hundredth time in my career, I asked myself, "Do these darn things do any good?" It occurred to me that I had my first evidence-based practice project right in front of me—or, more accurately, around my patient's ankles.

I did not find anything compelling in the literature, so I decided to conduct my own study. I approached our quality department and asked for help setting up a randomized trial, because I knew that it would provide the most compelling evidence. Our unit quality representative told me that I was unlikely to persuade any of the surgeons to let me forgo the hosiery without at least a pilot test, so we put our heads together and came up with a way to demonstrate that my question might have merit. The quality representative reminded me that we had several surgeons who did not use the hosiery routinely. We decided to do a retrospective chart review, and chose a causal-comparative design for the study. In other words, we found surgical patients who had received compression hosiery and those who had not, and compared the rates of postoperative deep vein thrombosis (DVT) for the two groups. We knew this design was weaker than a randomized trial, so we controlled the extraneous variables we could. Because we knew the risk factors for DVT could affect the outcome, we collected data about each individual patient's risk factors. A big extraneous variable was the surgeon—we knew that factor would exert an effect because the patients without hosiery would all belong to a single set of surgeons. Thus, we identified the surgeon for each patient as well, along with information about the surgical procedure performed and some basic demographic data.

The result was very satisfying for me: I was able to show that the pressure hosiery was effective in preventing DVT only in patients who had preexisting risk factors. Compression devices were the most effective intervention for this group of patients, followed by pressure hosiery. In contrast, the patients without risk factors did not benefit from either intervention. The quality representative took my findings to the medical care committee, and they endorsed a randomized trial to confirm what we found in the pilot test. It took a while, but now—two years later—we have a preoperative checklist of DVT risk factors that determines whether a patient is prescribed compression hosiery. Patients get the evidence-based care they need, and those without risk factors do not have an unnecessary charge for a treatment that will not help.

Janice Leeper, RN

No design is perfect. The researcher can predict some threats that will require attention during design; others may arrive, unanticipated, in the midst of the study. The design process entails a series of decisions, balancing research rigor with reality. If a researcher considers design options thoughtfully, makes decisions based on the goals of the study, and can provide a rationale for each decision, the final product will be valid.

Research design:
The overall approach to or outline of the study that details all the major components of the research.

What Is a Design?

A **research design** is an outline of the study, in both a macro sense and a micro sense. From a macro perspective, design refers to an overall approach to the study, grounded in a set of beliefs about knowledge and the question that must be answered. When this macro view is adopted, only a handful of research classifications are apparent. Each has specific characteristics that confer unique strengths and weaknesses in producing credible knowledge. These macro research approaches have specific kinds of questions that they best serve, and part of the researcher's job is to match the requirements of the question to the uniqueness of a study type.

Macro decisions are among the first to be made, but each large classification of studies encompasses numerous ways to conduct the study. Dealing with these choices requires a micro view of the research process, including decisions that will give the researcher specific guidance in implementing the study. This micro view is called research design. For quantitative studies, the design details how the subjects will be selected and assigned to groups, the way the intervention will be applied, a measurement strategy, and a plan for data analysis. The goal of design in a quantitative study is to minimize error, limit the potential for bias, and address clinical questions as well as statistical issues (McCusker & Gunaydin, 2015). In qualitative studies, the design describes the planned approach to data gathering, including the researcher's beliefs about the nature of the information to be generated. Criteria for selecting informants, general guides for data collection, and plans for data analysis may be explicit in a qualitative research design.

Both the macro and micro views of research design are focused on one outcome: answering the research question with the greatest level of credibility. Reflecting on this overriding purpose can guide the researcher in the decisions that must be made.

The Basis for Design Selection

Ultimately, the basis for selecting a design is the *demands of the research question*. If a research question has been carefully considered and purposefully constructed, then it can be matched to a specific design. This match between well-constructed question and best possible answer is the goal of the research design process (Delost & Nadder, 2014).

The *nature of the variables* of the study may keep the ethical researcher from manipulating the environment or the treatment situation. These ethical limitations are strong influences that may require implementation of a weaker design in exchange for stronger subject protections. For example, it would be unethical to intentionally inflict a disease on a patient so as to test a treatment for that disease.

Other factors affecting the design selected include the sampling plan and the measurements, which often present a challenge. A population may be inaccessible, or an instrument may possess low reliability. The *researcher* also brings his or her own strengths and limitations to the study. A specific researcher may not possess the skill and competence to conduct a wide range of study types; researchers often focus on one tradition, or even one design, for most of the studies they conduct. Even when the researcher has the skill and competence to conduct the type of research needed, he or she may not have the *resources* necessary to carry out a study in an ideal way. These resources may range from measurement instruments to data collection forms to software, all of which are often expensive and difficult to obtain. Almost all research studies require funding for expenses; all of them require time. Both may be in short supply for the nurse researcher. Without the necessary resources, even a strong design may be subject to compromises during execution. Thus, consideration of the available resources—people, money, and materials—should also be part of the research planning process.

The *time frame* is another important consideration in research design. The length of time available to the researcher from planning to implementation to write-up is a critical concern when finalizing design decisions. It would be unrealistic to plan a longitudinal study of the development patterns of infants as they mature into toddlers, for example, if the researcher has only a year for study.

The *amount of control* the researcher needs in the study provides guidance in the design of the study. Studies that require a high level of control (e.g., drug trials and intervention studies) will need a high level of structure. Threats to the validity of the results must be anticipated and dealt with *a priori*, or before the study begins. Quantitative studies are often concerned with managing threats to internal validity.

In some studies, particularly qualitative or descriptive ones, control is not much of an issue. The qualitative paradigm is a naturalistic one, requiring only that the researcher have a general direction in mind prior to starting the study. The research design may be planned, but is allowed to evolve as the study progresses. Emergent designs are expected in qualitative research. Qualitative researchers are less concerned with the effects of extraneous variables because they are not measuring effects at all, but rather attempting to understand phenomena. This understanding requires using the subject's frame of reference—not the researcher's perspective—as the guiding voice in the study. For these studies, very little may be prescribed *a priori*.

Finally, the researcher must consider the ultimate audience for the study results. Some clinical fields focus on specific designs; for example, the practice of pharmacy is based almost exclusively on evidence produced via randomized controlled trials. The profession of nursing uses a variety of research paradigms to answer questions about nursing care; yet even within the profession some audiences expect specific types of research. For example, critical care nursing, with its focus on data-driven decision making and managing physiological responses, relies heavily on the scientific method to produce evidence. Mental health nursing, in contrast, often seeks guidance from the results of qualitative studies. The expectations of the audience that will be reached with the study should be incorporated into the design decisions.

It is not always possible to control a research process as well as one might desire, because a host of practical issues may affect design. The subjects are human beings, after all, and they may behave in unpredictable ways. They may be difficult to recruit or to keep in a study. The researcher may have limited access to the subjects' information or may have to rely on secondary data. Subjects may be untruthful, behave unnaturally, or refuse treatment.

It is important to emphasize that all studies have strengths and weaknesses; no single study can be definitively and perfectly designed. In turn, it is the convergence of findings across a wealth of studies that adds knowledge to professional practice, not the perfection of a single design (Wallace & Clarke, 2012). Although the researcher should strive to control extraneous variables and threats to validity as much as possible, every study will have its limitations. If the nurse researcher waits until the perfect design is achieved, research will never get accomplished.

The Design Decisions

Design decisions paint the study in broad strokes first and then hone in on a more detailed level as the study is planned. Different decisions may be assigned different relative weights depending on the amount of structure needed in the study. For example, sampling might be more important in a case-control study, where matching of cases and controls is essential. Conversely, qualitative studies require more emphasis on the way information is elicited and checked with informants, so willingness to communicate verbally may be a primary concern.

Study design always involves tradeoffs. Some design flaws may have little impact on the study's outcome; others may fatally affect the credibility of the results. The researcher's obligation is to clarify the purpose of the study and design the study to achieve this purpose in a trustworthy way.

In the end, there is no single best design. Even expert researchers often disagree on the merits of a particular design decision. Although some designs provide stronger levels of evidence for nursing practice, all good designs share the virtues of being rigorous and systematic. The nature of the data collected may vary substantially, but a focus on finding truth should be unwavering in good research design. A great deal of a study's credibility is based not on the researcher making a single correct decision, but rather on the researcher making a sequence of defensible, rational decisions.

It is probably unrealistic to think of these decisions as occurring in a particular sequence. Researchers often move back and forth between decision levels that are interrelated, rather than mutually exclusive. In general, however, the decision-making process has three major phases:

1. Identify assumptions about the knowledge to be gained from the study.
2. Select a design that serves the purpose of the study.
3. Develop detailed plans for implementation of the study.

These phases start with a high-level, macro view of the problem and purpose of the study and hone in on more detailed decisions as the design plan unfolds. Think of these phases as looking at the study with a series of ever more powerful microscopes, focusing more tightly with each subsequent look.

Identify Assumptions About the Knowledge to Be Gained from the Study

When designing a research study, the researcher must reflect on any assumptions he or she has made regarding the nature of the knowledge needed to answer the question.

These assumptions will guide the researcher to a quantitative or qualitative design or may reveal that a mix of both methods is required.

Quantitative designs are appropriate when the purpose of the study is to measure the effect of an intervention, test a theory about relationships, or describe a phenomenon with precision. Quantitative designs involve measurement of some sort, so they will ultimately involve the analysis of numbers. Such studies require control of internal validity for trustworthiness and strong external validity for generalizability. Quantitative designs are appropriate when the results must reveal the true relationship between a cause and an effect or between two variables. Measurement gives the researcher a level of certainty about the relationship that is quantifiable, and the effects of error and random chance can be calculated (Khudyahov, Gorfine, Zucker, & Spiegelman, 2015). The control inherent in a quantitative design allows the researcher to rule out rival explanations for the results and quantify the amount of confidence the reader can place in the findings.

Qualitative approaches to design are appropriate when the purpose of the study is to understand the meaning of a phenomenon. The qualitative researcher has a goal of describing social reactions and interactions with such vividness that the reader can understand the meaning of the event, even if he or she has not experienced it. Qualitative research can also be used to develop theories, build models of relationships and inter-relationships, and develop instrumentation (Wener & Woodgate, 2013). Such research places little emphasis on control. The context for the study is a natural one, and the study is allowed to unfold as information is gathered and analyzed. Often, a qualitative study follows a path marked by twists and turns as the investigator strives to understand the phenomenon by exploring its meaning with informants. The design is an emergent one, with only general guidelines planned up front. This emergent design enables the qualitative researcher to follow leads provided by informants to understand the social context for the behavior being studied (Denzin & Lincoln, 2011).

A mixed method design is appropriate when a combination of meaning and control is needed. Frequently, this type of design is adopted when a qualitative approach is used to design an instrument or an intervention that is subsequently tested for effectiveness using quantitative methods. A mixed method study may also be indicated for evaluation research, where effectiveness, efficiency, and satisfaction are important elements (Terrell, 2012). The desirability of a treatment may be measured using qualitative measures, while the effectiveness of the treatment is documented quantitatively. Mixed methods seem attractive—it makes intuitive sense to consider the meaning of an event prior to testing its effectiveness—but they are complex, difficult designs to implement. The rigorous nature of both research methods must be reflected in the design, and the researcher must be competent in both traditions.

Although the quantitative and qualitative traditions may seem diametrically opposed, in actuality they have much in common. By their very nature, the characteristics of one may overlap with those of the other. Both quantitative and qualitative approaches are characterized by rigorous attention to the scholarly nature of the work. Both aim for reliability of results, confidence in the conclusions, and a focus on creating credible evidence. Both research traditions also have a single goal—to establish truth. Although the specific methods applied during these types of research may be quite different, the goal of each is to produce quality results that answer the question in a trustworthy way. In that way, quantitative and qualitative research approaches are very much alike.

Select a Design That Serves the Purpose of the Study

Once assumptions of the study question have been determined, the researcher selects an approach that will answer the research question and meet the goals of the study. This selection process is the result of a series of decisions based on reflection on the aim of the study, the concepts under study, and the nature of the research question. The researcher can make these decisions by answering a series of questions.

Is the Aim of the Study Exploratory or Confirmatory?

Exploratory studies are often qualitative or mixed methods studies, but they may also be quantitative if measurement is employed. Exploratory studies are classified as descriptive, even if they happen to describe relationships and associations. They explore and describe a given phenomenon. Survey methods are frequently used for exploratory studies; mixed methods are also popular choices for the initial exploration of a topic. For example, a study that explores the reasons that nurses choose a clinical specialty may determine the specific characteristics that the nurse was looking for, such as certifications required and work hours, but also examine the value-based reasons a particular selection was made. The former might be measured by a survey instrument, whereas the value-based information would be more appropriately gathered through an interview.

Confirmatory studies are those in which a relationship between variables has been proposed, and the study is designed to test the relationship statistically while minimizing bias. In this case, some form of study to determine relationships or examine causality is required. Confirmatory studies are more structured and controlled than exploratory studies. They require careful definition of the variables and concepts of interest so they can be adequately measured and analyzed. Confirmatory studies are often "next steps" from exploratory studies. For example, an analysis of the results of a knowledge-based questionnaire administered to patients with diabetes might be used to design a specific diabetic education program that is subsequently tested for effectiveness.

Which Concepts Will Be Studied?

A clear definition of the concepts that will be studied guides the design of a study and the subsequent measurement strategy. In quantitative research, the concepts that are of interest are translated into measurable characteristics called **variables**. A variable is a characteristic, event, or response that represents the elements of the research question in a detectable way. Variables are carefully described up front to guide the design of quantitative studies. Several types of variables may be used to represent the intent of the research question. **Table 6.1** depicts some research questions in terms of their respective variables and concepts.

Exploratory studies: Research to explore and describe a phenomenon of interest and generate new knowledge.

Confirmatory studies: Research in which a relationship between variables has been posed and the study is designed to examine this hypothesis.

Variable: Characteristic, event, or response that represents the elements of the research question in a detectable or measurable way.

Descriptive variables:
Characteristics that describe the sample and provide a composite picture of the subjects of the study; they are not manipulated or controlled by the researcher.

Independent variable:
A factor that is artificially introduced into a study explicitly to measure an expected effect; the "cause" of "cause and effect."

Table 6.1 Research Questions and Correlated Concepts/Variables

Research Question	Concepts/Variables
What is the perception of the effectiveness of complementary medicine among intensive care unit nurses?	Descriptive variable: perception of effectiveness
Is music therapy an effective treatment for patients who experience anxiety in the intensive care unit as compared to patients who receive no music therapy?	Research variables: independent—music therapy; dependent—anxiety Extraneous variables: sound level in the ICU; preexisting anxiety disorder
What are the emotional and psychological reactions of patients who have been patients in the intensive care unit for more than 5 days?	Concepts: emotional and psychological reactions

Descriptive Variables

As the name implies, **descriptive variables** describe the sample or some characteristic of the phenomenon under study. A descriptive variable may represent demographic data about the subjects (e.g., age, gender, and ethnicity) or measurable characteristics (e.g., blood pressure, weight, and hematocrit). The variables of interest may be perceptual, as in responses on a pain scale, or attitudinal, as in patient satisfaction. The primary characteristic of a descriptive variable is that it is used solely to provide a composite picture of the subjects of study. Descriptive variables are not considered part of a cause-and-effect equation, and although the researcher may look for associations between variables, no attempt is made to manipulate or control descriptive variables.

Research Variables

Research variables are introduced into a study explicitly to measure an expected effect. A research variable may be categorized as either independent or dependent. An **independent variable** is one that is applied to the experimental situation to measure its effects. Such a variable is independent of the naturally occurring situation and is introduced into the experiment so that its impact on a specified outcome can be quantified. In a true experiment, the independent variable is manipulated, meaning it is introduced by the researcher. It may also be called a treatment, experimental variable, or intervention. One can think of an independent variable as the "cause" in "cause and effect." For example, if a nurse is interested in studying the effects of therapeutic touch on postoperative pain, therapeutic touch is the independent variable—that is, it is artificially inserted into a situation to measure its effects.

Some designs consider causal variables to be independent even if they are not manipulated; in these cases, the variable of interest is found in its naturally occurring state, and subjects with the specified characteristic are compared to those without it to understand its potential effects. For example, a researcher might be interested in studying the effects of breast cancer on body image. Although breast cancer is not manipulated, its effects are of interest in this study, and it may be referred to as an independent variable. Technically, independent variables are only those that are artificially introduced to subjects, but the term is used loosely to apply to other types of causal variables.

A **dependent variable** is the outcome of interest. In an experiment, it is expected that an independent variable will have an effect on the dependent variable. In other words, the outcome is dependent on the independent variable having been introduced into the experiment. Thus the dependent variable can be considered the "effect" in "cause and effect."

In a specific type of design that is focused on prediction, the independent variable is more accurately called a predictor variable, and the dependent variable is referred to as an outcome variable. Although the terms *independent* and *dependent* are commonly used to describe the predictive relationship, technically the terms are not accurate descriptions of these variables because the predictor variable is not manipulated. Predictive studies are classified as descriptive, so these variables are more accurately referred to by their function, rather than by their dependent nature. For example, a nurse researcher may want to identify the characteristics of patients who present to the emergency department who are at high risk for multiple visits. In this case, demographic variables such as age, diagnoses, socioeconomic status, and family support might be studied to determine whether they are predictive of repeat admissions. In this example, age, diagnoses, socioeconomic status, and family support would accurately be described as predictor variables and repeat admissions identified as the outcome variable.

Extraneous Variables

One goal in study design is to control external influences on a process so that rival explanations for the outcome can be ruled out. These rival explanations are considered **extraneous variables**, meaning variables that exert an effect on the outcome but that are not part of the planned experiment. Realistically, extraneous variables exist in every study, but they are most problematic in experiments. Extraneous variables can be controlled if they are expected or recognized when they occur. The most problematic extraneous variables are those that cannot be predicted, are difficult to control, or go unrecognized until the study is complete. Extraneous variables confuse the interpretation of the results and may render an experiment so flawed that the results cannot be used in practice. A primary goal of research design, particularly experimental designs, is the elimination or control of extraneous variables.

A specific type of extraneous variable is a confounder. Confounding occurs when the association between cause and effect is partially or entirely due to a third factor that is not part of the experiment. For example, a study might show that alcoholism is a causative factor in lung cancer, when in reality the relationship is due to a confounder—smoking. Because smoking rates are higher among alcoholics, this third factor confounds the true relationship between alcoholism and lung disease. For a variable to be a true confounder, it must be associated with the independent variable and a true cause of the dependent variable (Nieswiadomy, 2012). When a confounder is suspected, the research design

Dependent variable: An outcome of interest that occurs after the introduction of an independent variable; the "effect" of "cause and effect."

Extraneous variables: Factors that exert an effect on the outcome but that are not part of the planned experiment and may confuse the interpretation of the results.

Descriptive studies:
Research designed to describe in detail some process, event, or outcome. Such a design is used when very little is known about the research question.

must be altered to control or account for its effects. The most common approaches used to control confounders are random sampling, matching subjects, and statistical analysis of covariates.

Qualitative Concepts

The term *variable* is rarely used in qualitative research. Its rarity in this setting occurs because a variable, by definition, is something that is measurable, and measurement is not typically part of qualitative designs. However, qualitative studies do have goals related to understanding a phenomenon, belief, perception, or set of values (Cooper, 2012). In the case of qualitative research, the design is driven by the nature of the information to be gained from the study, and establishing this relationship requires thoughtful consideration of the particular phenomenon of interest. Although it is not necessary to develop operational definitions for qualitative phenomena, the researcher should be able to articulate the concepts, theories, or processes that are of interest. In the case of grounded theory—a specific type of qualitative research design—the researcher may also plan to study relationships between these phenomena.

Whether the researcher plans to measure variables or study phenomena, consideration of these characteristics will help determine the specifics of the research design. Sometimes it is necessary to incorporate elements of both types of study. Identifying the variables and concepts in a study is an important precursor to design. By clarifying the conceptual focus of the study, the researcher can begin to implement the research question in a way that lends itself to study.

What Is the Nature of the Research Question?

Once the conceptual basis of the study has been articulated, the research question becomes the focus of more specific design decisions. The nature of the research question serves as the foundation for the next set of decisions—namely, classification of the specific research study design. Most research questions can be classified into one of four categories:

- Questions that seek to describe a phenomenon or population
- Questions that seek to quantify the nature of relationships between variables or between subjects
- Questions that seek to investigate causality or the effects of interventions or risk factors
- Questions that determine effectiveness of interventions as evidence for practice

Descriptive Research

Descriptive research is appropriate when very little is known about the question at hand. Often, researchers seek to fix problems without understanding the current problem as it exists. Descriptive research can help the investigator discover a baseline performance level, describe a subject's responses to treatment, or determine the desirability of a new service. Research questions that begin with "what" and "why" generally indicate that a descriptive study will be undertaken. **Descriptive studies** set out to describe in detail some process, event, or outcome; they document the characteristics of a "subject" of some sort. "Subject" appears in quotes here because it represents a broad range of possibilities other than individuals. For example, a subject may be a child, a patient, a patient care unit, an emergency department, a county's health, or a unit's adverse event rate. Once a subject of interest has been described, an exploratory study sets out to discover as much about the subject as possible and to find themes that can help the researcher effectively derive meaning from the study.

Descriptive qualitative studies rarely have detailed procedures identified up front; instead, the design of a qualitative study is "emergent" in that the details of the study become apparent as information is gathered and the nature of the information is evaluated. The qualitative researcher will identify a specific approach to data gathering and a philosophical basis for the approach, but rarely creates a detailed plan prior to initiating a qualitative study. In contrast, most quantitative descriptive studies feature a clear plan for implementation that outlines the sample, the measurement procedures, and statistical processes that will be used to summarize the data.

Descriptive studies are often exploratory, but they can also be confirmatory, meaning the researcher suspects that a phenomenon or event exists in a population, and he or she sets out to confirm those suspicions. Most often, however, descriptive studies are applied when very little is known about the situation, and baseline knowledge is required to be able to design effective nursing practices. **Table 6.2** highlights the commonly used descriptive designs and the characteristics of each; details of the various designs are described in depth later in this text.

Research That Examines Relationships

The research question often reflects a need to go beyond describing single characteristics to determining whether a relationship exists between variables or between subjects. This type of research can fall into either of two categories: correlation research or predictive research.

Correlation research involves the quantification of the strength and direction of the relationship between two variables in a single subject or the relationship between a single variable in two samples. For example, a researcher might want to determine if there is an association between anxiety and blood pressure in the preoperative patient, or the researcher may seek to compare the nature of anxiety between mothers and daughters.

The purpose of **predictive research** is to search for variables measured at one point in time that may predict an outcome that is measured at a different point in time. For example, given a patient's total cholesterol, can the occurrence of myocardial infarction be predicted?

Both correlation and predictive research are considered descriptive because the variables are not manipulated and the relationships are not controlled. Correlation and predictive research also may be used legitimately to search for suggested causal relationships that may subsequently be studied through experimental designs. Experimental designs are discussed in more detail later in this chapter. **Table 6.3** summarizes common designs that are used to describe relationships and their associated characteristics.

Correlation research: Research designed to quantify the strength and the direction of the relationship of two variables in a single subject or the relationship between a single variable in two samples.

Predictive research: Research designed to search for variables measured at one point in time that may forecast an outcome that is measured at a different point in time.

Table 6.2 Some Common Descriptive Designs

Design	Description	Example of a Research Question	Strengths	Limitations
Survey design	Describes the characteristics of a sample or event at a single point in time through self-report	Which coping strategies do adults use when diagnosed with cancer?	Description of current state provides a basis for planning interventions	Unable to determine causes of change or differences between groups
Cross-sectional study	Describes the characteristics of samples that differ on a key characteristic, measured at a single point in time	Which coping strategies do adults use when newly diagnosed with cancer?	Uncomplicated to manage Economical	Does not capture changes that occur over time
Longitudinal study	Data collected from a sample at selected points over time to describe changes in characteristics or events	Which coping strategies do adults use when managing their cancer in the 5 years after diagnosis?	Enables exploration of issues affected by human development	Affected by attrition of subjects Extended time period required for data collection
Case study	Explores in depth a single individual, program, event, or action through the collection of detailed information using a variety of data collection techniques	What are the responses of a group of adults to participating in a holistic treatment support group?	Enables evaluation of rare events or conditions Allows for the study of the uniqueness of individual people or situations	Time consuming, requiring extended study
Single subject design	Studies the response of a single individual to an intervention, based on measurement of a baseline and ongoing measurement after introducing a treatment	What are the responses of a 30-year-old woman diagnosed with breast cancer after introduction to a holistic treatment support group?	Allows for the study of the unique responses of individuals to interventions Enables the determination of timing of responses after an intervention	Does not permit generalization to larger populations
Phenomenology	Investigates the meaning of an experience among those who have experienced the same phenomenon	What is the meaning of the experience of receiving a diagnosis of cancer?	Produces rich data from the informant's perspective Can be used to study a wide range of phenomena	Requires a high level of analytic skill
Ethnography	Intensive study of the features and interactions of a given culture by immersion in the natural setting over an extended period of time	How do women in Muslim society respond to a diagnosis of breast cancer?	Produces rich data that enable the development of culturally sensitive interventions	Requires extensive contact over long periods of time

Table 6.3 Some Designs That Describe Relationships

Design	Description	Example of a Research Question	Strengths	Limitations
Correlation	Describes the relationship between two variables in a single population or the relationship between a single variable in two populations	Are coping skills and socioeconomic status related in a sample of adults newly diagnosed with cancer?	Enables scrutiny of a large number of variables in a single study Provides an evaluation of the strength of relationship between two variables Provides a basis for subsequent experimental testing	May be affected by extraneous variables Does not enable a conclusion to be drawn about causality
Predictive study	Describes the relationship between a predictor variable (or a group of predictor variables) and an outcome variable	Can coping skills in adults with newly diagnosed cancer predict their level of compliance with the treatment plan?	Describes the predictive capacity and quantifies the explanatory ability of a variable or group of variables	May be affected by extraneous variables
Grounded theory	Qualitative method in which the researcher attempts to develop a theory of process, action, or interaction based on in-depth analysis of the words of informants	How do social support systems affect the development and use of coping skills in adults newly diagnosed with cancer?	Enables development of theoretical models of action and interaction	Requires sophisticated analytic skills Involves collection of large amounts of data
Tests of model fit	Test theories of causal relationships between variables based on fitting data to a preconceived model	Does the introduction of a support group affect the type and effectiveness of coping skills used by adults with newly diagnosed cancer?	Enable quantification of the fit of a theoretical model to real life	Complex studies that require large samples, statistical sophistication, and specialized software

Research That Examines Causality

Evidence-based nursing practice commonly focuses on determining the effectiveness of nursing interventions—a quest that requires a research design that can establish and quantify causality. Measuring cause and effect is complex, however; several requirements must be met before a researcher can conclude that the cause did, indeed, result in the effect to the exclusion of all other causes. To establish that a causal relationship exists, several criteria must be met. These criteria form the basis for the elements that make up the set of research designs known as experimental and quasi-experimental methods. The criteria include the following considerations:

- *Temporality:* The time sequence between independent and dependent variables must support causation.
- *Influence:* The effect that the independent variable has on the dependent variable can be detected statistically, and the probability that the relationship was caused by chance is small.
- *Specificity:* Rival explanations for the specific relationship between independent and dependent variables have been eliminated or controlled (Hartung & Touchette, 2009).

Other sources of rival explanations are extraneous variables. For this reason, control of extraneous variables is a central part of experimental design. Accounting for rival explanations is an important concern in establishing that the independent variable—and only the independent variable—produced the effect that was observed.

A research question that requires establishing causality forces the researcher to consider how all these elements will be managed in an experiment. The more carefully thought out the details of a study, the stronger the design will be and the more confidently the nurse can apply the findings as evidence for practice. Once the considerations that are inherent in the research question have been made explicit, the researcher can begin focusing even more closely on the structure of the explicit design that will be used to answer the question. **Table 6.4** highlights the designs commonly used for examining causality and the characteristics of each; these designs are discussed in depth later in this text.

Research That Compares Effectiveness

New research designs have emerged specifically in response to the need to provide evidence for practice. These studies seek to compare the effectiveness of a set of interventions with the effectiveness of alternative or traditional practices. Comparative effectiveness studies assess competing interventions for efficacy, cost, and usefulness to specific populations. Such studies have many of the characteristics of randomized controlled trials but are adapted to allow for a more naturalistic approach, a shorter timeline, and easier translation into practice.

Comparative effectiveness research emerged in response to the necessity of answering real-world questions in settings in which a range of possible options are available, and the best choice may vary across patients, settings, and time (Armstrong, 2012). Oftentimes, double-blinded, randomized controlled trials are impractical, costly, and time consuming in these settings—yet the importance of generating evidence about clinical effectiveness

Table 6.4 Some Designs That Examine Causality

Design	Description	Example of a Research Question	Strengths	Limitations
Experimental design	Studies causality by introducing an intervention to one group (the treatment group) and comparing the outcome to that of another group that has not experienced the intervention (the control group); subjects are randomly assigned to groups	Does coaching to improve coping strategies result in increased compliance with the treatment program for adults with newly diagnosed cancer?	Provides the most rigorous test of effectiveness of interventions	Difficult to implement May be impossible or ethically undesirable to withhold treatment from the control group
Quasi-experimental design	A treatment is introduced to a group, but random assignment and/or a control group are missing	Does coaching improve coping strategies in adults with newly diagnosed cancer who are participating in a support group?	Enables scrutiny of causality	Cannot definitively determine causality Level of evidence provided is weaker than with experimental designs
Causal-comparative design/case control	Nonexperimental study in which groups are selected because they do or do not have a characteristic of interest and are examined for a dependent variable; groups are carefully matched based on the independent variable	Do adults with newly diagnosed cancer who have supportive spouses comply with their treatment plan more effectively than those without supportive spouses?	Useful when the independent variable cannot be manipulated Provides evidence that suggests causal relationships that can be tested experimentally	Inferences about causality are limited Extraneous variables may affect the outcome May be difficult to find matched controls
Time series analysis	Studies the effects of an intervention by measuring a baseline, implementing a treatment, and collecting data about an outcome at specified periods over time	Does coaching to enhance coping skills introduced after initial treatment improve compliance with the treatment plan for adults with cancer?	Treatment group serves as its own control group, so subjects' effects are minimized Extended time period for measurement strengthens the capacity to attribute effects to the intervention More powerful in detecting changes over time	May be affected by attrition of subjects Outcome may be affected by historical events or maturation of subjects No comparison group measured to determine the effects of extraneous variables

has never been more important. Comparative effectiveness research encompasses both the generation of evidence and its synthesis. Evidence is generated using both experimental and observational methods. Synthesis of the evidence uses systematic reviews, decision modeling, and cost-effectiveness analysis to draw conclusions.

While randomized trials are increasingly seen as artificial and difficult to implement, they will likely continue to form the cornerstone of any comparative effectiveness research. In addition, modifications of the randomized trial—such as pragmatic trials and adaptive trials—may render these studies more naturalistic and practical. Comparative effectiveness research also relies on observational studies, in which the population of interest is assigned to alternative interventions based on patient, provider, and system factors and observed for the natural occurrence of an outcome of interest.

Collectively, these adaptations are emerging in response to widespread demand for evidence that will be immediately useful, yet still rigorous. Such new designs are expected to become more acceptable and relevant for evidence-based practice as the field evolves. **Table 6.5** depicts some of the research designs used in comparative effectiveness research.

Develop Detailed Plans for Implementation of the Study

Many of the decisions that guide the research will be dictated by the type of design chosen. For example, an experimental design requires a random sample or random assignment of subjects to groups, whereas a qualitative study will engage in purposeful sampling. Even after an explicit design is chosen, however, many decisions remain to be made— for example, the procedures to be used for recruiting subjects, applying interventions, and measuring outcomes, to name a few. Other decisions are required to ensure that an adequate sample can be accessed and that ethical considerations are addressed.

A research plan guiding implementation of the study describes the following design elements:

- The sampling strategy
- The measurement strategy
- The data collection plan
- The data analysis plan

The research plan is used like a road map to ensure that all the steps of the research process are systematically and rigorously applied. The research plan provides documentation of steps that were taken and the rationale for specific decisions, and it represents the primary way a researcher can increase the study's replicability. A detailed research plan also helps the researcher recall the decisions that were made when the time comes for writing the final report of the research.

Reading Research for Evidence-Based Practice

The research report should provide a clear description of each step that was taken in the design and implementation of the research study. This description is often summarized in the abstract of the article under the heading "Methods." The methods section is relatively

Table 6.5 Some Comparative Effectiveness Designs

Design	Description	Example of a Research Question	Strengths	Limitations
Observational design	Population of interest is assigned to alternative interventions based on patient, provider, and system factors and observed for the outcome of interest	Does the effectiveness of treatment for postnatal depression vary by region of the country?	Incremental cost of adding subjects is low, so samples are usually large Easier to implement; a natural variation of care Naturalistic; not highly artificial, so easier to generalize	Low control of confounders Feasible only if the intervention is already being used Subject to selection bias and measurement error
Adaptive design	Patients are assigned to a treatment randomly, but accumulating evidence from the trials is used to modify the trial to increase efficiency and the probability that subjects will benefit from participation	Can postnatal depression that is partially treated with medication be improved by adding therapeutic counseling?	Can test whether sequential treatments will work Lessons learned can be incorporated into the trial Patients for whom initial treatments do not work may benefit from later treatments	More difficult to isolate the effects of a single intervention Subject to treatment effects
Pragmatic trials	Relaxes some of the traditional rules of randomized trials to maximize the relevance of the results (e.g., inclusion criteria may be broadened, flexibility in application of the intervention)	Does therapeutic counseling improve postnatal depression in those women who have physical comorbid conditions?	Easier to recruit and enroll subjects More naturalistic design so easier to generalize Lessons learned during the trial can be incorporated into future tests	Low control of selection error

standard. A good quantitative methods section, for example, will review the sampling strategy, design of the study, instruments, procedures, and analysis. A qualitative methods section should describe the sampling criteria, identify the method for gathering information, and provide an overview of data coding procedures. Although the length limitations imposed by journals may restrict the depth of detail an author can provide, the nurse reader should be able to find enough key elements to assess the validity or trustworthiness of the study.

Validity of the research is primarily a quantitative concern; a valid study is one in which enough control has been exerted so the effect of the concepts under study can be isolated from other effects. In contrast, trustworthiness of the research is the primary concern in qualitative studies; a trustworthy study is one in which the researcher has drawn the correct conclusions about the meaning of an event or phenomenon. Achieving validity and trustworthiness is not a minor task, but meeting each criterion is essential for the respective application of the evidence to practice. Judging the validity or trustworthiness of the data is primarily based on how well the study design accomplished the purpose of the study and how thoroughly the design allowed for the answer to the research question.

The nurse can follow several steps when evaluating the study design to determine the quality of the research report:

1. The methods section should be complete. It should present an accurate and thorough account of every important step in the design and conduct of the research. This thorough account allows the reader to make decisions about accepting the results of the study. Providing sufficient detail about the methods used in the study enables readers to decide for themselves how much confidence they have that the experimental treatment did, indeed, lead to the results.

2. A strong methods section supports replication—one of the hallmarks of sound research that makes a valuable contribution to the overall professional body of knowledge. In practical terms, the nurse should be able to get enough information from the description of the methods to conduct the study exactly as the author did, using different subjects, to determine whether the results can be generalized to another population.

3. A thorough methods section allows comparison of findings across studies. This is critical for the systematic review process, which is a key way that studies are transformed into evidence-based practice. A thorough account of the subjects, intervention, measurement, and analysis allows for a comparison across studies to draw conclusions about both the size of the treatment effect and the consistency with which outcomes are achieved (Fain, 2013).

The design section of a research study serves as the basis for the conclusions drawn about the validity and trustworthiness of the findings. A critical appraisal of study methods should lead the nurse to the conclusion that inconsistency in procedures is not an explanation for the results. In other words, can all other rival explanations for the outcome be eliminated, except that of the intervention? If the methods section is sound, the answer to this question should be an unequivocal "yes," giving the nurse confidence to apply the findings to practice.

WHERE TO LOOK

Where to look for information about the methods and procedures:

- The design of the study is usually described in the abstract of the study and again in the introduction. It should be identified in a straightforward way and clearly described. If not, it should be described early in the section labeled "Methods."
- The design section may be called "Research Design" or "Plan." Other words may appear in the heading, such as "Methods and Procedures" or "Methods and Materials."

- The description of the design should be easily identifiable and a major part of the research study write-up. The description may be concise, but it should provide enough detail that an informed reader could replicate the study.
- If the intervention or measurement is complex, the write-up may include a separate section for procedures, which may be labeled as such or called "Protocols." This section may describe the specific steps for applying the treatment, the specific steps for measuring its effects, or both.

CHECKLIST FOR EVALUATING THE DESIGN OF A RESEARCH ARTICLE

- ❑ The design is clearly identified and described using standard language.
- ❑ A rationale is provided, or can be easily inferred, for the choice of a design.
- ❑ The characteristics of the design can be clearly linked to the nature of the research question.

- ❑ The variables are explicitly identified and definitions are written for each.
- ❑ Enough detail is provided that an informed reader could replicate the study.
- ❑ If the study is qualitative in nature, the researcher has documented the basis for decisions as the design emerged.

Using Research in Evidence-Based Practice

All types of research designs are useful in application to practice. Although the hierarchy of evidence puts more weight on the results of experimental designs, all types of knowledge can, in fact, contribute to the effective practice of nursing. The task of the nurse is to choose the type of knowledge—and, therefore, the range of designs—that produces the kind of information needed to solve a clinical problem.

Descriptive research is useful when determining the characteristics of specific populations, identifying the practices that are used at other organizations, or measuring baseline performance. This type of research is helpful when little is known about the existing state of a phenomenon or when exploring perceptions, attitudes, or beliefs. Descriptive research focuses on what is, so it is not used for quantifying the effectiveness of interventions; nevertheless, it can provide valuable information about the status quo. This baseline information is often necessary to establish the overall desirability of a change in practice.

When the focus of the nurse is on improving a clinical intervention, then quantitative research is more valuable. Quantitative research enables the nurse to determine whether an intervention has produced a desired effect and to estimate the probability that it will continue to do so, even with different populations. If the nurse needs to change a procedure, standardize practices, measure relationships, or determine cause and effect, then quantitative studies are the most useful.

Often, the nurse also needs to determine the acceptability of a nursing intervention. If the goal is to provide emotional or social support for patients and their families, for example, then qualitative research is more likely to produce the evidence needed for practice. When design of an appropriate intervention requires that the nurse understand the meaning of a life event for a patient, then qualitative studies are more likely to provide the insight that is needed to design acceptable treatments.

The nurse should evaluate the soundness of the design for answering the specific research question to determine whether it can be applied to nursing practice. This includes an appraisal of the match between the purpose of the study and the kind of knowledge generated for it, the links between the nature of the research question and the explicit design chosen to answer it, and the appropriateness of the specific procedures put in place to carry out the study.

Creating Evidence for Practice

Creating an effective research plan involves a systematic process of considering the purpose of the study and the nature of the question and then making decisions about the way the study will be carried out to draw the correct conclusions. These designs are rarely clear cut; almost always the investigator is charged with weighing the relative strengths and weaknesses of various design elements to arrive at the best possible decision given the specific characteristics of the study at hand. That said, the researcher is well served by spending the time to consider and create a careful research plan, because it will serve as a blueprint for the study as well as its documentation.

SKILL BUILDER   Design a Stronger Study

Although the hierarchy of evidence-based practice identifies randomized controlled trials as the strongest designs, such studies are not always possible or even desirable. Although experimental designs do often yield strong evidence for nursing practice, it is difficult to conduct a pure experimental design. There may not be enough subjects to ensure that the study will attain sufficient power, and those subjects who are available may not consent to participate in the study. Extraneous variables abound, and it is often unethical to withhold treatment from a control group. Once the study has begun, it is difficult to ensure that the experimental group always gets the exact same treatment, particularly in an applied setting. Time constraints and availability

of individuals to collect data can hinder the validity of the experiment.

Although it may be challenging to conduct a true experiment in a nursing practice environment, there are still some measures that can be undertaken to strengthen the validity of a study:

1. Use a comparison group of some kind. Although it may be difficult to randomly assign patients to groups, the use of a comparison group does strengthen validity, even if it comes from a convenience sample.

2. If using a nonrandom comparison group, match the groups as closely as possible on potential extraneous variables (e.g., age, severity of illness, and number of comorbid conditions).

3. Measure a baseline in a group of subjects, which becomes the comparison group, and then repeat the measure as the treatment is applied. This design, called a repeated measure design, has a great deal of power.

4. If the sample is less than desirable, use a strong and valid measurement system. Sampling error can be balanced somewhat by a reduction in measurement error.

5. Clearly identify the variables of interest and write formal operational definitions of each. These definitions can help determine the criteria for inclusion in the study, treatment protocols, and measurement systems. For a qualitative study, explicitly identify the concepts that are of interest to the researcher.

6. Replicate the studies of others whenever possible. Finding a similar study can help jump-start your own study by describing procedures and measures that you might be able to use. The original author will likely be flattered; contact with him or her may garner you free advice as well.

7. Use standard designs, methods, and procedures whenever possible, even if they do not exactly match your question. Standardized approaches allow for the aggregation of similar studies into practical guidelines that make a contribution to the overall body of nursing knowledge.

The researcher needs to determine the answers to the following questions:

- What is the nature of the knowledge that will be required to address this research problem? Quantitative studies are needed to test interventions; qualitative studies are needed to discover the meaning of phenomena.
- Which concepts are involved in answering this question? Describing the variables that will be studied, or the phenomena of interest, guides the measurement strategy.
- What is the nature of the research question? A descriptive design is required for research questions that ask about what is or that are exploratory. If the question focuses on the nature of relationships, then correlation studies are needed. Questions related to causality or the effectiveness of interventions demand experimental designs. The specifics of the design will depend on the accessibility of the population, the skills and resources of the researcher, and the expectations of the ultimate audience for the research.
- Which specific procedures will be required to answer the question? Once a design is selected, the researcher must determine how the subjects or informants will be recruited, how the concepts will be measured, and how data will be analyzed.

Summary of Key Concepts

- A design is a plan that outlines the overall approach to a study, while being grounded in a set of beliefs about knowledge and inextricably linked to the nature of the research question.
- The research design focuses on answering the research question with the greatest level of credibility.
- Selection of a design is based on the purpose to be achieved by the study, the availability of subjects, ethical limitations, the skills and resources of the researcher, the time frame, the amount of control required, and the expectations of the audience for the research.

- The phases of the research process include identifying assumptions about the knowledge needed, selecting an overall approach that serves the purpose, specifying an explicit design for the study, and developing detailed plans for implementation.
- Assumptions about the knowledge needed to answer the research question will result in the choice of a quantitative, qualitative, or mixed methods approach.
- The overall approach of the study is determined by considering whether a study is exploratory (generating new knowledge) or confirmatory (testing theories or hypotheses).
- The concepts reflected in the research question are translated into measurable variables for a quantitative study; these variables may be descriptive, independent, dependent, or extraneous. The concepts in qualitative questions describe characteristics, experiences, or phenomena that are of interest to the researcher.
- Once these decisions have been made, the research design is translated into a specific plan of study—one that can be used to guide and replicate the study.
- Detailed plans for research implementation form a road map for the research and include specification of procedures for sampling, measurement, and analysis.
- The four major classifications of research designs are those that seek to describe a phenomenon or population, those that seek to quantify the nature of relationships, those that seek to investigate causality, and those that compare the effectiveness of interventions for application to practice.
- Three conditions must be met to establish causality: The cause must precede the effect; the probability that the cause influenced the effect must be established; and rival explanations for the effect must be ruled out.

For More Depth and Detail

For a more in-depth look at the concepts in this chapter, try these references:

Brouwers, M., Thabane, L., Moher, D., & Straus, S. (2012). Comparative effectiveness research paradigm: Implications for systematic reviews and clinical practice guidelines. *Journal of Clinical Oncology, 30*(34), 4202–4207.

Cantrell, M. (2011). Demystifying the research process: Understanding a descriptive comparative research design. *Pediatric Nursing, 37*(4), 188–189.

Higgins, J., Altman, D., Gotzsche, P., Juni, P., Oxman, D., Savovic, A., . . . Sterne, J. (2011). The Cochrane Collaboration's tool for assessing risk of bias in randomized trials. *British Medical Journal, 343*(7829), 1–9.

Levin, G., Emerson, S., & Emerson, S. (2013). Adaptive clinical trial designs with pre-specified rules for modifying the sample size: Understanding efficient types of adaptation. *Statistics in Medicine, 32*(8), 1259–1275.

Liodden, I., & Moen, A. (2012). Knowledge development in nursing: Pragmatic, randomized controlled trials as a methodological approach to support evidence-based practice. *Nordic Nursing Research, 2*(3), 233–246.

Ruggeri, M., Lasalvia, A., & Bonetto, C. (2013). A new generation of pragmatic trials of psychosocial interventions is needed. *Epidemiology and Psychiatric Sciences, 20*, 1–7.

CRITICAL APPRAISAL EXERCISE

Retrieve the following full text article from the Cumulative Index to Nursing and Allied Health Literature or similar search database:

Koli, R., Kohler, K., Tonteri, E., Peltonen, J., Tikkanen, H., & Fogelholm, M. (2015). Dark chocolate and reduced snack consumption in mildly hypertensive adults: An intervention study. *Nutrition Journal, 14*(84), 1–9.

Review the article, looking for information about the research design. Consider the following appraisal questions in your critical review of this element of the research article:

1. What is the specific design chosen for this research? Why is it the most appropriate design for this question?
2. Is the design clearly discernible early in the article? Is it described in such a way that the reader could replicate it?
3. Are the primary variables clearly identified and defined (independent and dependent)?
4. Why did the researchers ask subjects to reduce snack consumption during the study period?
5. Which extraneous effects did the cross-over aspect of this study control? Which others might be present and uncontrolled?
6. What are the strengths of this design for answering the research question? How could the nurse apply these findings in practice?

References

Armstrong, K. (2012). Methods in comparative effectiveness research. *Journal of Clinical Oncology, 30*(34), 4208–4214.

Cooper, K. (2012). *Qualitative research in the post modern era: Contexts of qualitative research.* Dordrecht, Netherlands: Spring Science.

Delost, M., & Nadder, T. (2014). Guidelines for initiating a research agenda: Research design and dissemination of results. *Clinical Laboratory Science, 27*(4), 237–244.

Denzin, N., & Lincoln, Y. (2011). *The Sage handbook of qualitative research.* Thousand Oaks, CA: Sage.

Fain, E. (2013). *Reading, understanding, and applying nursing research* (4th ed.). Philadelphia, PA: F. A. Davis.

Hartung, D., & Touchette, D. (2009). Overview of clinical research design. *American Journal of Health System Pharmacy, 66*(15), 398–408.

Khudyahov, P., Gorfine, M., Zucker, D., & Spiegelman, D. (2015). The impact of covariate measurement error on risk prediction. *Statistics in Medicine, 34*(15), 2353–2367.

McCusker, K., & Gunaydin, S. (2015). Research using qualitative, quantitative or mixed methods and choice based on the research. *Perfusion, 30*(7), 537–542.

Nieswiadomy, R. (2012). *Foundations of nursing research* (6th ed.). Boston, MA: Pearson.

Terrell, S. (2012). Mixed-methods research methodologies. *Qualitative Report, 17*(1), 254–280.

Wallace, J., & Clarke, C. (2012). Making evidence more wanted: A systematic review of facilitators to enhance the uptake of evidence from systematic reviews and meta-analysis. *International Journal of Evidence Based Healthcare, 10*(4), 338–346.

Wener, P., & Woodgate, R. (2013). Use of a qualitative methodological scaffolding process to design robust interprofessional studies. *Journal of Interprofessional Care, 27*(4), 305–312.

Part III

Research Process

Fotima Kazimova/Shutterstock

Chapter 7

The Sampling Strategy

CHAPTER OBJECTIVES

The study of this chapter will help the learner to

- Define a population and discuss the rationale for sampling.
- Contrast probability sampling with nonprobability sampling.
- Discuss sampling options and select an appropriate strategy.
- Describe methods for estimating necessary sample size.
- Discuss methods for avoiding selection bias.
- Appraise how the sampling method affects research as evidence.

KEY TERMS

Convenience sampling	Population	Sampling error
Ecological validity	Population validity	Sampling frame
Effect size	Power	Selection bias
Exclusion criteria	Probability or random sampling	Snowball sampling (referral sampling, respondent-driven sampling)
External validity	Purposeful selection	
Inclusion criteria	Random selection	Unit of analysis
Independence	Sample	

Introduction

No aspect of the research plan is more critical for ensuring the usefulness of a study than the sampling strategy. It determines whether the results of the study can be applied as evidence and contributes to the trustworthiness of the results. Good sampling is critical for the confident application of the study findings to other people, settings, or time periods.

Disasters produce stressors for everyone, but for women who are pregnant or who have a new baby, a disaster offers another layer of difficulty in staying healthy. We experienced Hurricane Katrina in 2005. We believed that pregnant and postpartum women had unique needs in postdisaster settings, and we wanted to measure those stressors so we could design services to help these patients. We quickly realized, however, that traditional sampling methods to find such subjects were not effective. In any case, finding pregnant or postpartum women is especially challenging because fewer than 5% of women are pregnant or postpartum at any time. In postdisaster periods, typical community surveys may not find any of them.

We began to look for ways to increase the number of pregnant or postpartum women whom we could include in our assessment of unmet needs after a disaster. We partnered with the University of North Carolina at Chapel Hill's Gillings School of Global Public Health to pilot test a new cluster sampling method that involved asking the people who responded to our survey to refer us to pregnant or postpartum neighbors. In the first stage, we randomly selected 10 census blocks proportionate to the population. In the second stage, we used geographical information systems (GIS) software to select 7 random households. Sampled households were asked, as part of the interview, to refer all pregnant or postpartum women they knew who lived close to them. Theoretically, the selection of individuals discovered in this way remains a random representation, even though it is technically a snowball sample.

We tried our system in three pilot tests: after flooding in Georgia and after hurricane-related flooding and tornadoes in North Carolina. In each of the three pilots, we were able to increase the proportion of our sample by twofold and even by fourfold. When we used the method again after Hurricane Irene, we were able to demonstrate that pregnant and postpartum women living in homes that had been damaged by the disaster reported significantly more stressors than their peers who lived in homes that were not damaged. We demonstrated that this process could be used to document unmet needs and subsequently target disaster recovery assistance to the women and children at greatest risk. Furthermore, we identified several factors that could be considered to improve efficiency, including using local official disaster information and census data to localize the assessment. We were able to begin thinking about services that could help these women cope better in the aftermath of a disaster.

We felt comfortable that the sampling methods were effective, but we also realized that there were challenges with their use. We had to dedicate substantial resources and staff time to the sampling process—both of which may be in short supply following a major disaster. We developed an online toolkit to help others use this method.

This sampling approach is novel and takes a lot of work, but it can help public health practitioners use a population-based sampling method when trying to reach a small, specific subgroup of the general population after a disaster. Our goal was to maximize generalizability by ensuring that our study included a representative sample, and it seems this method worked. This is the biggest benefit of this approach.

Jennifer A. Horney, PhD, MPH
Marianne Zotti, DrPH, MS

Population:
The entire set of subjects that are of interest to the researcher.

Samples are drawn to represent populations in a research study. A **population**, sometimes called the target population, is the entire set of subjects who are of interest to the researcher. It is rarely possible, or even necessary, to study the entire population of interest. Rather, it is more likely that the researcher will study a subset of the population, called a **sample**. Samples, if selected carefully, can effectively represent the broader population. Because samples are more efficient and economical to study, their use enables researchers to study phenomena when reaching the entire population would be impossible.

Sampling has a downside, however. Measures acquired from a sample cannot be as precise and accurate as those drawn from the entire population; that is, the results from a sample will never match the population perfectly. Researchers use statistics to measure and account for this difference, resulting in a value called **sampling error**. Sampling error is a critical consideration in statistical testing; sometimes referred to as "chance" or "standard error," it is the criterion used to determine whether statistical results reflect real effects. It is critical, then, to use a selection strategy that minimizes sampling error by maximizing the chance that the sample will represent the population.

The sampling plan is important whether the research is qualitative or quantitative; the plan serves different purposes, however, based on the type of research. In qualitative research, the sampling plan is central to establishing credibility. The individuals who participate in such a study are referred to as informants or respondents and are chosen specifically for their capacity to inform the research question. In a quantitative study, the sampling strategy aims to maximize the potential for generalization or the ability to apply the findings to larger groups. The individuals who participate are referred to as subjects and are chosen using methods that ensure the sample represents the overall population. Therefore, the way samples are recruited and selected will determine our overall confidence in the results.

The sampling strategy is the primary way that researchers control selection bias. **Selection bias** occurs when subjects are selected for the study or assigned to groups in a way that is not impartial. When subjects are assigned to treatment groups using a random method, selection bias is reduced. Selection bias poses a threat to the validity of a study and is controlled almost exclusively by a sound sampling strategy.

No less critical is the sample's capacity to detect the effects of the intervention. Having an adequate number of subjects provides the study with power, or the ability to detect effects. Power increases confidence in the results of the study and depends on an adequate sample size. The researcher controls a study's power by ensuring that an adequate number of subjects are represented in the sample.

These aspects of research design—the method for selecting subjects and assigning them to groups and the number of subjects studied—are the most important considerations in the sampling strategy. Nevertheless, the sampling strategy often is given little attention in a research study and may be the weakest aspect of otherwise well-designed projects. A recent systematic review of the sample size adequacy of nearly 900 health education research studies revealed that only two of the studies were of an adequate size to detect a small effect. Between 22% and 27% of the reviewed studies could detect a large effect (Cook & Hatala, 2015). The authors concluded that most health education research studies can detect only large effects, suggesting there should be a lack of confidence in those studies that find no differences at all.

Shortcomings in the sampling approach may not be a reflection of the skill of the researchers. Even when effort is spent to design an effective sampling strategy, conditions

Sample:
A carefully selected subset of the population that reflects the composition of that population.

Sampling error:
A number that indicates differences in results found in the sample when compared to the population from which the sample was drawn.

Selection bias:
Selecting subjects or assigning them to groups in a way that is not impartial. This type of bias may pose a threat to the validity of the study.

Sampling frame:
The potential participants who meet the definition of the population and are accessible to the researcher.

beyond the researcher's control may limit the capacity to apply the sampling strategy as planned. In one study of a nursing intervention in a population of HIV-positive persons, 639 clients were eligible for the study. Despite multiple attempts to recruit subjects, only 43 agreed to participate; of those, only 16 finished the study (Nokes & Nwakeze, 2007). The authors noted the multiple challenges of obtaining adequate samples from this highly marginalized population and concluded that less rigorous sampling strategies may be the only recourse for studying such persons' care. New ideas about sampling—such as service- or respondent-driven sampling for hard-to-recruit populations—are also being tested and bring a fresh perspective to the interpretation of "generalizable sampling."

When reading published research, the sampling strategy is assessed to determine the level of confidence that the results are accurate and potentially valuable to practice. A sampling strategy that is not representative limits the ability to apply the research results in nursing practice. Creating an adequate sampling strategy requires that the nurse researcher maximize the representativeness and size of the sample. This endeavor frequently requires creativity and persistence, but is critical to ensure that the results can be confidently applied to nursing practice.

GRAY MATTER

Selection bias may occur under the following conditions:
- The accessible sample is not an accurate representation of the population.
- The researcher is able to influence selection or assignment of subjects.
- Inclusion or exclusion criteria systematically leave out a key group.
- The ease of recruitment for various subpopulations skews subject characteristics.
- The subjects elect not to participate or drop out of the study.

Selection Strategy: How Were the Subjects Chosen?

The first step of a sampling strategy is to clearly define the population of interest. Often, this definition begins to emerge during development of the research question. The final definition should be clear, unambiguous, and detailed enough to avoid misinterpretation. Populations are frequently defined in terms of age (e.g., adults, children, and neonates), diagnosis, setting, or geographic location. The available population is called the **sampling frame**; it comprises the potential participants who meet the definition of the population and are accessible to the researcher. Here, the term "accessible" does not necessarily mean physically accessible; for example, the sampling frame for the population of critical care nurses in acute care might be the membership roster for the American Association of Critical-Care Nurses.

Once the population is clearly defined, a selection strategy is designed to choose the actual subjects from the sampling frame. The selection strategy involves making decisions about how subjects will be recruited, selected, and, if appropriate, assigned to groups.

The goal of the selection strategy is to prevent bias, support the validity of the study, and enhance the credibility of the results.

All samples may be threatened by selection bias, meaning the sample is not an accurate representation of the population. This divergence may occur for many reasons—some related to design of the study, but others related to its execution. Selection bias can occur when a researcher can influence the selection of the subjects for the study or the assignment of subjects to groups, perhaps resulting in a sample that is biased toward success of the experiment. For example, a researcher may select an intervention group consisting of individuals who are healthy and, therefore, more likely to improve, and select a control group of sicker patients who are unlikely to experience improvement. This bias may be conscious, but it is more commonly unconscious. The potential for selection bias is of particular concern when the researcher has preconceived ideas about how the study will turn out.

Inadequate sampling can also lead to sampling bias. A biased sample under-represents or over-represents some characteristic in the sample. Unfortunately, the samples that are the easiest to recruit may introduce sampling bias into a study. Convenience samples, in particular, run the risk of over-representing characteristics that are local to the study. For example, subjects who are recruited primarily from a tertiary care center may inherently include more seriously ill patients. Conversely, recruiting from outpatient settings may under-represent the severity of a condition. Sampling bias increases sampling error as well as the chance the researcher will draw misleading conclusions.

Even when the researcher has developed a rigorous sampling plan, certain segments of the population may refuse to participate or be unable to participate in the proposed study. Sampling bias may be present when a group is too homogeneous, such that it does not reflect the diversity in the broader population. A homogeneous sample is one in which the subjects are very similar in terms of their characteristics, and it makes generalizing the study results to other populations difficult. Historically, samples for medical research have been heavily weighted toward white males. In the past decade, researchers have become more sensitive to the need to include a broader scope of ethnic and gender groups in research, but gaps in this area still exist.

Another kind of selection bias occurs when subjects elect not to participate in a study. Systematic sampling error can occur when response rates are low or attrition is high. Many reasons explain why subjects might decline to participate in a study or drop out once it has started. A certain amount of refusal or nonresponse is to be expected in any study. However, the researcher should describe the reasons for refusal or attrition to ensure that systematic sampling error is not exhibited. For example, if all the individuals who refuse to participate are from a particular ethnic group, socioeconomic status, or educational level, then the final sample will not represent the entire population.

The Sample Selection Strategy

A sound selection strategy is one of the best ways to control bias in an experiment. Several aspects of this strategy may enhance validity and control bias. The use of objective selection criteria and sound recruitment methods is appropriate for all

Inclusion criteria:
Guidelines for choosing subjects with a set of characteristics that include major factors important to the research question.

Exclusion criteria:
Characteristics that eliminate a potential subject from the study to avoid extraneous effects.

Purposeful selection:
A technique used in qualitative research in which the subjects are selected because they possess certain characteristics that enhance the credibility of the study.

types of research. These should be some of the earliest decisions made about the study, because objective selection criteria help minimize bias in both qualitative and quantitative studies.

The sampling strategy for a qualitative study has a different goal than that for quantitative research; in turn, the sampling procedures for these two types of studies can be quite different. In the case of qualitative research, the goal is credibility rather than generalizability, so selection methods are purposeful in nature. This approach makes the sampling strategy less complicated for qualitative studies, but no less thoughtful. Careful attention to selection criteria can help minimize the effects of both researcher bias and selection bias in a qualitative study (Polit & Beck, 2014).

For quantitative studies, the use of probability in sample selection or group assignment reduces bias and enhances the representativeness of the results (Carman, Clark, Wolf, & Moon, 2015). In addition, subjects are recruited and selected for the study based on criteria that are carefully considered to represent the population under study while minimizing the effects of extraneous variables. The criteria are applied objectively, and all subjects who meet the criteria are generally invited to participate.

Objective selection criteria may consist of inclusion criteria, exclusion criteria, or both. **Inclusion criteria** provide guidelines for choosing subjects who match a predetermined set of characteristics. These criteria define the major factors that are important to the research question and may include clinical, demographic, geographic, and temporal criteria as appropriate. The primary function of inclusion criteria is to limit the potential for selection bias by objectively identifying who can be considered a subject.

Many authors also include **exclusion criteria**, meaning characteristics that are used to exclude a potential subject from the study. Some individuals are not suitable for the study, even though they may meet the inclusion criteria. These subjects might meet clinical exclusion criteria (e.g., comorbid conditions that might affect the study) or behavioral exclusion criteria (e.g., high likelihood of being lost to follow-up). Exclusion criteria fulfill the same function as inclusion criteria and help to control extraneous variables.

Sampling in Qualitative Studies

Although objective criteria for recruitment and selection strengthen the credibility of a qualitative study, informants in this type of research are selected from the potential pool of subjects in a way that is controlled and executed by the researcher. This **purposeful selection** has as its aim the selection of those subjects most likely to inform the research question. Criteria for selection of informants for a qualitative study often look quite different than criteria for selection of informants for a quantitative study. Qualitative selection criteria may include requirements that an individual has experienced a phenomenon, possesses a particular attribute, or even expresses a willingness to talk openly about sensitive issues. Qualitative selection criteria are formulated through a thoughtful reflection on the type of individual who is most likely to inform the research question. The researcher then seeks out these individuals and invites them to participate in the study. **FIGURE 7.1** depicts the general progress of a sampling strategy.

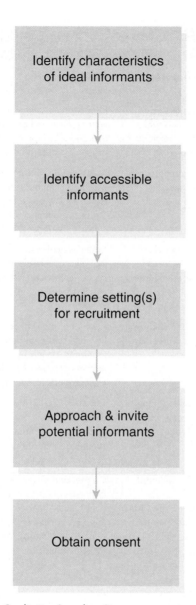

FIGURE 7.1 Stages of the Qualitative Sampling Strategy

A purposeful sample is in some ways easier to procure than a probabilistic one, but that does not imply the process is not systematic. A variety of techniques can be employed to achieve a purposeful sample, and each is appropriate under specific conditions to meet research objectives. Examples of strategies for purposeful selection appear in **Table 7.1**. Snowball sampling, also known as referral or respondent-driven sampling, violates many principles of quantitative research but is commonly used to generate qualitative samples. This type of networked sample, in which early respondents are asked to recruit subsequent subjects, is particularly appropriate when studying social structures and interpersonal relationships (Bhutta, 2012).

Table 7.1 Methods for Purposeful Selection

Strategy	Appropriate Use	Example
Typical case sampling	Used when the study requires subjects who have some characteristic in common	Pooe-Monyemore et al. (2012) selected Africans with an inherited disorder resulting in a lack of eye and skin pigment to determine their unique psychosocial and healthcare needs.
Homogeneous sampling	Used when concern arises that special or outlier cases may skew responses	Ko et al. (2014) recruited 15 participants who had schizophrenia but were not currently experiencing acute psychosis to determine how people with this chronic disease live with their illness experiences.
Criterion sampling	Used when the study requires subjects who have an experience in common	Matthew-Maich et al. (2013) studied strategies that clinical managers used to successfully implement evidence-based practices by recruiting health professionals who met four prespecified criteria.
Maximum variation sampling	Used when the study will benefit from a diversity of characteristics	Kurth et al. (2014) examined the practices of both first-time and experienced mothers in response to infants' crying by observing and interviewing mothers of diverse parity and educational backgrounds.
Extreme case sampling	Used to obtain a sample that has extreme target population characteristics	Tan et al. (2012) studied the bereavement needs of parents following the death of a child by finding a sample with variation in race, socioeconomic status, prenatal diagnosis, and number of gestations.
Theoretical sampling	Used when additional sources of data are needed during grounded theory development	Cognet and Coyer (2014) studied the practices of nurses discharging patients from the intensive care unit by interviewing focus groups, analyzing the data concurrently, and proposing a model of actions and interactions to explain problems with the procedure.

The researcher has an obligation to design a sound sampling strategy that will meet the goals of the research regardless of the nature of the research.

Sampling in Quantitative Studies

Quantitative samples have the best generalizability when subjects are selected and assigned to groups randomly. The resulting samples are often referred to as probability samples. In quantitative studies, the development and use of inclusion and exclusion criteria are only the first steps in a highly controlled, objective selection strategy. The goal of quantitative studies is excellent representation of the population, and the use of probability in sample selection or group assignment helps the researcher achieve this goal

(LoBiondo-Wood & Haber, 2014). **Probability sampling** (also called **random sampling**) refers to a sampling process in which every member of the available population has an equal probability of being selected for the sample. **FIGURE 7.2** depicts the general steps of the quantitative sampling strategy.

The only way to be sure a sample represents a population is to confirm that it meets two essential criteria: Each member of the population has an equal probability of selection for the sample, and each subject selection is an independent event. A random sample is one in which mathematical probability is used to ensure that selection of subjects is completely objective—a method called **random selection**. **Independence** is ensured when the

Probability or random sampling:
A sampling process used in quantitative research in which every member of the available population has an equal chance of being selected for the sample.

Random selection:
A method of choosing a random sample using mathematical probability to ensure the selection of subjects is completely objective.

Independence:
A condition that occurs when the selection of one subject has no influence on selection of other subjects; each member of the population has exactly the same chance of being in the sample.

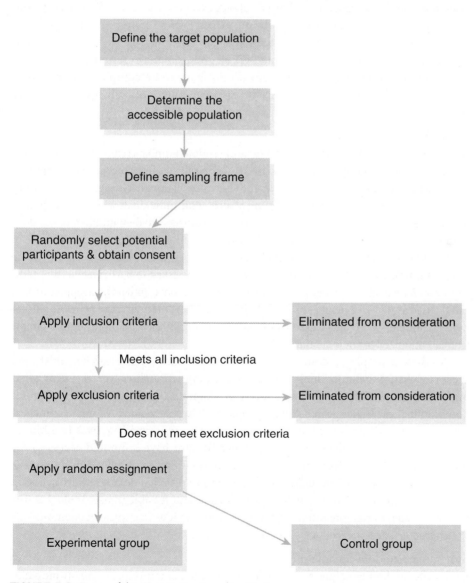

FIGURE 7.2 Stages of the Quantitative Sampling Strategy

selection of one subject has no effect on the selection of other subjects. In other words, each member of the population has exactly the same chance of being in the sample, and the selection of one subject has no influence on the selection of another. For example, if a subject were asked to recruit his or her friends and family members for the study, the assumption of independence has been violated. Randomness and independence are central to ensuring that a sample is representative of the population, and both are also underlying assumptions of most inferential statistical tests.

The strongest evidence is produced by quantitative studies conducted with samples that are either randomly selected or randomly assigned to experimental groups. In some cases, however, a researcher might have no choice except to ask accessible subjects to join the study—a practice that potentially introduces bias. Even so, if the researcher randomly assigns the subjects to experimental groups, then any differences between the sample and the population will be evenly spread out over all groups in the experiment.

Random sampling and assignment do not have to be complicated processes. Several types of random samples meet the essential criteria of both equal probability and independence.

Simple Random Sampling

Simple random sampling is used when a table of random numbers (either from a textbook or generated by a computer program) is used to select subjects from the sampling frame. As noted earlier, the sampling frame includes the entire population that is eligible for the study. The researcher must have access to a listing of all eligible individuals who both are part of the population and meet the selection criteria. The subjects are then numbered. Random numbers are drawn, and the subjects with the drawn numbers are asked to participate in the study. For example, if the drawn set of random numbers is "21, 11, 143, 86, . . .," then the 21st, 11th, 143rd, and 86th subjects on the list would be asked to participate in the study. Common statistical texts generally include a table of random numbers as an appendix that can be used as part of a manual process. Most spreadsheet programs can generate a list of random numbers, and statistical software can automatically select a simple random sample from an imported list of potential subjects.

To draw a simple random sample from a population, the researcher must have access to a list of the individuals who are in the population; however, access to a listing of the entire sampling frame is rarely available to the researcher. For example, how would a researcher get a list of all people with hypertension? All nurse managers who work in critical care units? All adolescents who are sexually active? In addition to these logistical problems, most researchers do not have unlimited access to the population. If nothing else, most studies are limited by geography or availability of resources. In these cases, other kinds of random samples that do not require access to a list of the sampling frame may be more efficient and feasible to use. Table 7.2 lists the major types of random sampling methods and provides examples that demonstrate the characteristics of each.

Systematic Random Sampling

Systematic random sampling is useful when the researcher is unsure how many individuals will eventually be in the population or when there is an indefinite sampling frame.

Table 7.2 Types of Random Samples and Examples

Type of Random Sample	Example
Simple random sample	The researcher wants to survey 40% of the nurses regarding their perceptions of the work environment. A list of all nurses who work on the patient care units is generated by the human resources department. This list is numbered. Random numbers are generated by computer, and the nurses with those numbers by their names on the list are invited to participate in the study.
Systematic random sample	The researcher is studying the relationship between time spent in an examining room and patient satisfaction, and wants a 10% random sample of patients who will present in the next 6 months. The nurse selects the number 5 from a table of random numbers. The 5th patient to present to the clinic is invited to participate. Every 10th patient who presents is invited to participate until the 6-month period has ended.
Stratified random sample	The researcher is studying the relationship between educational level and the identification of early symptoms of myocardial infarction. The researcher wants to ensure that neither gender is over-represented. A list of individuals who have presented to the emergency department with symptoms of myocardial infarction is generated by the health information management department. This list is divided by gender. A 20% random sample is selected from each list so that gender is represented equally in the sample.
Cluster random sample	The researcher is studying the baseline knowledge of school nurses relative to managing childhood diabetes. A list of all school districts in the state is generated, and the districts are numbered. Random numbers are generated, and the associated school districts are identified. All school nurses in the selected school districts are invited to participate in the study.

It is also a practical way to draw a sample from a prospective group—that is, a group that will be created in the future. In systematic random sampling, the first subject is drawn randomly, and remaining subjects are selected at predetermined intervals. For example, if a researcher needed a 10% random sample from the visitors to the emergency department over 12 months, the researcher might select the random number 6 from a table of random numbers. In this case, once the study began, the researcher would invite the 6th visitor (based on the initial random number, 6) to the emergency department and every 10th visitor (based on the random sample percentage, 10%) after that. Systematic random sampling does not produce a strict probability sample, but for all practical purposes it is usually just as good a method. It has the advantage that it is a relatively uncomplicated way to draw a representative sample.

Stratified Random Sampling

Stratified random samples are structured so that important characteristics are evenly distributed across all groups. Such sampling is a good way to reduce the probability that a subgroup will be under-represented or over-represented in some way. Stratification based on some important characteristic helps ensure that all subgroups are represented in proportion to their prevalence in the defined population. Stratified random samples are more difficult to accomplish than simple or systematic random samples, and their creation involves two steps. First, the researcher divides the population into groups based on some characteristic (e.g., gender, ethnicity, and diagnosis); then, the researcher picks a representative sample from each group. Often, a proportion from each subgroup is predetermined and is used to control a potential extraneous variable. For example, in a study of community-acquired pneumonia, the researcher might want to ensure that nonsmokers and smokers are represented in the sample in the same proportion as they appear in the general population. If the population had a 17% smoking rate, then the researcher would first identify the smokers and nonsmokers in the sampling frame, and then randomly select subjects from each group so that the sample had 83% nonsmokers and 17% smokers.

Cluster Random Sampling

Sometimes it is impossible to draw single subjects from groups, because of either geographic limitations or accessibility issues. In cluster sampling, the researcher randomly selects entire groups and then randomly selects subjects from only those groups. For example, an organizational researcher might want to study the effect of care delivery models on patient satisfaction within Magnet facilities. Instead of randomly selecting subjects from all patient care units in all Magnet facilities, the researcher would first randomly select Magnet facilities and then solicit participation from all the units in those facilities. Cluster random sampling is useful when subjects naturally fall into groups (e.g., schools, hospitals, and counties) and can be more economical in terms of time and money than other types of probability samples (LoBiondo-Wood & Haber, 2014).

Ensuring Independence

Independence, the second criterion for a probability sample, is a statistical concern rather than a representation issue. Independence is violated if subjects are related in some way or if more than one score is collected from the same subject. It would be expected that subjects who are not independent would share some characteristic. When data are not independent, then the score on one measure shares some of its variability with the score on another measure. As a consequence, the results might be correlated in a way that is unrelated to the study.

The most common nonindependent sample is a pretest/posttest design. Time series data, meaning data collected on the same sample over time, are also nonindependent. A researcher can compensate for nonindependence with specific statistical tests, but the nonindependent nature of the data must be recognized and dealt with.

The Most Common Sample: Convenience Sampling

When random sampling is not realistic, the researcher often relies on convenience sampling. **Convenience sampling** relies on subjects who are accessible to the researcher. Sometimes called accidental sampling, convenience samples have obvious advantages over probability samples, primarily with respect to logistics and cost. However, selection using convenience methods can introduce bias into the sample. Even greater potential for selection bias exists if the researcher is involved personally in selecting the subjects. In such a case, either consciously or unconsciously, the researcher's predetermined ideas about the research might affect subject inclusion.

A specific kind of convenience sample that violates both randomness and independence is **snowball sampling** (also called **referral sampling** or **respondent-driven sampling**). In snowball sampling, each subject is asked to identify and/or recruit other subjects. Although this may be the only way to reach some groups whose members possess sensitive characteristics (e.g., alcoholics, drug addicts, or sexually active teens), the subjects are not independent and randomly selected, so the ability to generalize the results of the study may be limited. Sadler et al. (2010) suggest that the weaknesses of snowball sampling can be compensated for, in part, by randomly selecting subjects from those who are referred. An additional quality control is to increase the sample size; for studies using respondent-driven sampling, the currently accepted practice is to collect a sample twice as large as the number needed for simple random sampling (Johnston, Chen, Silva-Santisteban, & Raymond, 2013).

Convenience sampling is often used in pilot studies when the specifics of a research study have yet to be completely determined. A small study conducted with a convenience sample can help guide the specifics for a larger study. In this situation, convenience sampling is acceptable and expected, because the intent is to inform the research design, not to generalize the results. However, even in pilot studies when convenience sampling is necessary, the researchers should take all steps possible to limit the bias that is inherent in this sampling method.

The best way to reduce bias in a convenience sample is to assign subjects to groups randomly once they have been recruited. A simple flip of a coin is considered a random event and can be used to assign subjects to groups. Using random assignment minimizes the bias of a convenience sample because it ensures extraneous variables are randomly spread over both groups.

Sampling Methods for Hard-to-Reach Populations

Some populations are inherently difficult to recruit. Members of those groups may avoid healthcare providers, or come from a vulnerable or marginalized population. Subjects may fear legal or immigration consequences, be ashamed of their condition, have difficulty reading or speaking English, or be compromised by addiction. These may be difficult populations to define and to access, yet they often have some of the most pressing healthcare needs that could benefit from evidence-based care. Sampling methods have been developed to compensate for these difficulties. **Table 7.3** outlines some contemporary sampling methods and their appropriate application.

Convenience sampling:
A nonprobability method of selecting a sample that includes subjects who are available conveniently to the researcher.

Snowball sampling (referral sampling, respondent-driven sampling):
A non-probability sampling method that relies on referrals from the initial subjects to recruit additional subjects. This method is best used for studies involving subjects who possess sensitive characteristics or who are difficult to find.

Table 7.3 Sampling Methods for Hard-to-Reach Populations

Strategy	Specialized Population	Example
Speak to potential subjects in their native tongue to promote response rates	When subjects have a native language other than English, such that they may be reticent to consent to studies	Mundt et al. (2012) used bilingual recruiters in one sample and English-only speakers in another when recruiting from a multiethnic population. The bilingual recruiters achieved a response rate nearly 6 times as high as did the English-only speakers.
Experience sampling methods, in which experiences are sampled individually over time	When the variable under study happens at random times that cannot be predicted	Moreno et al. (2012) asked adolescents to respond to text message surveys sent at 6 random times during the day to ask for recall of Internet use in the past 4 hours.
Respondent-driven sampling, in which respondents are incentivized both for participating and for recruiting their peers	When subjects are in marginalized or "hidden" populations due to shame or other interpersonal issues	Hope et al. (2015) used respondent-driven sampling to study injection-site infections and injuries in persons who were addicted to heroin.
Service-based sampling, in which individuals who seek out a service are recruited into a study	When subjects' only contact with the healthcare system is through accessing public or other services	Gunnell et al. (2015) studied the best way to provide recently resettled refugees with the Supplemental Nutrition Assistance Program (SNAP) by collecting data from refugee attendees at English as a second language classes at a worksite-training center.

Mixing Methods

Some studies have as their goal the study of phenomena that do not occur frequently in the lifespan or are uncommon in the general population. Good examples include the study of rare diseases in populations and the study of disaster response. At any given time, the chance of an individual having the condition is relatively small. Horney et al. (2012) demonstrated the effectiveness of combining strategies when the target is hard to reach by using a combination of cluster and referral sampling. These researchers randomly selected geographic areas (cluster sampling) and then asked respondents to identify others (referral sampling) in the area who had the condition. These kinds of combined methods may be the only practical alternatives for achieving both representativeness and a good response rate in the sample for studies of rare conditions.

Sampling in Survey Designs

Recruiting subjects to answer surveys can be particularly difficult. In the case of survey sampling, an additional complexity is added: the response rate. Traditionally, the response rate is measured by dividing the total number of surveys distributed by the number who returned the survey. Additionally, the usable response rate is a third measure of importance: Of the surveys returned, how many were usable and complete? The response rate is important, because it reflects the degree to which representativeness of the population exists for the study and, therefore, indicates the generalizability of the results. This consideration is particularly important when assessing the use of survey results as evidence for practice.

The most common flaw in survey sampling is basing conclusions on response rates that make answers nonrepresentative of the population. Nonresponse error occurs when the respondents to a survey differ from the population from which they are drawn. In other words, the individuals who are invited to participate in a survey differ on some characteristic from those who ultimately respond. These errors threaten the validity of results when important demographic groups—for example, the young, the institutionalized, or the poor—are under-represented in the sample (LaRose & Tsai, 2014).

Kramer et al. (2009) report that a 50% response rate is needed to draw accurate conclusions about a population from a surveyed sample; this is a commonly reported requirement. Although recommendations in the literature are variable and inconsistent (ranging from 15% to 80%), there are typically strong reservations about the adequacy of response rates less than 40%.

However, some thinking—specifically about Internet surveys—supports the contention that smaller response rates of 15% to 25% may be adequate if the overall sample size is sufficient to assume generalizability (Berger et al., 2005; Dillman et al., 2009). Davern et al. (2010) noted that the costs of attempting to get a larger response rate may not be worth the returns; these researchers found only incremental differences between statistical results before and after multiple attempts at increasing response rate. Their research showed that making multiple contacts increased the response rate, but did not change the outcome of the study. Jelinek and Weiland (2013) challenge the notion that representativeness necessarily and automatically increases with a greater response rate. They describe the challenges of administering surveys via the Internet—and recognize the "survey fatigue" created by the sheer number of solicitations received by healthcare providers—and conclude that response rates as small as 10% may be adequate if the sample size itself is large enough to detect the phenomenon of interest. Given the findings of Davern et al. (2010) and Jelinek and Weiland (2013) that "larger is not always better," researchers should consider whether the costs and efforts required to obtain a larger response are worth the amount of additional information they will receive. The term "effective sample size" was coined to reflect the final number of respondents needed to draw *representative* conclusions, rather than a strict response rate standard.

Web-based sampling has been demonstrated to be feasible, effective, and efficient in soliciting participation (Fan & Yan, 2010), yet current methods of assessing response rates have demonstrated lower overall rates from this method that may create response bias. Social networking sites and online questionnaires make it possible to do survey research quickly and inexpensively, with rapid growth now being seen in personal device-based sampling strategies (Bhutta, 2012). Research guidelines have not yet produced a method for determining the response rate for Internet and other

Unit of analysis:
The definition of the major entity that will be considered a "subject" for analysis.

electronic survey methods. One solution may be to issue a read receipt with the delivery of an email containing the survey link, with the number of openings then being used as the denominator for the calculation of the response rate. This method may be biased, however, toward younger respondents with better computer skills and greater access to technology.

Some researchers maintain that nonresponse error can be reduced only by using both paper and Internet surveys simultaneously. Funkhouser et al. (2014) found that the results of an electronic survey differed in significant ways from the results of an identical survey administered in paper form. They maintain that, even in an era of increasingly electronic communication, omitting a paper option altogether can result in the over- or under-estimation of certain age- and gender-related characteristics.

Other Sample Selection Considerations

Although the subjects in an experiment are most likely to be people, this is not always the case. Populations and samples are not restricted to human beings. Subjects might refer to documents (such as medical records), counties, or whole hospitals. In a particular kind of evidence-based research called meta-analysis, the subjects are actually research studies. When the subject is something other than an individual human being, it is referred to as the **unit of analysis**. If a researcher wants to study the relationship between socioeconomic status and teen pregnancy rates in counties, for example, then the researcher needs a sample made up of whole counties; in this case, the unit of analysis is a county. The unit of analysis may be groups of people, whole organizations, or cities. When the unit of analysis is quite large, then it becomes more difficult to recruit an adequate sample. For example, if the unit of analysis is a hospital, and the researcher needs a sample size of 60, then 60 hospitals must be recruited for the study. Careful consideration of the unit of analysis involves thought about the difficulty of recruitment as well as the characteristics that are needed in the sample.

IMPROVING RESPONSE RATES

Getting a good response rate is critical for determining the representativeness of the sample and, therefore, the generalizability of the study for practice. Several evidence-based ways to improve response rate have been developed.

Dillman et al. (2009) found that offering multiple means of data collection improved the response rate. In his study, members of the sample were offered one of four randomly selected data entry methods: telephone interview, mail, interactive voice response, or Internet. When nonrespondents were switched to a different means of answering the survey, the response rate went up.

Fan and Yan (2010) conducted a systematic review of elements that enhanced survey response rate. Their recommendations are grouped into four stages: (1) survey development (how to better format a survey); (2) survey delivery (how to better contact subjects); (3) survey completion (how to enhance completion of the survey); and (4) survey return (how to ensure completed surveys are submitted.) Attention to each stage of the process led to better response rates overall.

Li and colleagues (2015) found that text messages were an effective way of improving response rates, but noted that the rate declined over time. Multiple text messages on the same day were not effective in increasing responses; the researchers hypothesized that annoyance with the flood of messages likely contributed to nonresponse in such surveys. Using escalating rewards with the text messages (e.g., phone cards) improved response rates, but only nominally, and the additional information gathered was not unique.

O'Keeffe et al. (2015) were able to achieve a 65% response rate to a survey by using multiple modes of contact. Their efforts to get Irish women to respond to the Pregnancy Risk Assessment Monitoring System (PRAMS) involved an invitation letter, which was followed by three mailed surveys, a reminder letter, and text message reminders for remaining nonrespondents over a 90-day period.

LaRose and Tsai (2014) found that lottery incentives (e.g., "win an Amazon.com gift card") increased response rate beyond a solicitation with no incentive at all, but the highest response rates were achieved with the certainty of a prepaid cash card. Surveys using the latter reward achieved response rates nearing 60%.

Perez et al. (2013) also found that financial incentives improved response rates, but the increase in returns was driven by substantially higher per-person costs. A return rate of more than 40% was achieved with a $10 incentive. The survey completion rate increased twofold when the incentive was increased to $20, and threefold when $30 was offered. Clearly, this approach would be prohibitive for large samples, but it may be an effective means to target difficult-to-recruit samples.

Teclaw et al. (2012) found that asking demographic questions before nondemographic or sensitive questions improved the overall response rate. Starting a survey with less threatening or sensitive questions seems to encourage overall completion.

Boyd et al. (2015) determined that professionally designed information materials—as compared to standard printed brochures—resulted in higher response rates. When telephone reminders were added to these efforts, response rates were even higher. Mailed reminders had no effect on the ultimate response rate.

Jin (2011) used default settings effectively to improve response rates for Internet surveys. On each screen, the desirable outcome was used as the default setting (e.g., "take longer survey") and the completion rate was increased. In addition, more respondents were willing to participate in future surveys and accepted email invitations to do so when desirable defaults were set.

Finally, judicious use of questions can improve the response rate. Choudhury et al. (2012) demonstrated that shorter surveys had higher response rates, both in paper form and via telephone interview. Personalization also seems to help; more respondents participated in a randomized trial when invited with a handwritten envelope rather than a preprinted envelope.

Regardless of the unit of analysis, the sample should be selected based on preset criteria, using credible strategies. However, the sampling strategy is not of much use, no matter how well it is constructed, if an inadequate number of subjects agree to participate in the study.

Sample Size and Power: How Many Subjects Are in the Sample?

Although subject selection determines whether the results can be generalized to a larger population, the number of subjects in the sample affects whether the results can be trusted. Sample size influences the ability to detect significant findings and the level of confidence with which we can incorporate results into practice and expect a similar outcome.

Sample Size in Qualitative Studies

In qualitative studies, sample size is rarely predetermined. Although a researcher may have a general number of informants in mind—and although some standards have been set for particular kinds of qualitative studies such as phenomenology—criteria are generally not strict. The general standard for sample size in a qualitative study is the achievement of redundancy and saturation (Trotter, 2012). Saturation has been achieved when the researcher concludes that responses are repetitive and that no new information is being generated.

Power:
An analysis that indicates how large a sample is needed to adequately detect a difference in the outcome variable.

Determining when saturation has been achieved is based on the judgment of the researcher—there is no formula or calculation to detect when this point has been reached. Complicating the process is that there is little consistency in how saturation is determined, and the literature lacks clear guidelines on when to apply this standard, and how to identify and report it (Francis et al., 2010). Walker (2012) recommends the following standards for determining saturation based on the study design:

- Qualitative description: Redundancy is achieved.
- Phenomenology: Insight into the experience of the phenomenon becomes repetitive.
- Ethnography: No new information from the members of a cultural group is emerging.
- Narrative analysis: Similarity in types of stories is discovered in the analysis.

Saturation may be discovered during data collection or upon data analysis. The constant comparison analytic method—in which emerging themes are compared to those already detected—is particularly strong in supporting the detection of sampling adequacy.

Documenting saturation is one of the ways that qualitative researchers can improve the trustworthiness of a study. Saturation may be achieved with as few as six or eight subjects, or it may require much larger numbers. As the complexity of a phenomenon under study increases, it becomes more likely that a larger number of subjects will be required to achieve saturation.

Sample Size in Quantitative Studies

In quantitative studies, the standard for determining sample size is **power**. Adequate power means there are enough subjects to detect a difference in the outcome variable. The calculation of power is a mathematical process and may be done either prospectively (to determine how many subjects are needed) or retrospectively (to determine how much power a sample possessed). The ultimate sample size in a study is a function of three factors: the significance level needed, the power, and the magnitude of any differences found (i.e., effect size) (McCrum-Gardner, 2010).

The calculation of power involves making several decisions about accuracy and tolerable error, as well as consideration of some characteristics of the population. In general:

- Adequate power is more difficult to achieve when results must be very accurate. When the significance level is set very low—for example, at 0.01 or 0.001—then larger samples are needed to meet the more stringent standard.
- The number of variables to be examined simultaneously and the number of subgroups to be compared increase demands for power. When a large number of characteristics will be compared among several subgroups, then samples must be larger. Focusing a research question carefully can reduce the size of the sample needed to answer the question.
- A highly heterogeneous population—one that has a lot of diversity—is not represented well by a small sample, so the study will have less power. The chances are greater in a diverse population that some group will be under-represented or overrepresented, and larger samples can help ensure this does not happen.
- Very strong effects are easier to detect with small samples, but more subtle effects are more challenging to detect without large samples. In the phenomenon called

effect size, big effects are easier to see in the data, just as a large object is easier to see than a small one. When small effects are expected, then larger samples are needed to find them (Polit & Beck, 2014).

- Likewise, problems that are rare or uncommon are more difficult to detect with smaller samples. The power to detect a problem—sometimes called prevalence detection—does not rely on differences between groups, but rather existence in a population. Perneger et al. (2015) set out to determine the power of samples used for pretests and pilot studies. They found that a sample of 32 is sufficient to detect a problem that occurs 5% of the time, but 45 subjects are needed if the condition occurs in only 1% of the population. These samples are adequate to detect the problem once; if a problem must be observed twice, then 60 to 75 subjects are needed.
- Research designs that involve dependent data (e.g., repeated measures or pretest/ posttest design) are associated with greater statistical power than those involving independent groups.

> **Effect size:**
> The size of the differences between experimental and control groups compared to variability; an indication of the clinical importance of a finding.

Low power reduces the likelihood that the researcher will find significant results; it also affects the reader's level of confidence in the findings (Polit & Beck, 2014). The best samples are based on a power analysis that estimates the size of sample needed, taking into consideration the characteristics of the study and the population.

Researchers can use other methods to estimate sample size needs by applying some rules of thumb. It is generally considered sufficient to have 15 subjects per variable, although some researchers estimate this number to be as high as 50 (Hulley, Cummings, Browner, Grady, & Newman, 2013). A widely reported approach is to multiply the number of independent variables by 50 and add 8 (Fawcett & Garity, 2009). In general, samples with fewer than 30 subjects are not considered powerful enough to detect changes in an outcome variable.

If power is insufficient, then Type II error is more common. A Type II error occurs when there is a difference between groups but the researcher does not detect it. In other words, the intervention works, but the researchers do not conclude that it does. Power is primarily a function of sample size, so inadequate samples are most suspicious when results are *not* significant. The potential for a Type II error should be considered whenever a researcher is working with a small sample of subjects and cannot find any significant differences or relationships. This issue can be addressed by increasing the sample size until sufficient power is ensured. Of course, if findings were significant, then the sample obviously had enough power to detect them, and calculation of power retrospectively is not required.

In general, larger samples are more desirable from many perspectives. Larger samples are likely to have more power and less sampling error. They are also more likely to be normally distributed (to fall in a bell curve), which is an assumption of many statistical tests. More generally, larger samples tend to represent the population better, especially if it is a highly diverse population.

Nevertheless, when samples are very large, standard error—the basis for statistical significance—becomes very small. When standard error is very small, even inconsequential differences between groups may be statistically significant. Statistical significance ensures only that a difference is real—not that it is clinically important. This is a particularly important consideration when working with very large samples.

Reading the Sampling Section of a Research Study

The way a sample is selected allows for generalization of the results; the size of a sample allows confidence in the results. Both are considerations when reading and evaluating the sampling section of a research study. A representative sample may not be trustworthy if it is too small, but even a large sample may not be applicable if it does not represent the population well.

The most important considerations in evaluating a research sample are whether the sample is biased and whether the results can be trusted. Bias is minimized by the use of objective inclusion and exclusion criteria. Confidence in the results is based on an adequate sample size. When reading the sampling section of a research article, the nurse researcher should evaluate both sample selection methods and sample size.

When critically reading a quantitative research study, ask the following questions to guide the evaluation of the sampling strategy:

- Were the subjects selected in an objective way?
- Was the sampling strategy applied consistently?
- Were the subjects assigned to treatment groups in an impartial manner?
- Were enough subjects included for you to be comfortable with the conclusions?

When critically reading a qualitative research study, ask the following questions to guide the evaluation of the sampling strategy:

- Were criteria established for the characteristics that were desirable in informants?
- Did the researchers apply enough effort to find respondents who could best inform the question?
- Was saturation achieved and documented as a standard for sample size?

WHERE TO LOOK

Where to look for information about the sample:
- A description of the sampling strategy should appear in the methods section. It may be labeled "Sample," "Subjects," or "Participants." The researcher should describe the inclusion and exclusion criteria in this discussion.
- The descriptive characteristics of the actual sample will likely appear in the results section. If the researcher has conducted statistical tests of group equivalency, the results of those tests will appear with the overall results. The reporting of such data is intended to demonstrate that the

experimental and control groups have roughly the same characteristics. It is a good thing when these tests of group equivalency show no differences between groups; that outcome indicates the groups were alike in every way except group assignment. In other words, tests for group equivalency should *not* be statistically significant.
- The sampling strategy may not be described at all. This is particularly true if a convenience sample was used. If a description is not clear, then it is safe to assume the sample was not selected

randomly and is a convenience sample. Random samples can be complex and difficult to obtain, so the researcher will almost certainly report it if a random sample was accomplished.

- The terms "probability sample" and "random sample" mean the same thing. Conversely, the term "nonprobability sample" indicates the sample was one of convenience. This is the most common kind of sample in a qualitative study and is not a weakness in that context. Instead, the sample will appear to be one that best informs the research question.
- Specific calculation of power is becoming more common, but it may not be reported. Its omission is not a problem if the results are statistically significant; if the results are significant, then the sample had adequate power (even if the sample was small). If results are not statistically significant, however, then reporting of power calculation is essential to avoid a Type II error. It cannot be assumed that negative results are conclusive without calculated power of at least 80% or 0.80. Because power can be calculated retrospectively, there is no reason not to report it.
- The sampling plan is critical for generalization to other patients and settings. If the sampling plan is seriously flawed, then it is wise to be cautious in generalizing results unless they have been replicated in other, more representative samples.

The ideal sample for qualitative research is purposefully selected based on selection criteria, and saturation is documented. The ideal sample for a quantitative study has objective selection criteria, is randomly selected and/or assigned to groups, and has at least 80% power. The authors should report these elements of the sampling strategy in clear, straightforward terms in the methods section of the research article.

Using Research as Evidence for Practice

The sampling strategy is a key determinant of whether the research findings can be used in a specific patient care environment. The use of research as evidence for practice is based on studies that are well designed and that consider populations similar to the user's population. The appropriate use of research as evidence requires that the study possess external validity. **External validity** is the link between finding knowledge through research and using that knowledge in practice. In other words, whether a research project can be used in a specific situation with a specific group of patients is a function of external validity. External validity refers to the ability to generalize the findings from a research study to other populations, places, and situations. It is essential for the transformation of research into evidence.

It is obvious that the results of research studies done in limited settings or with small, convenience samples may not generalize well to other populations. However, external validity may be limited even in large, multisite studies. **Table 7.4** reviews common threats to external validity that are dealt with via the sampling strategy.

Two types of external validity are ecological and population. **Ecological validity** refers to findings that can be generalized to other settings. For example, a study has strong ecological validity if it is conducted in an acute care setting in a tertiary care center, and the findings will be applied in a similar setting. In contrast, that same study may have weak ecological validity for a small, rural skilled nursing facility. Ecological validity is evident if a study done in one geographic area can be generalized to other geographic areas. For example, findings from studies conducted in the Rocky Mountains of Colorado might reasonably be generalized to other western states at similar altitudes but may not apply as well to patients at sea level.

External validity: The ability to generalize the findings from a research study to other populations, places, and situations.

Ecological validity: A type of external validity where the findings can be generalized and applied to other settings.

Population validity:
The capacity to confidently generalize the results of a study from one group of subjects to another population group.

Table 7.4 Threats to External Validity Addressed with Sampling Strategies

Threat	What It Is	How It Is Controlled
Selection effects	The way subjects are recruited and selected may limit generalization to all populations (e.g., volunteers and compensated subjects may have motives that are different from the motives of the population in general).	Select samples randomly. Choose samples from real-world settings. Report descriptive data for subjects so external validity can be evaluated objectively.
Refusal and attrition	Subjects may refuse to participate or drop out of a study in a way that introduces systematic bias; those who refuse to participate may share some characteristic that would inform the study. As the proportion who do not participate increases, external validity decreases.	Limit the investment demands (time, effort, and discomfort) on subjects to improve participation. Report descriptive data for those who refuse to participate and those who do not complete the study to judge the impact on the generalization. Report overall refusal and attrition rates.
Setting bias	Settings that encourage research subjects to agree to participate may introduce bias via shared characteristics; research-resistant organizations may not be represented at all.	Consider the characteristics of the setting when discussing generalization of the study to other organizations. Use random selection when possible.

Population validity means that a study done in one group of subjects can be applied to other subjects. A study has strong population validity if it was conducted on a population that has characteristics similar to the nurse's patients. Age, gender, ethnicity, and diagnoses are examples of characteristics that might limit external generalization. Samples that are more diverse generally have more external population validity; highly homogeneous subjects, in contrast, limit generalization.

Although many considerations affect external validity, the strongest element is the sampling strategy. The sampling process determines whether subjects are representative of the larger population and whether they can reasonably be expected to represent all patients.

Unfortunately, many of the measures used to control internal validity (e.g., very tightly drawn inclusion and exclusion criteria, sample matching, and stratified random sampling) make it difficult to maximize external validity. When samples become so homogeneous that most extraneous variables are controlled, they no longer represent the real world very well. Creating research that is generalizable, then, requires a balance between control of internal validity and real-world sampling.

To determine whether a research study can be used in a specific setting, the nurse should consider these questions:

- How is the population defined?
- Could extraneous variables in the research situation affect the outcome?
- Is the setting one that is reasonably similar?
- Have the findings been replicated with a range of subjects in different settings?

To determine whether the study results can be used, evaluate whether the sample and environment of the study are similar enough to the current setting's characteristics that the results could reasonably be expected to apply in the current setting. If the defined population and environment are considerably different, then results that were achieved in the study may not be replicated.

How similar do the study specifics have to be for successful generalization? Sources of guidelines based on research rarely find studies that have exactly the same patient mix in an identical situation. As a consequence, critical judgment must be used to evaluate whether the results of a study can be applied in real-world practice. Although the authors might suggest extensions of the study or potential sites for application, final responsibility lies with the reader to decide whether a study can be translated from research into reality.

Creating an Adequate Sampling Strategy

Although the sampling strategy is critical to ensure that the study findings will be applicable, it does not have to be complicated. The researcher can take many steps to ensure that the sample is as unbiased as possible, achieves the best possible representation of the population, and is adequate to find statistical significance or achieve saturation. Most of the decisions affecting these outcomes are made during design of the study; careful consideration of the sampling strategy is well worth the effort.

Define the Population

A clear definition of the population of interest—often called the target population—drives the sampling strategy. This definition may include clinical, demographic, or behavioral characteristics. The target population is the whole set of people to whom the results will be generalized, although it may be defined broadly (e.g., all people with type 2 diabetes) or more narrowly (e.g., all people with type 2 diabetes who present to the emergency department with hyperglycemia).

CHECKLIST FOR EVALUATING THE SAMPLING STRATEGY

- ❑ The target population is clearly and objectively identified.
- ❑ Inclusion criteria are specific and relevant.
- ❑ Exclusion criteria are specified to control extraneous variables.
- ❑ Procedures for selecting the sample are specified. (If not, assume a convenience sample.)
- ❑ Sampling procedures are likely to produce a representative sample for a quantitative study.
- ❑ Sampling procedures are likely to produce the best informants to answer the qualitative research question.
- ❑ Potential for sampling bias has been identified and controlled by the researcher.
- ❑ The sample is unaffected by common sources of bias such as homogeneity, nonresponse, and systematic attrition.
- ❑ The sample is of adequate size, as documented by power for a quantitative study or by saturation for a qualitative study.
- ❑ Power analysis is conducted and reported and is at least 80% (unnecessary if results were statistically significant).

Create Inclusion Criteria

The inclusion criteria define the main characteristics of the desired population. The development of inclusion criteria often requires clinical judgment about which factors are most closely related to the research question. Inclusion criteria involve a tradeoff between generalizability and efficiency. Very specifically designed inclusion criteria will limit those aspects available for the study; very broad ones will increase the chance that extraneous variables are introduced.

To develop inclusion criteria, consider the factors that are most relevant to the research question:

- *Demographic characteristics:* Ethnicity, gender, socioeconomic status, and educational level are all examples of demographic characteristics that might define a desirable subject set.
- *Clinical characteristics:* The specific clinical conditions under study should be specified.
- *Temporal characteristics:* The specific time frame for the study is identified.
- *Behavioral characteristics:* Certain health behaviors (e.g., smoking or alcoholism) may be essential considerations for a study. In qualitative studies, a legitimate behavioral characteristic is the informant's willingness to talk with the researcher about the phenomenon under study.
- *Geographic characteristics:* Practical considerations generally form geographic criteria for a study.

Develop Exclusion Criteria

Exclusion criteria indicate subjects who are not suitable for the research question; thus these criteria eliminate individuals from consideration in the study rather than identify them for recruitment. Such criteria may improve the efficiency, feasibility, and internal validity of a study at the expense of its generalizability, so they should be used sparingly. Exclusion criteria are generally clinical (e.g., certain comorbid conditions) or behavioral (e.g., a high risk of loss to follow-up).

SKILL BUILDER   Strengthen a Convenience Sample

When selecting a random sample is not possible, the following methods enhance the validity and representativeness of a convenience sample:

- Develop inclusion and exclusion criteria and apply them consistently. This will lower the risk of selection bias.
- Use an element of randomness. Although the subjects may not be selected randomly, they can be assigned to groups randomly. The process used for this purpose does not have to be complicated; flipping a coin and rolling dice are both acceptable methods of randomization.
- Conduct a power calculation to determine adequate sample size. If it is not possible to prospectively identify the sample size, use a power calculation to determine how much power the sample did have, particularly if no significant findings were produced.

Design a Recruitment Plan

Once the eligible population has been identified, a specific plan is needed to recruit subjects for the study. The goals of recruitment are twofold:

- Represent the population.
- Recruit enough subjects to attain adequate power or saturation.

From a practical standpoint, recruitment of a sufficient sample depends on finding those individuals who are eligible and making contact with them. Nurses are commonly asked to help recruit patients for studies and provide information for patient consent. Clinical nurses are in a unique position to understand and influence the attitudes of patients toward participation in research, and nurses bring a broad range of skills that can be applied to recruitment for clinical research.

Recruiting a sample from a population that has sensitive characteristics (e.g., drug users) or from minority or immigrant populations may present a particular challenge. These populations are sometimes called "hidden" because it is rare that the sampling frame is available for random selection. Nevertheless, such patients make up a substantial part of the healthcare population, and these populations may be disproportionately affected by some important health problems. Designing culturally sensitive approaches to recruitment can enhance the potential for ensuring these populations are represented appropriately in healthcare research (Calamaro, 2009). Other factors such as cultural appropriateness, safety of the investigators, time, and expense also may pose barriers to random sampling. Furthermore, some members of these populations may be purposefully hidden for personal, legal, or social reasons. In these cases, a purposeful sample may be the only possible approach to gain access to an adequate sample.

Subjects also may be recruited through advertisements and flyers or by mailing surveys directly to them. Recruitment may include compensation if the study is burdensome or involves effort on the subject's part. Recruiting through compensation, however, adds bias because the most financially needy persons will be over-represented in the sample.

Determine the Number of Subjects Needed

The number of subjects needed for a qualitative study will be an emergent characteristic. Francis et al. (2010) recommend two general steps when determining this number: First, specify a minimum sample size that will provide information for initial analysis. Second, specify how many more interviews will be conducted without new ideas emerging. This *a priori* identification of the number of responses that are analyzed without detecting new themes strengthens the credibility of the sampling strategy and reduces the effects of bias.

As the study proceeds, an analytic method is generally used that involves continuously comparing results to those that have already been recorded. This method, called constant comparison, allows the researcher to evaluate when saturation has been achieved—that is, when no new information is being gathered. Generally, it is wise to continue collecting data for one or two additional subjects to confirm that saturation has truly been achieved.

The number required to reach saturation may be quite small, or a study may require a large number of informants to meet this goal. The researcher, using his or her knowledge of the population characteristics and the phenomenon under study, determines whether saturation has been achieved.

Determining the number of subjects needed for a quantitative study is part mathematics, part judgment. If power analysis is not available, an estimate can be achieved by applying the broad rule of thumb of using 15 subjects for every variable that will be studied. Include at least 30 subjects, but recognize that enrolling more than 400 subjects is rarely necessary. Although this rule of thumb produces a very general estimate, it can be useful as an initial projection of necessary sample size.

Calculating the sample size needed to carry out a strong study helps avoid wasting resources on studies that are unlikely to detect significant outcomes (particularly if the intervention is inconvenient or ineffective for the patient). An actual calculation of statistical power is superior to general rules of thumb in making this determination. Nevertheless, the researcher must make decisions and some "educated" guesses about the sample to complete a power analysis. Prior to calculating power, the researcher must know the planned analytic method, the level of acceptable error, the amount of power desired, and the effect size expected. A multitude of Internet sites provide free calculations of statistical power. Estimates of the amount of variability in the outcome variables must also be determined by finding similar or concurrent studies of the same phenomena.

Power calculation is more accurately called an "estimation," and it is mathematically complex. Determining which kind of analysis is needed and identifying the major elements of the calculation may prove difficult. As a result, some researchers use a rule of thumb to guide the number of subjects recruited and then calculate a retrospective power analysis based on the actual findings. This step is necessary only if no statistically significant findings were achieved; when significant differences are detected, the sample is considered to have possessed adequate power.

Apply the Selection Methodology

Once a potential sample has been recruited, then the specific selection methodology is used to identify the final participants. If a purposeful selection method is used for a qualitative study, the researcher invites participants directly from the eligible pool, based on a judgment as to the credibility of each informant.

For quantitative studies, some element of randomness either in selection or group assignment will strengthen the representativeness of the sample. As noted earlier, a table of random numbers can be used, either from a textbook or generated by computer. Simpler methods are also acceptable. For example, a systematic random sample can be determined using a roll of dice. Considered a random event, the roll of dice can be used each time a potential subject is recruited; it is a simple and straightforward way to determine whether that person should be part of the sample. Likewise, a flip of a coin is acceptable for assigning subjects to treatment groups randomly. One researcher, when studying the validity of a pain instrument in long-term care, stood in the doorway of each eligible patient's room and flipped a coin. If the coin landed on heads, the researcher entered the room and informed the patient about his or her eligibility for the study. If the coin landed on tails, the researcher moved on.

GRAY MATTER

The following methods reduce subject attrition in research samples:
- Keep procedures for data collection simple and hassle free.
- Design clear data collection methods.
- Minimize any inconvenience to the subject.
- Follow up with subjects using multiple methods.

Implement Strategies to Maximize Retention

When an adequate number of acceptable subjects have been identified, recruited, and enrolled in a study, the researcher maintains an adequate sample by implementing strategies that maximize retention. Subjects may move away, withdraw for personal reasons, or die during the course of the study. Attrition is particularly problematic in intervention studies and time series studies.

Subjects who have a personal interest in the study are more likely to complete it. In other cases, a combination of personal enthusiasm and nurturing by the researcher is often necessary to keep subjects in a study. Keeping procedures for data collection simple and hassle free, designing clear collection methods, and minimizing any inconvenience to the subjects may all reduce subject attrition. Efforts to follow up with subjects using multiple methods and reminders may also prevent loss of subjects. No matter which techniques are used, however, it is generally agreed that maintaining an adequate sample of subjects throughout the life of an experiment is challenging and requires effort and attention on the part of the researcher.

Summary of Key Concepts
- Sampling strategy is critical for application of research findings to larger or different populations.
- The way a sample is selected is the major control for selection bias and is the primary determinant of whether results from a sample can be generalized to a larger population.
- The goal of the sampling strategy for a qualitative study is credibility; it requires that the researcher use judgment in the purposeful selection of individuals who can best inform the research question.
- Objective inclusion and exclusion criteria can reduce the potential for selection bias in any type of study.
- An element of randomness in sample selection for a quantitative study strengthens the potential for generalizability of the study results.

- If random selection is impossible, random assignment may evenly distribute population characteristics across all treatment groups.
- Random selection is possible through several methods, including simple random, systematic random, stratified random, and cluster random sampling methods.
- Other methods, such as respondent- and service-driven sampling, may be necessary to enroll hard-to-reach or marginalized populations.
- In survey designs, response rate is an important consideration in drawing solid conclusions about the population.
- Sample size is an important consideration in determining the study's power, or the ability to detect differences using a sample. Samples with at least 80% power are desirable.
- Power is a concern only if no statistically significant results were reported; if statistical significance was achieved, the sample had sufficient power.
- Several characteristics of the design and the population affect how much power a study has, including effect size, variability in primary outcome measures, and the level of certainty required.
- The criterion for sample size in a qualitative study is saturation—that is, the point at which no new information is being generated.
- The sampling strategy should be clearly described in a research study, along with a rationale for each sampling decision. It is the basis for trusting the results and applying them to specific patients.

For More Depth and Detail

For a more in-depth look at the concepts in this chapter, try these references:

Cleary, M., Horsfall, J., & Hayter, M. (2014). Data collection and sampling in qualitative research: Does size matter? *Journal of Advanced Nursing, 70*(3):473–475.

Haas, J. (2012). Sample size and power. *American Journal of Infection Control, 40*(8), 766–767.

Kandola, D., Banner, D., O'Keefe-McCarthy, S., & Jassal, D. (2014). Sampling methods in cardiovascular nursing research: An overview. *Canadian Journal of Cardiovascular Nursing, 24*(3), 15–18.

Kelfve, S., Thorslund, M., & Lennartsson, C. (2013). Sampling and non-response bias on health outcomes in surveys of the oldest old. *European Journal of Ageing, 10*, 237–245.

Olson, C. (2014). Survey burden, response rates, and the tragedy of the commons. *Journal of Continuing Education in the Health Professions, 34*(2), 93–95.

O'Reilly, M., & Parker, N. (2012). "Unsatisfactory saturation": A critical exploration of the notion of saturated sample sizes in qualitative research. *Qualitative Research, 13*(2), 190–197.

Sauermann, H., & Roach, M. (2013). Increasing web survey response rates in innovation research: An experimental study of static and dynamic contact design features. *Research Policy, 42*, 273–280.

Turner, R., Walter, S., Macaskill, P., McCaffery, K., & Irwig, L. (2014). Sample size and power when designing a randomized trial for the estimation of treatment, selection and preference effects. *Medical Decision Making, 34*, 711–719.

CRITICAL **APPRAISAL EXERCISE**

Retrieve the following full-text article from the Cumulative Index to Nursing and Allied Health Literature or similar search database:

Tucker, J., Cheong, J., Chandler, S., Crawford, S., & Simpson, C. (2015). Social networks and substance use among at-risk emerging adults living in disadvantaged urban areas in the southern United States: A cross-sectional naturalistic study. *Addiction Research Report, 110*, 1524–1532.

Review the article, focusing on information about the sampling strategy. Consider the following appraisal questions in your critical review of this element of the research article:

1. What is the population for this study?
2. What was the sampling method used? Why did the authors select this technique?
3. Did this sampling method meet the criteria for a probability sample? Did it meet the criteria for independence?
4. What are indications that the sample size is adequate for this study?
5. What are the weaknesses of the way this sample was drawn? How did the authors attempt to compensate for these weaknesses?
6. In your opinion, can the sample be expected to represent the population? Are these findings generalizable?
7. How strong is the evidence generated from this study?
8. How could a public health nurse use the evidence generated from this study?

References

Berger, A., Berry, D., Christopher, K., Greene, A., Maliski, S., Swenson, K., . . . Hoyt, D. (2005). Oncology Nursing Society year 2004 research priorities survey. *Oncology Nursing Forum, 32*(3), 281–290.

Bhutta, C. (2012). Not by the book: Facebook as a sampling frame. *Sociological Methods & Research, 41*(1), 57–88.

Boyd, A., Tilling, K., Cornish, R., Davies, A., Humphries, K., & Macleod, J. (2015). Professionally designed information materials and telephone reminders improved consent response rates: Evidence from an RCT nested within a cohort study. *Journal of Clinical Epidemiology, 68*, 877–887.

Calamaro, C. (2009). Cultural competence in research: Research design and subject recruitment. *Journal of Pediatric Healthcare, 22*(5), 329–332.

Carman, M., Clark, P., Wolf, L., & Moon, M. (2015). Sampling considerations in emergency nursing research. *Journal of Emergency Nursing, 41*, 162–164.

Choudhury, Y., Hussain, I., Parsons, S., Rahman, A., Eldridge, S., & Underwood, M. (2012). Methodological challenges and approaches to improving response rates in population surveys in areas of extreme deprivation. *Primary Health Care Research and Development, 13*(3), 211–218.

Cognet, S., & Coyer, F. (2014). Discharge practices for the intensive care patient: A qualitative exploration in the general ward setting. *Intensive & Critical Care Nursing, 30*(5), 292–300.

Cook, D., & Hatala, R. (2015). Got power? A systematic review of sample size adequacy in health professions education research. *Advances in Health Sciences Education, 20,* 73–83.

Davern, M., McAlpine, D., Beebe, T., Ziegenfuss, J., Rockwood, T., & Call, K. (2010). Are lower response rates hazardous to your health survey? An analysis of three state telephone health surveys. *Health Services Research.* doi: 10.1111.j.1475–6773.2010.00129.x

Dillman, D., Phelps, G., Tortora, R., Swift, K., Berck, J., & Messer, B. (2009). Response rate and measurement differences in mixed-mode surveys using mail, telephone, interactive voice response (IVR) and the internet. *Social Science Research, 38*(1), 1–18.

Fan, W., & Yan, Z. (2010). Factors affecting response rates of the web survey: A systematic review. *Computers in Human Behavior, 26,* 132–139.

Fawcett, J., & Garity, J. (2009). *Evaluating research for evidence-based nursing practice.* Philadelphia, PA: F. A. Davis.

Francis, J., Johnston, M., Robertson, C., Glidewell, L., Entwistle, V., Eccles, M., & Grimshaw, J. (2010). What is an adequate sample size? Operationalising data saturation for theory-based interview studies. *Psychology and Health, 25*(10), 1229–1245.

Funkhouser, E., Fellows, J., Gordan, V., Rindal, D., Boy, P., & Gilbert, G. (2014). Supplementing online surveys with a mailed option to reduce bias and improve response rate: The National Dental Practice-Based Research Network. *Journal of Public Health Dentistry, 74,* 276–282.

Gunnell, S., Christensen, N., Jewkes, M., LeBlanc, H., & Christofferson, D. (2015). Providing nutrition education to recently resettled refugees: Piloting a collaborative model and evaluation methods. *Journal of Immigrant & Minority Health, 17*(2), 482–488.

Hope, V., Ncube, F., Parry, J., & Hickman, M. (2015). Healthcare seeking and hospital admissions by people who inject drugs in response to symptoms of injection site infections or injuries in three urban areas of England. *Epidemiology & Infection, 143*(1), 120–131.

Horney, J., Zotti, M., Williams, A., & Hsia, J. (2012). Cluster sampling with referral to improve the efficiency of estimating unmet needs among pregnant and postpartum women after disasters. *Women's Health Issues, 22*(3), e253–e257.

Hulley, S., Cummings, S., Browner, W., Grady, D., & Newman, T. (2013). *Designing clinical research* (4th ed.). Philadelphia, PA: Lippincott Williams & Wilkins.

Jelinek, G., & Weiland, T. (2013). Response to surveys: sample sizes and response rates. *Emergency Medicine Australia.* doi: 10.1111/1742–6723.12108

Jin, L. (2011). Improving response rates in web surveys with default setting: The effects of defaults on web survey participation and permission. *International Journal of Market Research, 53*(1), 75–94.

Johnston, L., Chen, Y., Silva-Santisteban, A., & Raymond, H. (2013). An empirical examination of respondent driven sampling design effects among HIV risk groups from studies conducted around the world. *AIDS and Behavior, 17,* 2202–2210.

Ko, C., Smith, P., Liao, H., & Chiang, H. (2014). Searching for reintegration: Life experiences of people with schizophrenia. *Journal of Clinical Nursing, 23*(3–4), 394–401.

Kramer, M., Schmalenberg, C., Brewer, B., Verran, J., & Keller-Unger, J. (2009). Accurate assessment of clinical nurses' work environments: Response rate needed. *Research in Nursing and Health, 32*(3), 229–240.

Kurth, E., Kennedy, H., Stutz, E., Kesselring, A., Fornaro, I., & Spichiger, E. (2014). Responding to a crying infant—you do not learn it overnight: A phenomenological study. *Midwifery, 30*(6), 742–749.

LaRose, R., & Tsai, H. (2014). Completion rates and non-response error in online surveys: Comparing sweepstakes and pre-paid cash incentives in studies of online behavior. *Computer in Human Behavior, 34,* 110–119.

Li, Y., Wang, W., Wu, Q., VanVelthoven, M., Chen, L., Cu, X.,...Car, J. (2015). Increasing the response rate of text messaging data collection: A delayed randomized controlled trial. *Journal of the American Medical Informatics Association, 22,* 51–64.

LoBiondo-Wood, G., & Haber, J. (2014). *Nursing research methods and critical appraisal for evidence-based practice* (8th ed.). St. Louis, MO: Elsevier.

Matthew-Maich, N., Ploeg, J., Jack, S., & Dobbins, M. (2013). Leading on the frontlines with passion and persistence: A necessary condition for breastfeeding best practice guideline uptake. *Journal of Advanced Nursing, 22*(11/12), 1759–1770.

McCrum-Gardner, E. (2010). Sample size and power calculation made simple. *International Journal of Therapy and Rehabilitation, 17*(1), 10–14.

Moreno, M., Jelenchick, L., Koff, R., Eikoff, J., Diermeyer, C., & Christakis, D. (2012). Internet use and multitasking among older adolescents: An experience sampling approach. *Computers in Human Behavior, 29,* 1097–1102.

Mundt, A., Aichberger, M., Kliewe, T., Ignatyev, U., Yayla, S., Heimann, H.,...Heinz, A. (2012). Random sampling for a mental health survey in a deprived multi-ethnic area of Berlin. *Community Mental Health Journal, 48*(6), 792–797.

Nokes, K., & Nwakeze, P. (2007). Exploring research issues: In using a random sampling plan with highly marginalized populations. *Journal of Multicultural Nursing and Health, 13*(1), 6–9.

O'Keeffe, L., Kearney, P., & Greene, R. (2015). Pregnancy risk assessment monitoring system in Ireland: Methods and response rates. *Maternal–Child Health Journal, 19,* 480–486.

Perez, D., Nie, J., Ardern, C., Radhu, N., & Ritvo, P. (2013). Impact of participant incentives and direct and snowball sampling on survey response rate in an ethnically diverse community: Results from a pilot study of physical activity and the built environment. *Journal of Immigrant and Minority Health, 15*(1), 207–214.

Perneger, T., Courvoisier, D., Judelson, P., & Gayet-Ageron, A. (2015). Sample size for pre-tests of questionnaires. *Quality of Life Research, 24,* 147–151.

Polit, D., & Beck, C. (2014). *Essentials of nursing research appraising evidence for nursing practice* (8th ed.). Philadelphia, PA: Lippincott Williams & Wilkins.

Pooe-Monyemore, M., Mavundla, T., & Christianson, A. (2012). The experience of people with oculocutaneous albinism. *Health SA Gesondheid, 17*(1), 1–8.

Sadler, G., Lee, H., Lim, R., & Fullerton, J. (2010). Recruitment of hard-to-reach population subgroups via adaptations of the snowball sampling strategy. *Nursing & Health Sciences, 12*(3), 369–374.

Tan, J., Docherty, S., Barfield, R., & Brandon, D. (2012). Addressing parental bereavement support needs at the end of life for infants with complex chronic conditions. *Journal of Palliative Medicine, 15*(5), 579–584.

Teclaw, R., Price, M., & Osatuke, K. (2012). Demographic question placement: Effect on item response rates and means of a Veterans Health Administration survey. *Journal of Business and Psychology, 27*(3), 281–290.

Trotter, R. (2012). Qualitative research sample design and sample size: Resolving and unresolved issues and inferential imperatives. *Preventive Medicine, 55,* 298–400.

Walker, J. (2012). The use of saturation in qualitative research. *Canadian Journal of Cardiovascular Nursing, 22*(2), 37–41.

Chapter 8

Measurement and Data Collection

CHAPTER OBJECTIVES

The study of this chapter will help the learner to

- Discuss the link between the research question and the measurement strategy.
- Describe the types of reliability and validity and explain how they are assessed.
- Evaluate sources of measurement error and plan strategies to minimize their effects.
- Compare the advantages and disadvantages of data collection methods.
- Discuss the importance of having clearly prescribed data management procedures.
- Determine how the measurement strategy supports application of the data to evidence-based practice.

KEY TERMS

Calibration	Measurement error	Scales
Closed questions	Open-ended questions	Secondary data
Codebook	Operational definition	Sensitivity
Conceptual definition	Photovoice	Specificity
Guttman scale	Precision	Systematic error
Internal reliability	Primary data	Test blueprint
Inter-rater reliability	Psychometric instruments	Validity
Likert scale	Random error	Visual analog scale (VAS)
Measurement	Responsiveness	

Introduction

There is an old saying in performance management: You get what you measure. This is never truer than with the measurement strategy employed in nursing research. The credibility of a study as evidence for practice is almost completely dependent on identifying and measuring the right things. A strong measurement strategy is critical for good evidence. The process of measurement allows the researcher to determine if and in what quantity a characteristic is present, and to provide evidence of that characteristic, usually represented by a number. If that measurement is not correct, or if it is

Measurement: Determination of the quantity of a characteristic that is present; it involves assigning of numbers or some other classification.

inconsistent, then the researcher may draw the wrong conclusions. The conclusions from a research study will be only as good as the data that were used to draw them. A research study can be beautifully designed, well controlled, and impeccably executed, but if the data that are collected are not consistent and accurate, then the results will be suspect.

Measurement

Measurement is based on rules. Often, measurement is about assigning numbers or some other classification to subjects in a way that represents the quantity of the attribute numerically. When we think of measurement, that concept often brings to mind equipment or tools applied to some concrete physical manifestation. Indeed, measures used for the sciences involve very strict rules about assigning numbers to characteristics in a completely unbiased way. Not all measurement, though, is quite so straightforward.

Many forms of measurement exist, not all of which involve quantifying a trait; a considerable number of measures involve sorting subjects into categories based on their characteristics. For example, using a thermometer measures the amount of heat in the body, whereas asking about religious affiliation seeks to classify the subject based on his or her belief system. Classification measures are frequently used in nursing. Subjects may be classified by some neutral observer, or they may classify themselves by completing an instrument that asks for a self-rating of perception of attributes.

Rules are used to guide the determination of measures, whether they are collected by instrumentation or classification. Such rules may specify the way a measure is administered, the timing of the procedure, the exact protocol for collecting the result, and even such details as how questions are worded and how the interviewer should read a question.

Whether data are collected by calculation of a value or by classification into groups, they will likely be represented by a number. Numbers are key elements of measurement in nursing for several reasons. Numbers are objective and often standardized, so that they are consistent. Numbers can serve as a universal language and as a means of communication in an increasingly global world. Statistical tests can be applied to numbers, resulting in quantification of how much error a measure represents. Numbers are precise and can accurately represent attributes.

Regardless of the type of measure, numbers are useful only to the extent that they represent the underlying characteristic they are intended to represent. To have value, they must be clearly linked to the research question, appropriate to represent the variable of interest, and consistently accurate.

GRAY MATTER

Numbers are a key element of measurement in nursing because they are:
- Objective
- Standard
- Consistent
- Precise
- Statistically testable
- An accurate representation of attributes

VOICES FROM THE FIELD

I became interested in the topic of teamwork very early in my career. Even when I was a novice nurse, I vividly remember that there were times when the people I worked with seemed to "click," and we were able to get an enormous amount of work done without any unit strife. At other times, when there were particular groups of nurses working together, we could not even get an average amount of work done without conflict of some sort. I began wondering about the effects of teamwork on productivity and whether improving teamwork would result in a more efficient unit. When I later became a department manager myself, it was important to me to build and maintain good team relations, and I believe that is why I had a unit that had a reputation for getting a lot of work done.

I did one study in particular that focused on how teams function at night versus during the day. I have worked both shifts and I know the environment, the way people relate, and the work to be done—it is radically different on the two shifts. It is literally like night and day. I wanted to see if I could differentiate team behaviors that happen at night from those that occur during the day.

I could not find exactly the instrument I wanted; I did not find any, in fact, that broke teamwork down into the behaviors I was interested in. There were some that came close, but none that I thought asked the specific questions I had. I was a bit cocky, I guess, when I decided I would just write my own. I had looked at quite a few instruments, and I thought, "How hard can it be?" So I set out to develop my own instrument for measuring team behaviors.

I did it quite logically. I consulted a friend who was a nursing faculty member, and she helped me develop a test outline and gave me advice on the wording of questions. Still, it took me almost a month to get a first draft done. I knew I had to test it for reliability, and my faculty friend helped me find a statistician. I was really excited up to this point. I thought I might try to copyright my instrument, use it as a team-building basis, that kind of thing. We gave the instrument to about a dozen nurses and the statistician ran reliability statistics for me. What a nightmare! The number came back at 46%, which is woefully inadequate for any kind of research. I was really crestfallen; I thought I had done a pretty good job.

The statistician was really nice about it. He showed me how some of the questions were written in a confusing way. I had some double negatives in the questions; they were confusing even to me when I reread them. Some of the words could be interpreted several different ways, and there were some typographical errors that I just flat-out overlooked. It was a humbling experience. I persisted, but it took a couple of revisions and about 6 months before I could get my little instrument where I was comfortable using it.

After I had the results, there was a bit more of a disappointment, because I did not have anything to which I could compare the numbers. Because it was a totally unique instrument, the numbers I produced were isolated; I had no way to put them into context. In retrospect, it would have been much easier and led to stronger results if I had just used an existing instrument, even if it was not exactly what I needed. "Close enough" actually would have been better than what I wound up with. In hindsight, I should have balanced the weaknesses of a unique tool with the little bit I would have lost from using a standard one.

Since then, I have done quite a bit of work measuring teamwork. I found a standard tool that enables me to measure teamwork reliably while having a large, national database to which I can compare my scores. It also means that studies I have done can be replicated and that some of my studies have been used in meta-analyses and integrative reviews.

Overall, developing my own tool was a good experience. Painful but good; I learned a lot. I would say my strongest lesson was this: If you need to write your own instrument—and you may—then be sure it is for a really good reason and that you have the time, energy, and know-how to put into it. Measurement is not as easy as it looks.

Janet Houser, PhD, RN

Conceptual definition: Clearly stated meaning of an abstract idea or concept used by a researcher in a study.

Operational definition: An explanation of the procedures that must be performed to accurately represent the concepts.

The Measurement Strategy

The actual measure of an attribute is only one part of a measurement strategy. The complete measurement strategy is critical to the design of a valid research study, so both time and energy should be applied to its planning and execution. The measurement strategy involves the following steps:

1. Thoughtful determination of the most relevant attributes that demonstrate the answer to the research question
2. Definition of the attributes in terms of the operations used to demonstrate them
3. Selection of an instrument that will reliably capture an accurate representation of the attribute
4. Documentation that the instrument and the measurement procedure are reliable and valid
5. Development of protocols to guide the process of gathering data
6. Quality checks to ensure the data collection process results in an accurate and complete data set

Define the Research Variables

The first step of the measurement strategy is to give careful thought to the concepts represented in the research question. The research question will describe the phenomena or characteristics of interest in a study, which then must be translated into observable attributes so that they can be measured (Morrow, Mood, Disch, & Kang, 2015). Eventually, these concepts may be represented as a physical attribute (for example, blood sugar), a perception (for example, pain), a behavior (for example, a gait), or a response (for example, recall). These factors are called, logically enough, attribute variables. To ensure that everyone is interpreting the attribute in the same way, the researcher must write definitions that represent the characteristic in such a way that it cannot be misinterpreted.

GRAY MATTER

To represent the underlying characteristics, numbers used in research measurements must be:
- Clearly linked to the research question
- Appropriate to represent the variable of interest
- Consistently accurate

There are two kinds of definitions for attribute variables: conceptual and operational. A **conceptual definition** describes the concept that is the foundation of the variable by using other concepts. For example, a conceptual definition of depression might include the presence of sadness, lack of pleasure, and changes in eating or sleep habits. An **operational definition** defines the operations that must be performed to accurately represent the concepts. An operational definition of depression might include using a scale to record weight loss or gain in kilograms or using a log to record hours of sleep per night. It is useful to begin the process of defining the research variables by describing conceptual definitions because they can help ensure the researcher is measuring the right things. Operational definitions ensure that the researcher is measuring attributes reliably.

Determine a Measurement

After writing an operational definition, the researcher defines the procedure for collecting and recording the data. Measurements may be either primary or secondary. **Primary data** are recorded by the researcher directly from a subject. That is, the researcher uses specific rules to collect the data and makes and maintains a record of the responses. Measures for primary data can involve the following tools:

- Calibrated instruments, such as a thermometer
- Equipment, such as a digital camera
- Paper-and-pencil or online tests, questionnaires, surveys, or rating scales, such as a pain scale
- Observation, rating, and reporting characteristics or behaviors, such as a skin assessment
- Counting the frequency of an attribute or exhibited action, such as the number of falls on a unit

Primary data are considered most reliable because the data are collected by the researcher for a single, specific purpose, but they do have some limitations. Primary data are time consuming to collect, and the quality of the data depends on many factors. Some of these factors are related to the subjects, but others are due to the data collectors who are administering the measure. Sometimes a subject's recall of a physical reaction or an event may be quite different from reality. Some subjects may not be able to communicate clearly, or language barriers may be present that distort reporting. A subject may have a mental condition that prohibits accurate and clear reporting of data. Subjects may misrepresent sensitive data, respond dishonestly, or simply give the answer they think the researcher wants to hear. However, although self-reports of behavior, beliefs, and attitudes are prone to biases, there are no acceptable alternative means of measurement for many constructs of interest to nurse researchers, such as satisfaction, pain, depression, and quality of life (Walford, Tucker, & Viswanathan, 2013).

The data collectors can also affect the accuracy of primary data. For example, the data collector may use equipment or instruments incorrectly. When collecting perceptual data, the individual making the recording may not use consistent language or a consistent approach. Inflection or wording may inadvertently lead a subject to give an inaccurate answer. For example, the question "Do you abuse alcohol?" will elicit a far different response than "How many alcoholic drinks do you have in a week?" The response to either question can also be affected by the tone of voice of the questioner. Those doing the data recording must be carefully trained in data collection techniques. The consistency of data captured by multiple raters must be checked by measures of inter-rater reliability; this is important with any measure for which different individuals will be asked to score observations (McHugh, 2012).

Primary data: Data collected directly from the subject for the purpose of the research study. Examples include surveys, questionnaires, observations, and physiologic studies.

Psychometric instruments: Instruments used to collect subjective information directly from subjects.

The measurement methods most commonly used for collecting primary data are physiologic measurements, psychometric instrumentation, surveys, and questionnaires. Because the credibility of the resulting data depends so heavily on the quality of the instrument, these data collection methods warrant the use of clear strategies to minimize measurement error.

GRAY MATTER

Effective data collection must be designed to:
- Be clear
- Be unbiased
- Be reliable
- Be valid
- Answer the research question

Physiologic Measurement

Evidence-based practice focuses attention on the use of physiologic measurements from patients for clinical research efforts. Physiologic measurement involves the assignment of a number or value to an individual's biological functioning. Such a measure can be self-reported, observed, directly measured, indirectly measured, electronically monitored, or obtained through diagnostic tests.

Nurses commonly rely on physiologic measurements to make patient care decisions. For example, they take vital signs, read lab results, and measure blood glucose. The measurement of a patient's biological functioning involves the use of specialized equipment and often requires specific training in the use of that equipment. The specialized equipment used to measure a patient's biological functioning must be accurate, precise, and sensitive. In turn, it can provide valid measures for variables related to physical functions. Physiologic measurements, then, are readily available for the clinician researcher and provide objective data. To use such data for research purposes, the data must be collected from each participant in exactly the same way. Consistency in the data collection process is very important; the researcher's goal is to have minimal variability in the data collection procedure by ensuring all data collectors follow the same steps.

Physiologic measurement can also be self-reported for variables such as pain, nausea, and dizziness. These variables are often a critical part of research but are subjective in nature, so that their measurement depends on the participant understanding what is being asked of him or her. Such data are usually collected using instruments, but of a different nature than the ones used for measuring biological functioning. Specifically, the instruments used to collect this kind of subjective information directly from subjects are referred to as **psychometric instruments**.

Psychometric Instrumentation

Psychometric instrumentation is applied to measure subjective or conceptual information. Examples of psychometric instruments include tools that measure coping, stress, self-concept, self-esteem, motivation, and similar psychosocial elements (Fain, 2014). To provide valid data for a study, the instrument chosen for measuring the variables must fit closely with the conceptual definition of those variables; indeed, it will likely become the operational definition for some of them.

Many instruments exist that have been determined to measure subjective characteristics reliably. Finding an acceptable instrument is critical to a strong measurement strategy. Before a researcher begins to develop his or her own data collection tool, a literature review is justified to see whether an existing instrument might be applied to answer the research question. If one does, permission must be obtained from the original author before the instrument can be used in a publishable research study. The psychometric properties of the instrument are documented in the research write-up to assure the reader that measurement error is not responsible for the findings; they are described later in this chapter.

There are many advantages of using an existing instrument rather than developing a new one. Doing so saves the researcher the time needed to develop and validate a new instrument. Development of a new instrument for a research study involves developing a test blueprint, creating questions, soliciting feedback about the fidelity of the instrument to the blueprint, pilot testing the instrument, and making revisions. This process can be burdensome, can delay the research, and should be undertaken only when a thorough review of the literature reveals that there are no acceptable existing instruments.

The use of existing measurement tools also allows for the replication of a study and its inclusion in subsequent aggregate studies. The results of the research can be compared to the work of others if the procedure uses the same instrument.

Limitations of using a previously developed instrument include the cost of the instrument, failure of the instrument to address all the research interests, the feasibility of administering the instrument, and an inability to locate psychometric information or the original author.

Psychometric instruments encompass a variety of methods and may vary widely in complexity. Surveys, questionnaires, and scales are all examples of instruments that may measure psychosocial characteristics.

Surveys and Questionnaires

The most commonly used data collection method is the survey. In the survey method, a systematic tool is used to gather information directly from respondents about their experiences, behaviors, attitudes, or perceptions (DeVellis, 2011). Depending on the types of questions used, survey research can rely on a quantitative design, a qualitative design, or a mixture of both. Surveys may be personally distributed, distributed through the mail, or delivered online. They can be administered during a face-to-face interview or in a telephone survey, or the respondents may complete the surveys on their own. Responses of participants are described in numeric terms and/or in words. A systematic approach to developing survey questions appears in **Table 8.1**. **FIGURE 8.1** depicts a decision-tree approach to determining the survey method and outlines the qualities of a good question.

Open-ended questions:
Questions with no predetermined set of responses.

Table 8.1 Guidelines for Creating a Survey	
Step 1	Identify the objectives of the survey. Identify demographic characteristics. Identify the dependent variable (if applicable). Identify variables of interest or the independent variables (if applicable).
Step 2	Envision how the data will be analyzed. Create data definitions. Design a data tabulation form.
Step 3	Draft a set of questions. Make sure all the variables are addressed. Modify the wording of questions.
Step 4	Group the questions to reflect each major topic of the survey. Organize questions from general to specific. Format the survey so it is easy to follow. Write clear instructions for completion of the survey.
Step 5	Distribute a preliminary draft of the survey to a group of colleagues. Solicit their review of the document and identify problems with questions, including how the questions and the directions are worded. Provide the group of reviewers with a copy of the objectives so they can determine whether the questions address each of the objectives.
Step 6	Revise the survey. Test the survey on a pilot group of subjects. Measure the reliability of the survey and make any changes necessary based on the statistical analysis and the feedback of the pilot group. Analyze the results from the pilot group, looking for patterns of missing answers or inconsistency in responses, and make final revisions. Record the amount of time the subjects take to complete the survey. Revise the data tabulation form.
Step 7	Write instructions for the participants. Write an introductory letter. Write a consent form, if applicable. Distribute the survey. Give the participants clear instructions for returning the completed instrument.

Questions used in surveys can be either open-ended or closed questions. **Open-ended questions** are used when the researcher does not know all of the possible responses or when the researcher wants participants to respond in their own words. Typically, open-ended questions are characteristic of qualitative research, but they may be included as part of an otherwise quantitative data collection tool. Responses are analyzed using content analysis to find themes in the words of respondents. Disadvantages of open-ended questions are that it takes the respondent longer to complete each question, the respondent may misinterpret the question, and analysis of the data takes longer. Examples of open-ended questions appear in **Table 8.2**.

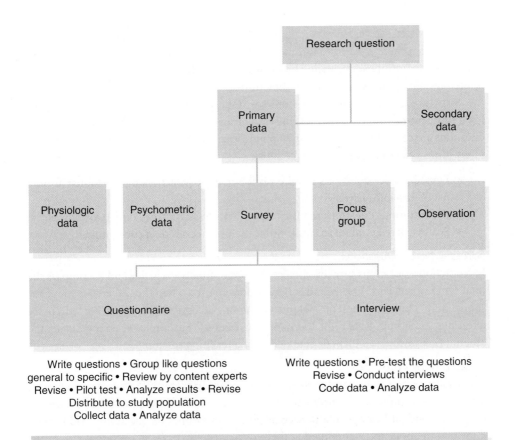

Write questions • Group like questions
general to specific • Review by content experts
Revise • Pilot test • Analyze results • Revise
Distribute to study population
Collect data • Analyze data

Write questions • Pre-test the questions
Revise • Conduct interviews
Code data • Analyze data

Qualities of a Good Question

• Will answer the research question • Written at a fifth-grade language level
• Uses language that is unambiguous • Uses words that are familiar
• Does not use words with more than one meaning
• Asks for an answer on only one dimension
• Is nonthreatening • Does not imply a certain type of answer
• Avoids words that might create a negative reaction in some people
regardless of the content of the statement

FIGURE 8.1 Steps in Survey Design

Table 8.2 Examples of Open-Ended Questions

What were your emotional reactions to the initial ultrasound that indicated there was a problem with your baby?

How did you deal with those emotional reactions?

How did the nurse practitioner help you deal with the birth of your baby?

Which strategies have you used to deal with the stress of caring for a baby with a significant health problem?

Closed questions:
Questions that have a fixed number of alternative responses. Respondents are forced to select answers or ratings on a scale provided by the researcher.

Scales:
Type of closed-question format in which respondents put responses in rank order on a continuum.

Likert scale:
A scale that uses attitude statements ranked on a five- or seven-point scale. The degree of agreement or disagreement is given a numerical value, and a total can be calculated.

Guttman scale:
A scale with a set of items on a continuum or statements ranging from one extreme to another. Responses are progressive and cumulative.

Sets of closed questions are commonly referred to as questionnaires. Such questions are used when there are a fixed number of alternative responses; the respondent has to select from the responses provided by the researcher. This may involve selecting from a limited number of answers or rating something on a scale.

Structured, fixed-response questions are best used when the researcher is investigating a finite number of potential responses. Compared to open-ended questions, closed questions are easier both for the respondent to answer and for the researcher to analyze. Many kinds of closed questions are possible:

- Forced-choice questions require respondents to select a single response from a list of possible answers.
- Dichotomous questions require respondents to select from only two choices.
- Scales ask respondents to rank-order their responses on a continuum.

Forced-Choice Questions

Forced-choice questions provide choices that are mutually exclusive and encompass the total range of answers. These kinds of questions are used when the researcher wants respondents to choose the best possible answer among all options presented. Forced-choice questions sometimes have right and wrong answers—for example, when measuring the amount of knowledge a diabetic retained after a teaching session.

Dichotomous Questions

Dichotomous questions can be answered by selecting from only one of two choices. These types of questions typically are used to determine if a characteristic is present or if a respondent belongs to a particular group. Dichotomous questions yield limited information about the respondent and are difficult to analyze. Because only a limited range of tests are available for their analysis, the use of dichotomous questions should be limited to those situations in which no other type of question is appropriate.

Scales

Scales ask respondents to rank some trait or ability on a continuum of possible responses. The individual entries on the scale correspond to variations in the strength of the response. The most commonly used types of scales include Likert scales, Guttman scales, and visual analog scales.

The Likert scale presents a set of attitude statements, with respondents then being asked to express agreement or disagreement with each statement on a five-point or seven-point scale (Likert & Hayes, 1957). Each degree of agreement is given a numerical value, so a total numerical value can be calculated from all the responses.

The Guttman scale presents a set of items on a continuum, but it may also use statements ranging from one extreme to the other (Guttman, 1947). When a person agrees with one statement, it can be assumed that he or she agrees with all previous questions in the scale. In other words, the responses are progressive. Each item on the scale is worth a point, and the total score is cumulative. Thus, if a respondent's score is 5, it means that the respondent agreed with all of the item statements from 1 through 5. Examples of closed questions and scales appear in **Table 8.3**.

Table 8.3 Examples of Closed Questions

Forced-Choice Question

What is your current marital status? (Select one.)

- Single
- Married
- Divorced
- Separated
- Widowed

Dichotomous Questions

What is your gender?

- Male
- Female

Were you born in the United States?

- Yes
- No

Likert Scale

The physical layout of my patient care unit is efficient.

1. Strongly disagree	2. Disagree	3. Neither agree nor disagree	4. Agree	5. Strongly agree

Guttman Scale

Please mark whether you agree with the following statements.	Yes	No
1. Anyone needing health care should pay out of pocket for the services rendered. (Least extreme)		
2. There should be health insurance for anyone who can afford to pay for it.		
3. Employers should be required to offer healthcare coverage for any employee.		
4. Employers should be required to pay for the healthcare premium of any employee.		
5. Employers should be required to pay for the healthcare premium of any employee and his or her family.		
6. Individuals below the poverty level should have their health care subsidized by the government.		
7. There should be universal healthcare coverage for all, subsidized by the government. (Most extreme)		

Visual analog scale (VAS):
A rating-type scale in which respondents mark a location on the scale corresponding to their perception of a phenomenon on a continuum.

The **visual analog scale (VAS)** is one of the scales most commonly used in health care for measuring perceptual variables such as pain or nausea. The VAS is designed to present the respondent with a rating scale that has few constraints and is easy to use. Respondents mark the location on the continuum corresponding to their perceptions of the phenomenon. The Wong-Baker Faces Pain Rating Scale, depicted later in this chapter, is an example of a VAS.

SKILL BUILDER   Design Better Questionnaires

Questionnaires are not easy to construct; their development requires a thoughtful, systematic approach. Despite the challenges, these instruments can be invaluable as data collection tools for both quantitative and qualitative research. Here are some simple suggestions for designing strong questionnaires that are more likely to be answered accurately and completely, making for stronger research conclusions:

- Keep the questions simple, clear, and easy to answer. Consider the value of each question before including it in the final survey. Write the questions in an unbiased way that does not imply there is one "correct" answer.
- Assess the reading level of the questionnaire. Unless the reading capacity of the potential subjects is known (for example, all respondents are college educated), write the items at a fifth-grade reading level.
- Keep the overall survey short, and ask the pilot-test subjects to estimate the amount of time it took them to complete it. Include this time estimate in the introductory letter so subjects will know when they have time to respond.
- Know how each question will be analyzed, and be sure the way the data are collected can be subjected to the specific analytic test. For example, a very limited range of statistical tests can be used

for analysis of yes/no questions; by comparison, questions that offer respondents multiple options arrayed along a scale can be subjected to a broader range of potential analytic procedures.
- Have a plan for handling missing data consistently. Determine ahead of time if you will allow analysis of incomplete responses.
- Group similar questions together. Start with nonthreatening questions, such as demographic information, and work up to more sensitive information at the end of the questionnaire. Avoid emotionally laden words that may imply a judgment.
- Avoid questions that ask about more than one characteristic or dimension. Limit each question to a single concept.
- Write scales so that they have no "neutral" or midpoint response. Often, respondents use the "neutral" category for many meanings—including "this doesn't apply," "I don't know," or "I don't want to tell you." If you need a neutral category, include a separate category that has no numerical value for "not applicable/no answer."
- Provide a well-written cover letter with explicit instructions for both completing and submitting the questionnaire. The instructions should be clear and concise. Make it a convenient process to respond and get the answers back to the researcher.

Writing Survey Questions

Whether the questions are closed or open-ended, some specific issues should be considered when writing questionnaires. Primary among these issues is clarity: Questions must be clear, succinct, and unambiguous. The goal is for all respondents who answer the question to interpret its meaning the same way.

The second issue concerns the use of leading questions or emotionally laden words. A leading question is phrased in such a way that it suggests to the respondent that the researcher expects a certain answer. The adjectives, verbs, and nouns used in a question can have positive or negative meanings and may influence the responder unintentionally. An emotionally laden question is one that contains words that can create a negative reaction in some people regardless of the content of the statement. Some words also have more than one meaning and should be avoided.

Regardless of which type of data is collected, which measurement instrument is used, or whether the responses constitute primary or secondary data, the information must be recorded in a way that minimizes the potential for measurement error.

Strategies to Minimize Measurement Error

Measurement error is the amount of difference between the true score (i.e., the actual amount of the attribute) and the observed score (i.e., the amount of the attribute that was represented by the measure). Measurement error is a threat to the internal validity of a research study, so minimizing measurement error means that the overall study results are more credible (Moses, 2012).

Measurement error is present in every instrument to some degree or another, and may be either random or systematic. **Random error** is expected and is affected by a host of influences that may be present in an experiment. Random error may be due to human factors, confusion, bias, and normal environmental variations. While these sources of error are not preventable, the researcher should avoid them whenever possible.

Systematic error has a more serious effect on the results of a research study, because measures with systematic error may appear to be accurate. **Systematic error** is any error that is consistently biased. In other words, the measure is consistent but not accurate. Such a measure may consistently underestimate the effect, overestimate it, or miss data in a way that is not random. For example, subjects with poor literacy skills may not participate in a study that involves reading a questionnaire. In this case, the missing data are not random; rather, they are systematically attributed to individuals who cannot read well. In the case of systematic error, results under-represent a key group that could provide information but does not. This type of error is of particular concern in vulnerable populations or when investigating sensitive issues. For example, Carle (2010) discovered systematic measurement bias across multiple studies related to self-reported educational attainment, poverty status, and minority status.

Systematic error may be a result of the following factors:

- *Measures that are consistent but inaccurate.* An example is a tape measure that has been used so often that it has stretched. Although it may still record length consistently, the tape measure will routinely overestimate the length.
- *Measures that have complicated or onerous procedures for the subject.* Individuals who are greatly inconvenienced by the measure or who have to expend substantial energy to respond may drop out, leaving only the most motivated subjects in the study. For example, asking a subject to maintain a daily diary will likely result in incomplete or hastily collected data.
- *Measures that reflect sensitive or socially taboo topics.* The subject may be able but unwilling to respond, and missing data may affect the results. For example, self-reports of tobacco and alcohol abuse often under-represent the prevalence of these behaviors in the population.

Measurement error: The difference between the actual attribute (true score) and the amount of attribute that was represented by the measure (observed score).

Random error: A nonreproducible error that can arise from a variety of factors in measurement.

Systematic error: Any error that is consistently biased; the measure is consistent but not accurate.

Calibration:
The use of procedures to minimize measurement error associated with physical instruments by objectively verifying that the instrument is measuring a characteristic accurately.

Precision:
The degree of reproducibility or the generation of consistent values every time an instrument is used.

Internal reliability:
The extent to which an instrument is consistent within itself as measured with the alpha coefficient statistic.

Variability that is due to anything other than a change in the underlying attribute represents error. It is important, then, to find instruments that measure characteristics consistently and with minimal unexplained variability. An instrument is not reliable when there is a discrepancy between the real attribute and its representation by the results.

Measurement error is minimized when reliability is high. In turn, when measures are highly reliable and precise, it becomes easier to detect the true effects of an intervention. The most common means of minimizing measurement error are calibrating instruments and ensuring instrument reliability.

Use Properly Calibrated Equipment and Instruments

Calibration of an instrument reduces the discrepancy between the true score and the observed score. **Calibration,** or the use of objective procedures to verify that an instrument is measuring a characteristic accurately, is a highly structured process. Laboratory instruments may be calibrated using samples with known quantities; for example, blood glucose monitors often come with calibration samples for quality assurance. These procedures ensure that the instrument is consistent (reliable) and accurate (valid).

However, not all instruments are easily calibrated. For example, how do you calibrate an instrument to measure depression? In the case of instruments that measure characteristics or traits, the calibration concern is replaced with an emphasis on reliability and validity. These are the most important issues to consider when selecting an instrument to measure nonphysiologic characteristics.

Ensure Reliability: A Focus on Consistency

Instruments are considered reliable if they consistently measure a given trait with **precision.** When a measure is reproducible—that is, when it generates a consistently accurate value every time it is used appropriately—it is considered precise. When a measure is precise, then the reader of a research report has a level of confidence that differences between groups are not explained by differences in the way the trait was measured. Reliability statistics document the degree to which an instrument is stable internally, among individuals, between raters, and over time.

Stability Within an Instrument
Stability within an instrument is called **internal reliability,** and it is measured with the alpha coefficient statistic. This coefficient may be called Cronbach's alpha, coefficient alpha, or internal reliability, and it should have a value of 0.7 or greater. Cronbach's alpha represents the extent to which the variability of individual items represents the variability in the overall instrument (Cronbach, 1951). In other words, the way that responses vary on one item should demonstrate the same pattern as the way that responses vary on the entire instrument. A high level of internal reliability indicates that changes from item to item represent real changes in the subject, rather than simply changes in the way the questions are interpreted (Connelly, 2011).

The coefficient alpha has an additional use: It allows the researcher to calculate the amount of measurement error inherent in the instrument (Buonaccorsi, 2012). Subtracting the coefficient alpha from the value 1 quantifies the error for this sample using this instrument. For example, if the coefficient alpha were 0.92, then measurement error would be equal to 1 minus 0.92, or 8% (0.08). The smaller the amount of measurement error, the stronger the internal validity of a research study. The reverse is also true: When measurement error is high—in general, more than 20% to 25%—then the conclusions of the study may be suspect.

> **Inter-rater reliability:** The extent to which an instrument is consistent across raters, as measured with a percentage agreement or a kappa statistic.

If differences are found, a question arises: Are those differences due to the intervention, or do they reflect inconsistencies in the measurement procedure? From the researcher's perspective, it is desirable to use an instrument that has as large a coefficient alpha as possible so as to minimize the measurement-related differences, thereby ensuring that any differences truly reflect the subjects' responses to the intervention.

Stability Among Individuals

Stability among individuals is measured by an item–total correlation, which should have a positive sign and an absolute value close to 0.5. An item–total correlation indicates whether performance on a single item is consistent with the individual's performance on all items.

Stability Between Raters

Stability between raters is documented as inter-rater reliability or scorer agreement. This specific type of reliability assessment is indicated when multiple raters observe and record a variable. **Inter-rater reliability** quantifies the stability of a measure across raters. For example, the degree of agreement between two or more nurses who are staging a pressure ulcer should be documented.

A simple percentage agreement can be used to document inter-rater reliability, but a kappa statistic is even better. Specifically called Cohen's kappa, this statistic focuses on the degree of agreement between raters and generates a p value, reflecting the statistical significance of the agreement (Cohen, 1968). A kappa value can be interpreted like a percentage, and in either case (percentage agreement or kappa) a value less than 0.40 is considered poor, 0.41 to 0.75 is considered acceptable, and a value greater than 0.75 is considered excellent (Shultz, Whitney, & Zickar, 2014). An associated small p value indicates the agreement was not due to chance. A high kappa (greater than 0.75) with a low p value (less than 0.05) reflects good reliability between multiple raters in an experiment. This finding is particularly important when reviewing evidence for practice, because the same nurse will rarely conduct all assessments on a single patient. Ongoing training and monitoring of raters can improve agreement and reliability between raters over time.

Stability over Time

Stability over time is quantified by a test–retest correlation coefficient. Although the usual standard for any reliability coefficient is 0.7, some measurement experts argue that a lower standard—as low as 0.5—can be applied to test–retest correlations because of the attenuation that naturally occurs over time (Shultz et al., 2014). Test–retest correlation is accomplished by administering an instrument, waiting a reasonable period of time, and then readministering the same instrument. A correlation coefficient may then be calculated between the two sets of item scores.

At least one test of reliability should be performed and reported for the instruments used in an experiment. **Table 8.4** summarizes the primary reliability tests and their

Table 8.4 Reliability Statistics		
Test	**What It Means**	**Interpretation**
Cronbach's alpha/ coefficient alpha	Internal reliability: Are the individual items consistent with the overall test results?	Coefficient alpha should exceed 0.7 as a minimum • < 0.4 is unacceptable • 0.4 to 0.7 is weak reliability • 0.7 to 0.9 is moderate reliability • > 0.9 is strong reliability
Guttman split half/split half alpha	Internal reliability: Is the first half of the test as reliable as the second half, or are odd-numbered items as reliable as even-numbered items?	Split half will be lower than coefficient alpha but should exceed 0.6 as a minimum
Test–retest reliability	Is the instrument stable over time? If the instrument is used repeatedly, are the results due to actual changes in the subject, not due to the instrument?	Yields a correlation coefficient, which should equal or exceed 0.5
Criterion related	Does the instrument measure actual performance or presence of the characteristic it is intended to measure?	Yields a correlation coefficient, which should exceed 0.5
Inter-rater reliability	Do two or more raters agree on the ratings?	Percentage agreement of 0.85 or greater; Cohen's kappa ≥ 0.80 with a p value < 0.05

interpretation. The gold standard is to assess consistency within the instrument and among individuals over time. Efficiency, resources, and time, however, often limit the capacity to run multiple tests of reliability.

If the instrument has been developed by the researcher, it should be pilot tested on a small group of subjects for assessment of reliability. These pilot tests should be performed and reported as part of the methods section of the study report. If a subject participates in the pilot, he or she should be excluded from the primary study to avoid a potential pretesting effect.

An instrument will be only as strong as its reliability. If an instrument does not measure a characteristic reliably, then it cannot be expected to represent the true score for an individual subject (Furr & Bacharach, 2014). Measuring the characteristic accurately requires validity, or assurance that the instrument measures the concept it is supposed to measure.

Ensure Validity: A Focus on Accuracy and Truth

An instrument has to be consistent to be precise, but a measure can consistently measure the wrong thing. For example, it is difficult to measure the length of a neonate.

A squirming baby is measured from the tip of the heel to the crown of the head, which is not exactly a precise description. Measuring over the head to the tip of the nose would be more reliable—it is easy to find the end of the nose—but it would not be an accurate representation of the baby's length. Reliability tells us that an instrument will be consistent; validity tells us that the instrument will consistently measure the right thing.

Reliability constrains, but does not ensure, validity. An instrument cannot be more valid than it is reliable. For example, a scale may weigh kilograms and accurately represent the concept of weight. If the scale consistently weighs light or heavy, however, then the observed score is not matching the true score, no matter how relevant the measure itself. Simply possessing reliability does not ensure validity; separate tests of each attribute are required to draw a comprehensive conclusion about the usefulness of an instrument. Even so, it is not uncommon for reliability to be reported without any comment on validity. In fact, both characteristics are required for a measure if we are to trust the outcome of a study that uses the measure.

The search for a valid measure begins by determining all of the most important aspects of the phenomenon under study. For example, a study of quality of life in hospice patients might include instruments to measure physical symptoms, social support, spirituality, and mental state. Such a study might require multiple instruments to confidently measure all the concepts related to the research question, and each instrument must be reliable and valid.

Validity is more challenging to test than reliability. Complicating this process is the need to test validity on multiple populations to determine who it is valid for and under which conditions. Consider the pain scale shown in **FIGURE 8.2**. This scale shows six faces, with the lowest end being a smile and the upper end being a face with a frown and tears. This instrument is intended to represent the quantity and nature of pain reported by pediatric patients. Is the instrument interpreted the same way by children and by adults? Might some groups of patients interpret the crying face as sadness instead of pain? Does the instrument represent pain for someone with dementia or in rehabilitation or from

> **Validity:**
> The ability of an instrument to consistently measure what it is supposed to measure.

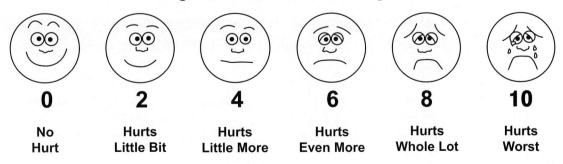

Wong-Baker FACES® Pain Rating Scale

0	2	4	6	8	10
No Hurt	Hurts Little Bit	Hurts Little More	Hurts Even More	Hurts Whole Lot	Hurts Worst

©1983 Wong-Baker FACES® Foundation. www.WongBakerFACES.org
Used with permission. Originally published in *Whaley & Wong's Nursing Care of Infants and Children.* ©Elsevier Inc.

FIGURE 8.2 Wong-Baker Faces Pain Rating Scale

another culture? The validity of the instrument must be tested and retested to ensure it is effective across settings and situations.

A researcher can use several methods to document validity. One or all types may be used in the same study.

Content Validity

Content validity involves a subjective judgment about whether a measurement makes sense. Content validity can mean that face validity has been assessed ("This instrument looks like it should measure pain") or that a panel of experts has verified that the correct concepts are included in the measure.

A helpful tool in determining content validity is the test blueprint. A test blueprint can help the researcher determine if items in the instrument represent all the basic content that must be represented. Often, the test blueprint and the instrument are reviewed by an impartial reviewer, who evaluates whether all the items in the blueprint are reflected in the content of the instrument. Table 8.5 shows a test blueprint for the measurement of fatigue in oncology patients.

Construct Validity

Construct validity indicates that a measurement captures the hypothetical basis for the variable. This type of validity is, as it sounds, abstract and very difficult to confirm, but extremely valuable. Construct validity may be the most important type of validity test to ensure that results will represent reality. Researchers can take years to validate the constructs represented by an instrument.

A common method of construct validation is factor analysis, which groups items within the instrument according to their shared variability (Shultz et al., 2014). The researcher can then review the factor groups and determine whether they represent the conceptual basis of the instrument.

Criterion-Related Validity

Criterion-related validity is the correlation of the instrument to some external manifestation of the characteristic. For example, a newer instrument may be compared with an

Table 8.5 A Test Blueprint for Measurement of Fatigue

Critical Concepts

Physical manifestations	Feeling tired	Drowsiness	Naps in daytime	Nauseated
Emotional reactions	Anxiety	Depression	Shortness of breath	Irritability
Mental state	Difficulty concentrating	Lack of interest	Lack of pleasure	Withdrawn
Vigor and energy	Lack of appetite	Sedentary behavior	Boredom	Lack of well-being

older, more established instrument. There are several ways to measure criterion-related validity:

- Concurrent validity is present when an instrument reflects actual performance. For example, the reading from a temporal thermometer might be correlated with the reading from a rectal thermometer.
- Predictive validity indicates that a measure can predict future performance. For example, an instrument measuring professional competency for a new graduate would have predictive validity if its measurements correlated with the actual competency of the nurse as measured by appraisal at the end of orientation.
- Discriminant validity demonstrates the capacity to differentiate those who have a characteristic from those who do not. An instrument has good discriminant validity if it can successfully sort subjects into classifications. For example, an instrument to measure the presence of a disease would have discriminant validity if it could accurately diagnose a disease when present and also definitively confirm when the same disease is absent.

Sensitivity:
A measure of discriminant validity in the biomedical sciences that indicates an instrument has the capacity to detect disease if it is present.

Specificity:
A measure of discriminant validity in the biomedical sciences that indicates an instrument has the capacity to determine when the disease is not present.

Most validity tests use the correlation coefficient to represent the degree of relationship between the instrument and the reference. Unlike reliability, for which a value of 0.7 is considered the cutoff for acceptability, it is uncommon for a validity coefficient to be greater than 0.5 (Shultz et al., 2014). This outcome may occur for a number of reasons, including inadequate sample size or attenuation due to reliability errors. The seminal work of Cohen (1988) established the standard for interpretation of a validity coefficient: Greater than 0.5 is strong, 0.3 to 0.5 is moderate, 0.1 to 0.3 is small, and less than 0.1 is trivial.

Table 8.6 depicts the various types of validity tests, provides a description of each, and explains the implications for its use.

The correlation coefficient has the added advantage of being the basis for the coefficient of determination, or the amount of variance in the criterion that is explained by this instrument. This value is calculated by squaring the correlation coefficient, represented as r^2. For example, if the correlation coefficient between a reading on a thermometer and a reading of core body temperature were 0.9, then 0.9^2 or 81% of the variance in core body temperature will be explained by this instrument.

Taken together, reliability and validity tests ensure that results are consistent and accurate. Both are key to supporting the internal validity of a research study.

Sensitivity and Specificity

Sensitivity and specificity are measures of validity used in the biomedical sciences because they measure characteristics of diagnostic tools used to detect disease. Sensitivity and specificity are types of discriminant validity. **Sensitivity** is the capacity of an instrument to detect a disease if it is present. A diagnostic tool such as a mammogram, for example, must be sensitive enough to detect breast cancer if it is present. **Specificity** is the capacity of an instrument to determine when the disease is *not* present. A diagnostic tool is specific if it can definitively conclude that the disease is not present when it is not. In other words, sensitivity helps the researcher avoid false negatives, and specificity helps

Table 8.6 Tests of Measurement Validity

Test	How It Is Done	Implications
Face validity	Subject-matter experts review the instrument and conclude that it appears valid.	Accurate conclusions are heavily reliant on the competence of the subject-matter expert. Is considered an essential element of validity testing.
Content validity	Subject-matter experts review the instrument and conclude that the content of the instrument represents the concepts of interest. Often, raters are asked to rate each item as "essential," "useful," or "not necessary" and to give feedback about the usefulness of the overall instrument.	Accurate conclusions are heavily reliant on the competence of the subject-matter expert. Helps determine which items should be included in the final instrument and which may be deleted. Results in feedback on both the content and the form of the instrument.
Criterion related: predictive validity	Correlation or regression statistical analysis is applied to determine if the instrument is correlated to or can predict an objective measure of performance.	Is important for tests that will be used to predict who will be successful (e.g., pre-employment tests or college admission tests) or who will exhibit a condition in the future (e.g., cardiac risk assessment).
Criterion related: concurrent validity	Collect test and criterion scores at the same time. Correlation analysis is applied to determine if the instrument reflects current performance.	Is important for tests of conditions that are difficult, expensive, or painful to detect (e.g., heart disease) or when tests are not available in an appropriate form (e.g., patients for whom English is a second language).
Criterion related: discriminant validity	Collect test and criterion scores. Discriminant analysis is applied to determine if the instrument can accurately sort subjects into groups that do and do not have the criterion condition.	Is important for tests of sensitivity and specificity of diagnostic tests. Is useful when differences between groups are subtle or difficult to detect (e.g., between a B+ and an A– score).
Construct validity	Difficult to evaluate but may be based on studies of group differences, studies of internal structure, factor analysis for subscale structure, or studies of the stability of test scores.	Is best suited to the instances when test scores assess an attribute or a quality that is not easily or objectively measured. Is often used for psychological or social conditions.

the researcher avoid false positives. Both sensitivity and specificity are needed to be confident that the study results accurately represent the distribution of the disease in the sample (Rothman, 2012).

In general, the larger the values of the sensitivity and specificity statistics, the better the test. However, there are tradeoffs: When sensitivity becomes very high, then specificity often suffers, and vice versa. An ideal test will balance sensitivity and specificity, with high scores on each.

Responsiveness

A final assessment of validity for clinical measurements is responsiveness. **Responsiveness** is the ability of a measure to detect change over time in the construct of interest (Cleland, Whitman, Houser, Wainner, & Childs, 2012). When an outcome measure is intended to capture the effect of an intervention, the capability to detect changes in the subject over time is critical. There are multiple ways to measure responsiveness, including the standardized response mean, Cohen's *d*, and responsiveness indices (Jewell, 2010). Responsiveness is a highly desirable characteristic in a measure, particularly when it will be used to determine the effect of interventions over time, and as such is of great interest when developing evidence-based practices.

Collecting Data Using Instruments

Once the specific measures have been selected and their reliability and validity documented, then the data must be collected using the measures. The conclusions from a research study will be only as good as the data on which they are based. The data collection plan, then, is an important step in producing findings that serve as reliable evidence for nursing practice.

Multiple methods are available for data collection. Traditional methods include paper-and-pencil surveys, whose results are subsequently manually entered into analytic software packages. Although paper-and-pencil surveys are still widely used, the contemporary researcher has a wide variety of options for collecting data efficiently and conveniently from subjects, including online and technology-based data collection, interviews, focus groups, and observation.

Online Data Collection

Today's technology enables the researcher to access millions of potential research subjects in geographically diverse sites. The online environment creates opportunities to collect data globally, especially among difficult-to-access populations. Web-based data entry is efficient and effective, and delivered in a way that is convenient for subjects (Walker, 2013). Data processing and analysis are expedited when web-based surveys are used because data can be directly downloaded into analytic software. In addition, the need for data tracking and transfer are eliminated with online data submission processes.

Weigold, Weigold, and Russell (2013) found that online survey distribution resulted in statistically equivalent responses to paper-and-pencil surveys, with reliability, validity, and completeness similar to those of standardized methods. Delivery of surveys as well

Responsiveness: A measure that indicates change in the subject's condition when an intervention is effective.

as receipt of responses is faster with online data collection (Balch, 2010). Callegaro, Manfreda, and Vehovar (2015) identified some of the many advantages of web-based surveys.

- They are low-cost means of delivering surveys.
- The cost does not generally increase with larger sample sizes.
- Web survey software increasingly enables convenient, user-friendly survey design and data collection.
- Data are more likely to be accurately retrieved and analyzed.
- Multimedia use is possible and can make surveys dynamic.
- Online administration provides flexibility in terms of both time and geography.
- Web surveys are convenient for respondents.
- The anonymity of a web survey may encourage more truthful responses, particularly when the subject is a sensitive one.

Online data collection is not without drawbacks, however. When data are submitted remotely, the researcher is unavailable to answer questions, deal with concerns, or troubleshoot problems. Participants may be confused by online data submission systems, resulting in inaccurate or unusable submissions. The researcher may be unable to prevent multiple submissions, or surveys may be abandoned before they are complete. Online systems may ultimately result in systematic sampling error because only those subjects with some level of technological literacy are able to participate effectively in the study (Hsiao & Moore, 2009). Critical problems in using online data submission systems include difficulty in accessing the electronic mail addresses needed to create a sampling frame and the challenges of determining response rates when the actual number of recipients is unknown.

The design and collection of online survey data have been made easier through user-friendly survey applications such as Survey Monkey. With such applications, the survey tool itself is created by using web-based tools, and the data are then downloaded directly into an Excel spreadsheet or a statistical software package for analysis, minimizing data entry error.

Collecting Data Through Social Media

The use of social media and virtual networks to collect data is controversial. The primary concern is the selection bias inherent in using a platform for data collection that is constructed *by* the subject for social purposes, and to which multiple groups will not have access. For example, potential subjects may not have access to the technology required to use social media, may lack Internet connectivity, or may be disinterested in social media applications.

In the best-case scenario, using social media can expand the geographical scope of a study and has been shown to be superior in gaining access to hard-to-reach populations. In particular, snowball sampling—that is, connecting to potential subjects through existing subjects' referrals—is enhanced by access to social media. Social media–based data collection has also demonstrated value in collecting data during disasters or when other means of communicating with subjects are not available.

Even when measurement is not conducted via social media, this platform may enable researchers to recruit subjects through paid advertisements on social media sites. Fenner and colleagues (2012) found a high response rate and relatively low costs for recruitment into a study using social media advertisements, and noted that subjects were highly engaged once recruited in this manner. Thus, there appears to be potential in using contemporary technology and media to access potential subjects, recruit them to the study, and—in some cases—conduct direct data collection via online sites. Until privacy considerations, ethical issues, and self-selection error are reduced, however, social media will remain controversial when used as the sole data collection method for studies. Clearly, although this platform has potential for enhancing access to potential subjects, its ability to facilitate valid data collection requires further exploration.

Technology-Based Delivery

Other technology-based data collection systems are also available to the nurse researcher. Many of these alternative device-based methods are ideal for achieving wide geographic coverage of the target population, are less resource intensive than other data collection methods, and may be superior options for collecting data that deal with sensitive topics (Belisario et al., 2015).

Laptop computers, for example, can allow subjects to respond to surveys or questionnaires efficiently and accurately. The provision of laptop computers may be particularly helpful when data are recorded in association with an interview, or during group meetings, or when it is suspected the subjects will not have access to the Internet. Haller and colleagues (2009) found that laptop data entry was fast and accurate, resulted in fewer errors, and led to less missing data than use of handheld devices or paper-and-pencil surveys for data collection. In addition, technology-based methods have been shown to elicit higher response rates than other methods in reporting risky or sensitive items (Wu & Newfield, 2007) and in rugged or remote environments (Caviglia-Harris et al., 2012). Wireless data collection using tablet devices also holds promise; early data indicate that the convenience of tablet-based data entry makes this method effective for both self-administered and researcher-entered data collection (Singleton et al., 2011).

Handheld digital devices hold promise as means to reach wide audiences and produce valid data. These devices are particularly useful in studies in which frequent—even daily—data collection is required to detect outcomes. Some researchers are using text message reminders to motivate subjects to record activity throughout the day; this method has been successful in gathering longitudinal and experiential data (Moreno, Grant, Kacvinsky, Moreno, & Fleming, 2012). When Belisario et al. (2015) conducted a systematic review comparing survey responses collected using mobile apps versus other methods, they discovered a wide range of implications for mobile data collection. In general, though, apps were shown to improve data completeness more than other types of web-based data collection.

Nevertheless, these novel data collection methods also have some distinct drawbacks. The devices can be expensive, subjects may have devices with widely varying capabilities, and not all individuals will find the devices user-friendly. Researchers have shown that data collection via handheld devices lengthens the duration of data entry while increasing the number of typing errors and the quantity of missing data. Most of the problems with handheld devices are attributable to technical difficulties, typing errors, and loss or theft of the device.

Handheld clicker technology may be an innovative approach to research data collection. Solecki et al. (2010) studied the integration of an audience response system (clickers)

Photovoice:
A method used in participatory action research in which subjects take pictures to exemplify their lived experiences, and record accompanying reflections.

into a presentation asking for participant opinions. Major advantages of this handheld data entry included ease of data collection, real-time analysis, and active engagement of participants. Most clicker technologies also provide summary data and graphics.

A relatively new method for collecting qualitative data about lived experiences is photovoice. Photovoice is a method used with participatory action research, in which subjects take pictures that exemplify their lived experiences. Each photograph is accompanied by reflective writing that describes the participant's thoughts and feelings (Evans-Agnew and Rosemberg, 2016). Photovoice is unique in that it purposefully connects the researcher and the participant in analyzing what is going on in each photograph, and actually engages the subject in determining overall themes from their experiences. It has become an effective means of studying the lived experiences of individuals in the context of their community and daily life (Han & Oliffe, 2016).

Other technologies available for data collection include audio computer-assisted self-interview (ACASI). ACASI is used in place of a personal interview. These systems achieve the advantages of an interview without the time or investment required for real-time, face-to-face data collection. In ACASI, the subject is fed a series of questions by an audio-enhanced computer application, and responses are recorded verbatim. ACASI has been found to be better than face-to-face interviews in eliciting accurate information when the data recorded are sensitive or embarrassing. In one study, individuals who used ACASI were compared to those who participated in face-to-face interviews and those who self-administered a paper-and-pencil survey. The individuals who used ACASI were less likely to have missing data, particularly on measures of sexual risk and alcohol abuse (Anastario, Chun, Soto, & Montano, 2013). This data collection method has also been shown to enhance the validity of self-report data in research and clinical settings by reducing measurement bias and error—a problem that plagues self-reports of all kinds (Brown, Swartzendruber, & Diclemente, 2013).

Although data collection may be maximized by using technology-based data collection, these methods are limited to predetermined surveys, questionnaires, or scales. When exploratory or qualitative data are required to answer the research question, the researcher must use more traditional methods of data collection. Asking questions directly of informants, followed by probing questions (i.e., delving more deeply into the meaning of experiences) requires a face-to-face means of data collection.

When the Data Collector Is the Instrument

Some quantitative studies and almost all qualitative designs require that the researcher collect primary data directly from subjects in the form of words. The most common methods for collecting these kinds of data are interviews, focus groups, and direct observation. In these studies, the researcher is the instrument, and the quality of the data collected depends on the skill of the interviewer, focus group leader, or observer. These techniques are not subject to measures of reliability and validity, but they are still methods in search of truth; thus they require rigor to learn and use effectively.

Interviews are a data collection technique in which the researcher interacts directly with the participant one-on-one via the telephone or in person. The format of the interview can be either highly structured or loosely structured, depending on the information needed. Types of questions may be closed, open-ended, or probing. Each question that is asked should relate back to the research question. Types of questions that might be asked in an interview include the following:

- Information or knowledge questions ("How much do you know about mandatory staffing ratios?")
- Opinion questions ("What do you think about states mandating nurse staffing ratios?")
- Application questions ("How do you develop a schedule that allows for equitable staffing to meet the mandatory levels?")
- Analysis questions ("What do you see as the relationship between staffing levels and patient safety?")
- Synthesis questions ("Which changes would you make to provide an equitable solution to the staffing problem?")

Wording of questions is as important in an unstructured interview as it is in a structured interview or in a questionnaire (Creswell, 2013). In a highly structured interview, questions are developed in the same way as for a questionnaire. For interviews that are less structured, the use of open-ended questions allows the respondent to provide more detailed information. Wording of the questions should be clear and words with double meanings should be avoided. To provide an environment that allows the respondent to answer in a truthful manner, the questions should be as neutral as possible.

The sequence of questions is also important and can set the tone for the interview as a whole. After the introductions, it is important to put the respondent at ease so that he or she is comfortable when responding to the questions. This may be accomplished by asking informational or factual questions that the participant can easily answer. Ask questions about the present before asking questions about either the past or the future. It is often easier to talk about what is current than to recall the past or predict the future.

As the interview progresses, the interviewer should remain as neutral as possible. Once a question is asked, the interviewer should be sure that the respondent has completely

---

SKILL BUILDER Conduct Better Interviews

- Use open-ended words such as "how," "why," or "what."
- Avoid questions that can be answered with a "yes" or "no."
- Avoid words with double meanings.
- Pose questions using neutral words.
- Start with questions that will put the respondent at ease.
- Use initial questions that involve informational or factual questions.
- Intersperse opinion, analysis, application, or synthesis questions with factual questions.

- Ask questions about the present before asking questions about either the past or the future.
- Remain as neutral as possible in both verbal and nonverbal communication.
- Ask only one question at a time.
- Allow the respondent plenty of time, but keep the interview on track.
- Take notes inconspicuously or use a recorder.
- Review notes and make additions or revisions immediately.

answered the question before moving on to ask a new question. Any note taking should be as inconspicuous as possible. Interviews are more personal than questionnaires. Unlike the questionnaire that the respondent completes, interviews give the interviewer the opportunity to ask follow-up questions.

Interviews can be very time consuming, and they are certainly resource intensive. The individual conducting the interview needs to be trained to ask the questions properly, to ask the questions in the proper sequence, and to handle any unanticipated possibilities that might arise during the interview process. Interviews are often used in qualitative studies and provide rich information about the respondents' perceptions and beliefs.

Focus Groups

A focus group is an in-depth, qualitative interview with a small group of people (generally between 6 and 12) who have been specifically selected to represent a target audience. The aim of a focus group is to understand the social dynamic and interaction between the participants through the collection of both verbal and observational data. These interactions often result in richer qualitative data because members of the focus groups can consider their own views in the context of the views of others. Indeed, the interplay of participants in a focus group may reveal ideas, experiences, and meaning that are not apparent when individuals are interviewed in isolation (Liamputtong, 2011). Other advantages of a focus group are as follows:

- The discussion can be recorded with audio, video, or both for later review and transcription.
- The facilitator can observe and note nonverbal behavior, reactions, and interactions of group members.
- Misunderstandings can be clarified immediately.
- Unanticipated but related topics can be explored, and the data from the interview are available immediately.

Although the data gathered through focus group interviews are rich in meaning, focus groups are time consuming and expensive to conduct. Coenen et al. (2012) compared focus groups and individual interviews and found that focus groups took more time than any other face-to-face data collection method. They require a skillful facilitator and often require the presence of two individuals—one to facilitate the discussion and one to record observations and nonverbal behaviors. Focus groups may not elicit accurate information if the facilitator is inexperienced or introduces his or her bias into the discussion. Recording of the group session may feel intrusive to participants and inhibit them from sharing their opinions, and respondents may hesitate to share sensitive information in a group setting. As with qualitative data in general, the results cannot be generalized to larger groups without careful sample selection and reliable content analysis procedures.

Observation

Observational research is used for studying observable behaviors and is generally a noninvasive method for gathering information (Gravetter & Forzano, 2011). There are two types of observation: direct and indirect (sometimes called unobtrusive). With direct observation, participants agree to be part of the research and know that the researcher will be watching them. Indirect observation involves recording data unobtrusively so that the subjects either are unaware of or become accustomed to the observation.

Observations can be made continuously or in specific time periods. Both of these methods involve extended contact with the subjects of the study. Continuous monitoring entails observing a participant or participants and recording in minute detail (manually, electronically, or both) as much of their behavior as possible. One of the drawbacks of this method of data collection is that individuals who know their behavior is being watched will not behave as they normally would until there has been a great deal of exposure. This comfort level—called habituation—takes a long period of time to elicit. As a result, a large amount of data is generated and must be managed. Time periods may be randomly selected for observation so that fewer resources are needed for data collection. With this approach, unlike with continuous monitoring, participants do not know the time or the place that the researcher will be collecting the data, so they are more likely to behave normally. In either case, ethical conduct dictates that the participants be informed that they will be observed, even if they do not know the particulars of where or when.

Table 8.7 summarizes the various methods of collecting data for research studies.

> **Secondary data:** Data collected for other purposes and used in the research study. Examples include electronic health records, employee or patient satisfaction surveys, organizational business reports, and governmental databases.

Secondary Data

Secondary data are often easier and quicker to collect than primary data. **Secondary data** are retrieved from data sets that have already been collected, usually for another reason. Examples of secondary data sources include the following data sets:

- Information documented in the electronic health record (for example, laboratory values or operative reports)
- Public or commercial databases of health data (for example, the renal dialysis data set or the behavioral risk factor data set)
- Registries or other outcomes measurement systems (for example, the National Database of Nursing Quality Indicators or tumor registries)
- Government sources of health data (for example, the Census Bureau or the *Healthy People 2020* database)

Many times, secondary data are recorded for specific research purposes and then made available to the research community after the primary research is complete. Secondary data can reveal important relationships and offer a good way to retrieve data efficiently and effectively.

The key consideration when deciding whether secondary data can be used is to verify that the data set includes measures of the specific variables needed to answer the research question. Secondary data can also improve the quality of subject recruitment and may reduce the time needed for data acquisition (Kopcke et al., 2013).

Although secondary data are attractive owing to their convenience, their use is also hampered by several limitations. Secondary data may be incomplete or inaccurate, and the researcher cannot control the conditions and rules under which they were collected. In addition, the data are necessarily retrospective because they have been collected in the past (Wade & Branningan, 2010).

Table 8.7 Comparison of Data Collection Methods

Method	Advantage	Limitation(s)
Primary Data		
Physiologic	Objective data	Calibration of equipment
Psychometric	Quantifiable data	Access to instrument acceptable for study
		Objective
Survey and questionnaire	Cost effective	Impersonal
	Anonymous	Biased wording
	Easy to administer	Low return rate
	Works with large groups	Literacy barriers
	Familiar	Time consuming
	Allows generalization	
Interview	Flexible	Costly
	Personal	Small numbers
	Nonverbal behaviors	Results cannot be generalized
	Immediate follow-up	
Focus group	In-depth information	Time consuming
	Nonverbal behaviors	Costly
	Trained facilitators	Training time
	Rich data	Results cannot be generalized
		Not useful for sensitive subjects
Observation	Detailed information	Time consuming
	Trained observers	Labor intensive
	Less biased	Training time
Secondary Data	Efficient	Costly
	Increases breadth of the study	Unknown issues with primary data collection
	Multiple uses of data	Concern for accuracy and completeness

The validity of secondary data collection may be enhanced in several ways. The individuals who are retrieving the data should be thoroughly trained in the data collection process. Processes such as quality checks and periodic reassessment of inter-rater reliability should be in place to sustain a high level of reliability. Development of a glossary or data dictionary can help the data collector identify equivalent forms of a single variable and is helpful in maintaining data integrity. For example, the glossary might note that "dyspnea," "SOB," and "shortness of breath" are all acceptable representations of the concept *difficulty breathing.*

In general, the patient record is the best and most sensitive source of objective data regarding patient conditions. Laboratory values, procedures, vital signs, and other documentation of physiologic processes may be accurately retrieved from the record and are highly useful as outcome measures. Electronic health records (EHRs) present unprecedented opportunities for aggregate data mining and reporting. The EHR is a critical component of evidence development and implementation; such systems are capable of supporting comparative effectiveness research. Patient-level data stored electronically can support the processes of generating research questions, conducting comparative assessments, and providing evidence for personalized care (Miriovsky, Shulman, & Abernathy, 2012). Even electronic records, however, must be subjected to quality measures. If the reuse of EHR data for clinical research is to be valid, the researcher must adopt a systematic method of ensuring the record contains accurate and reliable data (Weiskopf & Went, 2013).

Processes that are more subjective may be unavailable or unrecorded in the patient record and are more accurately retrieved via primary data collection. For example, patient education, discharge planning, and counseling may not be recorded consistently in the patient record, but such information can be retrieved directly from patients.

Big Data

The Internet and cloud computing have enabled the collection, storage, and transmission of an enormous quantity of data, which are collectively referred to as "big data." Applying data science methods to these massive amounts of data may produce insights about the patient experience that have not been available in the past (Brennan & Bakken, 2015). These data may originate from a variety of sources: Insurance claims, EHRs, diagnostic images, genomic information, social media, home-based physiologic monitors, and personal fitness devices are just some examples. The exciting potential for obtaining information and data about the health and behaviors of large populations of individuals has stimulated the growth of a new and influential field in evidence-based practice—the fast and flexible association of patient characteristics with patient outcomes.

"Big data" is first and foremost a metric of size, reflecting the idea that today's electronic data sets far exceed those commonly found in research or practice. These data sets reflect a diversity of data types, are collected in near real time, have low error rates, and are of high value to researchers. It is commonly believed that the future of evidence-based practice will experience quantum leaps as analysis of these large-scale data sets accelerates and communication of these results becomes more widespread (Brennan & Brakken, 2015).

The process of using big data begins—as does most evidence-based research—with asking a researchable question. The next step, though, differs from other studies. Rather than defining variables carefully *a priori,* the data schema is defined at the point of use, as data are retrieved and evaluated. Data exploration is a characteristic of data science-driven studies, whereas it is generally not a formal step in a randomized trial. Conclusions are iterative, rather than summative, and are designed to identify convergence rather than to confirm or reject a predetermined hypothesis. The purpose of interpretation in these large data sets is to gain insight, rather than to make a prediction, so these studies resemble descriptive or correlation studies more than experiments.

Codebook:
A guide for the qualitative analysis that outlines individual codes with definitions, criteria for inclusion, and examples.

Baldwin et al. (2015) identify three ways that big data can support evidence-based practice:

- Personalized medicine can be based on the integration of genomics information with EHR data.
- Knowledge dissemination can be optimized when real-time patient data analysis is available to the clinician.
- Big data analytics may eventually allow delivery of information directly to patients, encouraging them to take a more active role in directing their own care.

In the future, the role of big data will become increasingly more important in guiding practice as the characteristics of patients and effects of treatments are assessed on a large scale across whole populations of patients. While these large data sets do not enable researchers to perform true randomized trials, they do provide data about relationships, correlations, associations, and costs that can be invaluable in guiding patient care choices.

Data Management Procedures

During the development of the data collection tool, the researcher makes decisions about the way data will be recorded, including the forms that will be used and the procedures that the data collector will follow. Adequate time should be allocated for data collection. Data collection inevitably takes longer and is more difficult than anticipated. Problems should be expected by the researcher, and procedures put in place to handle common issues that will arise. For example, the data collectors need a procedure to handle incomplete or incorrectly completed forms and questionnaires.

Before initiating data collection, the researcher must develop a **codebook** for data definitions. Coding is the process of transforming data into numerical symbols that can be easily entered into the computer. For example, a researcher might code "gender male" as 1 and "gender female" as 2. Included in the codebook are definitions of variables, abbreviations for variables, and the range of possible values for the variables. In addition to the codebook, a file is established that contains copies of all scales, questionnaires, and forms used in the study.

The original data forms as well as a copy of the database should be stored for 5 years. Storage of data serves several purposes. Most importantly, the data are available to document the validity of the analysis and the published results of the study. The data also may be used as secondary data for subsequent studies or aggregate analyses.

Reading About Measurement and Data Collection

In the report of a study, the measurement section is generally identified in a straightforward way and labeled "measures." Other words may appear in the heading, such as "methods and measures" or "measures and materials." The measures may be called "instrumentation" or "tests." In any event, the measurement section should be an easily identifiable part of the write-up. If the measurement is complex, the write-up may have a separate section for measurement procedures, which may be labeled as such or called "protocols." This section may describe the specific steps for measuring variables and may include photographs or figures to support an objective process.

The researcher should summarize the concepts that were the focus of the measurement. The instruments and their content should be clearly linked to the research question and to the conceptual and operational definitions of the variables. It is helpful to make a list of all variables, identifying those that are descriptive, independent, and dependent.

At a minimum, calibration and/or internal reliability should be reported for any instruments used in the experiment. The study becomes stronger as more documentation of the reliability and validity of the instrument are provided. The tests and their actual results should be reported; jointly they are called the *psychometric properties* of the instrument.

If a survey is used, a separate section should describe the development of the instrument as well as its pilot testing. Unless the properties of the instrument have been determined, the results obtained with its use are suspect. Author-developed instruments should be subjected to the same scrutiny as publicly available tests. If the instrument has been used before, then information about its reliability and validity should be provided with the description of the instrument. The actual statistics should be reported, along with the names of the tests that were run.

It is not uncommon to see instruments that, from a statistical standpoint, are considered borderline acceptable. This does not mean that the researcher has designed the measurement strategy poorly, but rather that strengths and weaknesses of the measures have, by necessity, been balanced against each other. Many factors in instrument use should be considered in addition to the reliability and validity properties. Feasibility of administration, costs of instruments, and the type of measures considered professionally acceptable also drive the selection of an instrument.

The author of the research report may describe the instrument rather than provide a copy, but this practice is not considered a weakness. The instrument may be copyrighted or proprietary, or limitations on the length of publication may preclude its inclusion. The author should give enough information that the reader could determine how to obtain a copy of the instrument. The source of instrument or a citation for its publication should be included.

Finding the data collection section of a research report should be relatively easy. It is usually labeled "methods," "procedures," or "protocols." The description of the data collection procedure should be clear and complete enough that a relatively well-informed reader should be able to replicate it.

Each protocol—whether it deals with the measurement process or the documentation of the results—should be outlined. It is here that the researcher should identify the data as primary or secondary. The protocol should outline what was collected, who collected it, which instrument or questionnaire was used, and how the data were recorded. If the researcher was not the individual doing the actual data collection, the methods for training the data collectors should be described.

Using Measurements from a Research Study

Research procedures may be applied to practice just as research findings are. For example, instruments for measuring patient responses to interventions may be used by the clinician to monitor the effectiveness of nursing interventions, diagnose patient problems, and measure outcomes.

Bolton et al. (2009) conducted a literature search and reviewed the use of measurement instruments as evidence in nursing practice. The evidence commonly supported the use of patient risk-assessment tools to detect complications and prevent patient harm.

For example, prediction rules for risk of falls or for early signs of oversedation can be extremely helpful in clinical nursing practice.

Instruments should be reevaluated if they are applied to radically different problems, populations, or practice settings than those for which they were originally developed. For example, an instrument intended for the measurement of anxiety may not be useful in a study of panic disorder. Conversely, this instrument may measure preoperative anxiety as well as anxiety disorder. Repeated use and testing of the instrument strengthens the ability to apply the instrument to different problems.

An instrument should also be reevaluated before it is used in a different setting than the original one. For example, an instrument intended for use in acute care may not be applicable in a skilled nursing care setting; measures used in inpatient settings may not be relevant to outpatient settings. Testing the instrument's properties in a new setting prior to its use can verify its applicability in diverse settings.

Finally, an instrument should be rechecked before it is used in a different population. Instruments written in English may not be reliable when translated into another language, for example, and tests used with one age group may not be effective with younger or older groups. Because the reliability and validity of an instrument are specific to the sample used, these attributes should be checked with a pilot test before application of the instrument to practice.

Of course, the instrument itself should be acceptably reliable and valid before its use is considered in any setting—either research or practice. Finding suitable measures is also critical to creating valid nursing research projects.

WHERE TO LOOK FOR INFORMATION ABOUT THE MEASUREMENT STRATEGY

- A thorough description of the measurement procedures should appear in the methods section.
- The measures may be called "instrumentation," "tools," or "tests." If the measurement procedure is complex, it may have its own section called "protocols" or "procedures."
- Physiologic measures that are not standard may have accompanying photographs or figures to depict the measurement procedure.
- If a survey is used, a separate section may describe the development of the instrument, any pilot tests that were conducted, and the procedures for its completion by subjects.
- Information about reliability and validity should be provided with the description of the instrument.
- Description of the psychometric properties of the instrument should appear regardless of whether the instrument was developed specifically for the study or was an existing tool.
- It is not unusual for the author to describe the instrument rather than providing a copy; this is not a weakness. The survey may be copyrighted or proprietary, or limitations on the length of the article may preclude its inclusion.
- The measurement strategy should be explained in sufficient depth that the reader could re-create the measure with accuracy. If the instrument is a survey, an explanation of content and scales should enable the reader to grasp the concepts measured by the survey.
- Data collection methods should be easily identifiable and included as a major part of the research study write-up. The description may be concise, but it should provide enough detail that an informed reader could replicate the data collection procedure.
- If the data collection was complex, there may be a separate section for procedures, which may be labeled as such or may be called "protocols." This section should describe the specific steps followed for collecting and recording the data. On occasion, photographs may be used if procedures are not easily described with words.

GRAY MATTER

The following considerations drive selection of instruments used in research studies:

- Reliability properties
- Validity properties
- Feasibility of administration
- Acceptability for the subjects
- Instrument costs
- Professional acceptance of types of measures

CHECKLIST FOR EVALUATING THE MEASUREMENT STRATEGY

- ❏ The instruments are clearly linked to concepts in the research question.
- ❏ Instruments and measures are described objectively.
- ❏ The reliability of the instrumentation is described and supporting statistics are provided.
- ❏ The validity of the instrumentation is described and supporting statistics are provided.
- ❏ A detailed protocol for the use of each instrument in the measurement is described.

Creating Measures and Collecting Data

A strong measurement strategy involves a systematic approach to linking the concepts in the research question to a specific manifestation as a measure. This process begins by breaking down the research question into underlying concepts. For each concept, an operational definition is written. An operational definition gives a clear, unambiguous description of the steps needed to quantify the characteristics of a population. Table 8.8 depicts the process of translating a research question into operational definitions.

Table 8.8 Translation of a Research Question into Operational Variables		
Research Question	**Concepts**	**Operational Variables**
Do patients in hospice care who report fatigue have more physical symptoms than similar patients who do not report fatigue?	Hospice care Fatigue Physical symptoms	Hospice care: Patients who have been admitted to a home-based hospice care service based on a physician's assessment that their condition is terminal and they are within 6 months of death Fatigue: Reports of feeling tired and/or drowsy that disrupt the subject's life, as measured by the Fatigue Disruption Score of the Fatigue Symptom Inventory Physical symptoms: The number of symptoms reported, as manifested by physical, emotional, mental, or vigor scales of the Edmonton Symptom Assessment Scale

Once the concepts in a question are defined, a search for an existing instrument is carried out. Although instruments may be found in many locations, it is always best to start with a literature review. The literature can help identify potential instruments and their psychometric characteristics as well as point to experts in the field. The ideal situation is the discovery of a suitable instrument that has already been validated and determined to be reliable. When actual test statistics are reported, the researcher can be comfortable using the instrument for measurement of similar concepts in similar settings and patients. Finding an existing instrument is a highly efficient tactic that reduces the complexity of a study. Using an existing instrument makes the study consistent with previous studies and, therefore, easier to compare via the systematic review process. Using standard measures helps the study make a strong contribution to evidence-based practice. In addition, grants and publications are often based on having credible procedures, represented by strong, established measures.

It is rare, however, to find an instrument that meets the exact purposes of the researcher. As a consequence, the efficiencies of existing, imperfectly matched instruments must be balanced with the fact that they may be outdated or may not measure the concepts of interest exactly. The selection of an instrument always entails a balance between efficiency and accuracy.

The choice of the data collection method depends on the specific information needed to answer the research question and the resources available to the researcher. Given the wide variety of data collection methods available, the nurse researcher must use a systematic approach to navigate the choices that must be made in developing a strong data collection system. Harwood and Hutchinson (2009) recommended the following steps, which can help the researcher develop a sound data collection approach:

- Define the purpose of collecting the data.
- Select a feasible data collection approach.
- Select a delivery method that is appropriate for the study design and the subjects.
- Write realistic, reliable, and thorough protocols for collecting the data.
- Design forms and instruments for collecting valid and reliable data.
- Train staff in data collection methods and/or write clear instructions for subjects to guide data submission.
- Develop a plan to manage data and transfer them to analytic software.

SKILL BUILDER   Develop a Strong Measurement Strategy

Every measurement system has some inherent error—particularly when the measure is applied to unique human beings in applied settings. The following list highlights ways to minimize measurement error through instrument selection and research design:

- Select measurement instruments that have been developed and tested over time. Look for measures that have been administered to large,

diverse samples and in multiple studies. Continued testing and refinement of an instrument tend to decrease measurement error, increase reliability, and ensure validity. Standard measurement instruments also allow aggregation of results into evidence-based practice.

- Develop a custom instrument only as a last resort. Attempt to find an existing instrument, even if it does not match the study goals exactly. An existing instrument may be modified, a subset of items or scales may be used, or questions may be added to customize the instrument to the study. Be sure to contact the author for permission before altering an instrument. These actions require that the revised instrument be pilot tested again for reliability and validity.

- Standardize the measurement methods. Develop guidelines for using the measurement instrument, including verbatim instructions to be given to subjects who complete surveys individually. Use photographs and drawings if necessary; in addition, media such as video demonstrations may be used to train data collectors. The smaller the variability within measures, the stronger the reliability of the measure.
- Train and certify observers and data collectors. Minimize the risk of error from multiple raters by ensuring they maintain a consistent and complete approach to data collection. Measure inter-rater reliability and do not allow data collectors to conduct measures independently until they have achieved a preset competency level.
- Automate data collection. Use data from existing sources for efficiency and quality. Develop data definitions to ensure the data retrieved from different databases are identical in content.
- Repeat measures. Efficiency can be increased even more if the data collector has the capacity to measure several times and take a mean value. This advantage must be balanced with the disadvantage of the pretesting effect, which affects repeated administrations of a test.
- Blind the data collectors. The Hawthorne and testing effects can contribute to rater bias just as they can affect subject responses. Data collectors who are unaware of group assignment will yield more objective results with less inter-rater error.

The feasibility of a data collection approach is a practical, yet critical aspect of measurement to be considered. The complexity of the study, the resources available to the nurse researcher, the characteristics of the target population, and the skills of the research team are all important when determining whether a particular data collection system will be a realistic option.

The delivery method for data collection should be consistent with the goals of the study and the research question. Qualitative studies typically involve focus groups, interviews, or participant observation. Quantitative studies may use biological measurements, surveys, questionnaires, or observation. Responses to surveys and questionnaires may be collected via laptop computer, handheld data device, paper-and-pencil tools, online data submissions, or social media.

Once a feasible approach and delivery method have been selected, the researcher must write thorough protocols for the data collectors to follow. These protocols should be clear and unambiguous; all steps of the data collection process should be spelled out in detail. Asking an individual who is unfamiliar with the research plan to carry out the data collection procedure can be a useful exercise that reveals where the instructions are confusing or unclear. The plan should be tested until the researcher is sure it cannot be misinterpreted.

If the data are to be self-reported or an instrument will be self-administered, then clear directions should be developed for the subjects. Writing the directions in simple, straightforward language will support the completeness and accuracy of the responses.

Forms for collecting the data also need to be developed. These may range from questionnaires to surveys to entry logs. The forms should be self-explanatory and efficient to complete. Training data collectors in the procedures and use of the forms is essential to ensure the accuracy and completeness of the data collected via these forms. Periodic monitoring for quality control is necessary even when data collectors have been trained; measures to ensure ongoing accuracy and completeness are particularly critical in lengthy studies (Harwood & Hutchinson, 2009).

The final step of the data collection plan is the transfer of raw data for analysis. The content of web-based or computer-based data entry systems is often directly transferrable to analytic software programs. In contrast, data from paper-and-pencil surveys and questionnaires must be entered manually to be prepared for analysis. Quality monitoring for data entry errors should be a part of the data management plan.

A NOTE ABOUT QUALITATIVE DATA

Qualitative research is generally not concerned with a measurement strategy. In qualitative research processes, the researcher is the measurement instrument, so reliability is directly related to his or her skill at eliciting and describing information. Qualitative data are the outcome of a naturalistic inquiry that bases results on the analysis of meaning, generally in words; thus, there is little reliance on numbers. Nevertheless, qualitative researchers are interested in the pursuit of truth, and to the extent that data collection represents truth, qualitative research is also concerned with sound data collection.

Summary of Key Concepts

- Measurement is the process of quantifying characteristics that can answer the research question. The measurement strategy involves defining the research question in conceptual and operational terms and finding instruments to express these characteristics as variables.
- Data collected as primary data are solicited directly from the subject for the specific purpose of the research study. Secondary data collection involves retrieving information from data sets that were originally collected for purposes other than the research.
- Measurement error can be random or systematic. It may be due to human factors, problems with the instrument, variation in procedures, or data processing error. Random error is expected in a research study, but systematic error will bias the results.
- Reliability is a reflection of the consistency with which the instrument records the measure. It may take the form of calibration with technology or tests of reliability with other kinds of instruments. Instruments may have internal reliability, reliability across subjects, reliability among raters, or reliability over time.
- Instruments must be reliable if they are to be valid. Validity indicates the extent to which a measure accurately measures what it is supposed to measure. Types of validity testing include content validity, construct validity, and criterion-related validity.
- The reliability and validity of an instrument are the most important characteristics, and they should be documented in the research report. Using an existing instrument

is desirable for its efficiency and the capacity to provide a comparison with existing studies.

- Data collection methods are employed to gather information in a systematic way. Data used in quantitative studies will be of a numeric nature and subject to statistical analysis. Data used in qualitative studies will be of a text-based nature and subject to coding.

- The most commonly used types of data collection are physiologic measurement, psychometric instrumentation, surveys and questionnaires, interviews, focus groups, and observation.

- The most widely used data collection method is the survey. In this approach, a systematic measurement instrument is used to gather information directly from respondents about their experiences, behaviors, attitudes, or perceptions.

- Other data collection methods include paper-and-pencil tools, online means, computer-based technologies, social media, handheld devices, audio-delivery devices, and mining of "big data." Each has specific advantages and disadvantages that should be aligned with the goals of the research study.

- Interviews and focus groups can help the researcher gather rich data directly from the respondent and allow the researcher to explore topics as they arise. The drawbacks of these methods are their time-consuming nature and the demands they place on the facilitator's skill level.

- Qualitative research is concerned with discovering truth, so it focuses on the trustworthiness of the data.

CRITICAL **APPRAISAL EXERCISE**

Retrieve the following full-text article from the Cumulative Index to Nursing and Allied Health Literature or similar search database:

Girgin, B., & Cimete, G. (2016). Validity and reliability of the neonatal discharge assessment tool. *Journal for Specialists in Pediatric Nursing, 21,* 74–83.

Review the article, focusing on the section that describes the testing of the instrument. Consider the following appraisal questions in your critical review of this research article:

1. How did the authors determine the sample size needed for an adequate test? Did they achieve an adequate sample size?
2. Which descriptive data were collected to test the instrument? How did the authors minimize error in this phase of data collection?
3. Which elements of reliability were tested? Were these the appropriate tests for the proposed use of this instrument? Why or why not?
4. The authors tested reliability more thoroughly than they tested validity. Was the validity testing plan adequate? Why or why not?
5. Was the reliability of the instrument acceptable for application as evidence for practice? Was the validity of the instrument acceptable for application as evidence for practice?
6. How might this information be used to affect nursing practice?

References

Anastario, M., Chun, H., Soto, E., & Montano, S. (2013). A trial of questionnaire administration modalities for measures of sexual risk behavior in the uniformed services of Peru. *International Journal of STD & AIDS, 24*(7), 573–577.

Balch, C. (2010). *Internet survey methodology.* Boston, MA: Cambridge Scholars Publishing.

Baldwin, J., Bootman, J., Carter, R., Crabtree, B., Piascik, P., Edoma, J., & Maine, L. (2015). Pharmacy practice, education, and research in the era of big data: 2014–15 Argus Commission Report. *American Journal of Pharmaceutical Education, 79*(10), 1–11.

Belisario, M., Jamsek, J., Huckvale, K., O'Donoghue, J., Morrison, C., & Car, J. (2015). Comparison of self-administered survey questionnaire responses collected using mobile apps versus other methods. *Cochrane Database of Systematic Review,* Issue 7. Art. No.: MR000042. doi: 10.1002/14651858.MR000042.pub2

Bolton, L., Donaldson, N., Rutledge, D., Bennett, C., & Brown, D. (2009). The impact of nursing interventions: Overview of effective interventions, outcomes, measures, and priorities for future research. *Medical Care Research and Review, 64*(2 suppl), 123S–124S.

Brennan, P., & Bakken, S. (2015). Nursing needs big data and big data needs nursing. *Journal of Nursing Scholarship, 47*(5), 477–484.

Brown, J., Swartzendruber, A., & Diclemente, R. (2013). Application of audio computer assisted self-interviews to collect self-reported health data. *Caries Research, 47*(1), 40–45.

Buonaccorsi, J. (2012). *Measurement error: Models, methods, and applications.* Norway: Chapman & Hall.

Callegaro, M., Manfreda, K., & Vehovar, V. (2015.) *Web survey methodology.* Los Angeles, CA: Sage.

Carle, A. (2010). Mitigating systematic measurement error in comparative effectiveness research in heterogeneous populations. *Medical Care, 48*(6 suppl), S68–S74.

Caviglia-Harris, J., Hall, S., Mullan, K., Macintyre, C., Bauch, S., Harris, D., . . . Cha, H. (2012). Improving household surveys through computer-assisted data collection: Use of touch-screen laptops in challenging environments. *Field Methods, 24*(1), 74–94.

Cleland, J., Whitman, J., Houser, J., Wainner, R., & Childs, J. (2012). Psychometric properties of selected tests in patients with lumbar spinal stenosis. *Spine Journal, 12*(10), 921–931.

Coenen, M., Stamm, T., Stucki, G., & Cieze, A. (2012). Individual interviews and focus groups in patients with rheumatoid arthritis: A comparison of two qualitative methods. *Quality of Life Research, 21*(2), 359–370.

Cohen, J. (1968). Weighted kappa: Nominal scale agreement with provision for scaled disagreement or partial credit. *Psychological Bulletin, 70*(4), 213–220.

Cohen, J. (1988). *Statistical power analysis for the behavioral sciences* (2nd ed.). Hillsdale, NJ: Lawrence Erlbaum.

Connelly, L. (2011). Research roundtable: Cronbach's alpha. *MedSurg Nursing, 20*(1), 45–46.

Creswell, J. (2013). *Research design: Qualitative, quantitative, and mixed methods approaches* (4th ed.). Thousand Oaks, CA: Sage.

Cronbach, L. (1951). Coefficient alpha and the internal structure of tests. *Psychometrika, 16,* 297–334.

DeVellis, R. (2011). *Scale development: Theory and applications.* Thousand Oaks, CA: Sage.

Evans-Agnew, R., & Rosemberg, M. (2016). Questioning photovoice research: whose voice? *Qualitative Health Research, 26*(8), 1019–1030.

Fain, D. (2014). *Reading, understanding, and applying nursing research* (4th ed.). Philadelphia, PA: F. A. Davis.

Fenner, Y., Garland, M., Moore, E., Jayasinghe, Y., Fletcher, A., Tabrizi, N., & Wark, D. (2012). Web based recruiting for health research using a social networking site: An exploratory study. *Journal of Medical Internet Research, 14*(1), e20.

Furr, R., & Bacharach, V. (2014). *Psychometrics: An introduction.* Thousand Oaks, CA: Sage.

Gravetter, F., & Forzano, L. (2011). *Research methods for the behavioral sciences.* Independence, KY: Engage Learning.

Guttman, L. (1947). Scale and intensive analysis for attitude, opinion, and achievement. In G. Kelly (Ed.), *New methods in applied psychology* (pp. 173–180). Baltimore, MD: University of Maryland.

Haller, G., Haller, D., Courvoisier, D., & Lovis, C. (2009). Handheld vs laptop computers for electronic data collection in clinical research: A crossover randomized trial. *Journal of the American Medical Informatics Association, 16*(5), 651–659.

Han, C., & Oliffe, J. (2016). Photovoice in mental illness research: A review and recommendations. *Health, 20*(2), 110–126.

Harwood, E., & Hutchinson, E. (2009). Data collection methods series: Part 5: Training for data collection. *Journal of Wound, Ostomy, and Continence Nursing, 36*(5), 476–481.

Hsiao, E., & Moore, D. (2009). Web-based data collection. *TechTrends, 53*(6), 56–60.

Jewell, D. (2010). *Guide to evidence-based physical therapist practice* (2nd ed.). Sudbury, MA: Jones and Bartlett.

Kopcke, F., Kraus, S., Scholler, A., Nau, C., Schuttler, J., Prokosch, H., & Ganslandt, T. (2013). Secondary use of routinely collected patient data in a clinical trial: An evaluation of the effects on patient recruitment and data acquisition. *International Journal of Medical Informatics, 82*(3), 185–192.

Liamputtong, P. (2011). *Focus group methodology: Principles and practice.* Thousand Oaks, CA: Sage.

Likert, R., & Hayes, S. (1957). *Some applications of behavioral research.* Paris, France: UNESCO.

McHugh, M. (2012). Interrater reliability: The kappa statistic. *Biochemical Medicine, 22*(3), 276–282.

Miriovsky, B., Shulman, L., & Abernathy, A. (2012). Importance of health information technology, electronic health records, and continuously aggregating data to comparative effectiveness research and learning health care. *Journal of Clinical Oncology, 30*(34), 4243–4248.

Moreno, M., Grant, A., Kacvinsky, L., Moreno, P., & Fleming. M. (2012). Older adolescents' views regarding participation in Facebook research. *Journal of Adolescent Health, 51*(5), 439–444.

Morrow, J., Mood, D., Disch, J., & Kang, M. (2015). *Measurement and evaluation in human performance* (5th ed.). Champaign, IL: Human Kinetics.

Moses, T. (2012). Relationships of measurement error and prediction error in observed-score regression. *Journal of Educational Measurement, 49*(4), 380–398.

Rothman, K. (2012). *Epidemiology: An introduction.* New York, NY: Oxford University Press.

Shultz, K., Whitney, D., & Zickar, M. (2014). *Measurement theory in action: Case studies and exercises* (2nd ed.). Thousand Oaks, CA: Sage.

Singleton, K., Lan, M., Arnold, C., Vahidi, M., Arangua, L., & Gelberg, L. (2011). Wireless data collection of self-administered surveys using tablet computers. *Annual Symposium Proceedings/AMIA Symposium Proceedings,* 1261–1269.

Solecki, S., Cornelius, F., Draper, J., & Fisher, K. (2010). Integrating clicker technology at nursing conferences: An innovative approach to research data collection. *International Journal of Nursing Practice, 16*(3), 268–273.

Wade, T., & Branningan, S. (2010). Estimating population trends through secondary data: Attractions and limitations of national surveys. In J. Cairney (Ed.), *Mental disorder in Canada: An epidemiological perspective* (pp. 73–91). Toronto, ON: University of Toronto Press.

Walford, G., Tucker, E., & Viswanathan, M. (2013). *The Sage handbook of measurement.* Thousand Oaks, CA: Sage.

Walker, D. (2013). The Internet as a medium for health service research. *Nurse Researcher, 20*(4), 18–21.

Weigold, A., Weigold, I., & Russell, E. (2013). Examination of the equivalence of self-report survey based paper and pencil and internet data collection methods. *Psychological Methods, 18*(1), 53–70.

Weiskopf, N., & Went, C. (2013). Methods and dimensions of electronic health record data quality assessment: Enabling reuse for clinical research. *Journal of the American Medical Informatics Association, 20*(1), 144–151.

Wu, Y., & Newfield, S. (2007). Comparing data collected by computerized and written surveys for adolescence health research. *Journal of School Health, 77*(1), 23–28.

Chapter 9

Enhancing the Validity of Research

CHAPTER OBJECTIVES

The study of this chapter will help the learner to

- Define internal and external validity as applied to research.
- Explain why validity is an essential component of research that is to be used as evidence.
- Compare the concept of validity in quantitative research to the concept of trustworthiness in qualitative research.
- Identify threats to internal and external validity in quantitative studies.
- Determine threats to trustworthiness in qualitative studies.
- Appraise strategies that will control threats to the validity or trustworthiness of a research study.

KEY TERMS

Applicability and transferability	Historical threats	Replicability
Attrition	Instrumentation	Subject selection
Audit trail	Internal validity	Testing
Bracketing	Maturation	Treatment effect
Consent effect	Member checking	Triangulation
Effect size	Multiple-treatment effect	Type I error
Experimenter effect	Novelty effect	Type II error
External validity	Population validity	

Introduction

Whether developing a research study, reading a research report, or contemplating the use of research findings, the challenge is to determine whether the intervention or manipulation of the variables actually causes the desired outcome or result. **Internal validity** refers specifically to whether the researcher and the reader can be confident that an experimental treatment or condition made a difference—and whether rival explanations for the difference can be systematically ruled out. Internal validity is about the strength of the design and the controls that were placed on the experimental situation. In

Internal validity:
The confidence that an experimental treatment or condition made a difference and that rival explanations were systematically ruled out through study design and control.

External validity:
The ability to generalize the findings from a research study to other populations, places, and situations.

contrast, **external validity** refers to how generalizable the results are and to whom. External validity is about applicability and usefulness of the findings.

For example, we might want to know if a particular exercise and diet program results in a significant weight loss, and that no other reasons account for the weight loss except the exercise and diet program. If the findings of this research are credible and trustworthy, we will also want to know if the results can be generalized to a different or larger population.

The seminal work on the minimal conditions necessary to provide adequate evidence of a causal relationship between an intervention and an outcome was first published in 1965. Called the Bradford Hill Criteria, or Hill's criteria for causation, this list of requirements can be daunting. While Hill's criteria are still widely accepted, their application is debated. **Table 9.1** provides the full list of Hill's criteria.

To be used as evidence, research need not meet all of these criteria, as long as some fundamental conditions are met. Before determining if a causal relationship exists between the outcome and the intervention, these three most important conditions must be met:

- *Changes in the presumed cause must be related to changes in the presumed effect.* If the treatment is changed in any way, the outcome will change. In the example, if the exercise and dietary program are changed in any way, the weight loss will change.
- *The presumed cause must occur before the presumed effect.* In other words, the treatment or intervention must occur before the outcome. The weight loss must occur after the exercise and dietary program is introduced. This may seem obvious, but many researchers hold up correlational research as evidence of causal

Table 9.1 The Classic Hill's Criteria for Causality

Criteria	Meaning
Strength (effect size)	While a small change does not mean there is no causality, a big change is more likely to be causal.
Consistency (reproducibility)	Replication of findings by different researchers with different samples strengthens the likelihood of an effect.
Specificity	The more specific an association between an intervention and its effect, the greater the probability it is a causal relationship.
Temporality	The intervention has to precede the outcome.
Biologic gradient	Greater levels of intervention lead to greater levels of an outcome.
Plausibility	A theoretical link between the intervention and the outcome can be articulated.
Coherence	Consistency between highly controlled laboratory results and those in applied settings indicate causality.
Experiment	Documented experimental evidence as demonstrated by statistical analysis leads to a causal conclusion.
Analogy	If similar factors have similar effects, causality is supported.

Data from Hill, A. (1965). The environment and disease: Association or causation? *Proceedings of the Royal Society of Medicine, 58*(5), 295–300.

relationships. A correlation means two events are related to each other—but tells us nothing about sequence. This sequence must be verified before a causal relationship can be established.

- *There are no plausible alternative explanations.* No other factors could be responsible for the outcomes. In the example, nothing can have occurred that might have caused the weight loss except the prescribed exercise and dietary intervention (Hartung & Touchette, 2009).

Minimizing Threats to Internal Validity

Good research designs reduce the possibility that alternative explanations for the results might exist. These alternative explanations for the outcome are often referred to as threats to internal validity. Several methods can be used to minimize threats to internal validity:

- Measurement or observation
- Use of appropriate design
- Control of bias
- Statistical analysis

Measurement or Observation

Measurement or observation is one possible method to rule out threats to internal validity. This method can demonstrate that the threat either does not occur at all or occurs so infrequently that it is not a significant alternative explanation. In a study designed to determine the effects of music on agitation in a sample of hospitalized patients with dementia, for example, the music did reduce agitation. An alternative explanation for this outcome may have been the effect of visitors on these patients. However, observation and measurement of the number and frequency of visitors could reveal that this was a rare event for this sample.

Use of Appropriate Design

Most research questions can be examined using various designs. However, some designs are not appropriate for dealing with the specific requirements of a research problem. If the researcher wishes to determine whether music is effective in reducing anxiety in patients undergoing radiation therapy over time, a repeated-measures design might be effective, whereas a survey might not reveal any significant effects of the music intervention. An observational study might be appropriate if the researcher is concerned about the effects of ibuprofen on activity levels in a population of senior citizens; however, the same design will not be appropriate if the researcher is concerned with the subjects' perceptions of pain with activity. Choosing the correct design to answer the research questions is fundamentally necessary to control threats to internal and external validity.

Control of Bias

Good design is also dependent on the control of bias. Bias exists in all research. It can occur at any time in the process and in any research designs, and is difficult to eliminate—but it can be controlled (Smith & Noble, 2014). Controlling for bias requires careful

VOICES FROM THE FIELD

As part of my graduate work, I participated in a research grant project that examined the role of risk taking in work-based injury. The eventual goal was to figure out a public health intervention to reduce risky behaviors. We designed a descriptive study; the study was planned by an interdisciplinary group of mental health therapists, public health nurses, and occupational health physicians. Phase I of the study involved recruiting men and women to assess their attraction to risk behaviors so that we could establish a baseline of typical behaviors. The baseline measures, then, would become the basis for determining whether an intervention had an effect in Phase II of the study. The first study was intended just to gather a descriptive baseline, so it seemed pretty straightforward.

Subjects were recruited through a newspaper ad. We were offering a small stipend in exchange for about an hour of time with noninvasive data collection, so we expected we would get a pretty good response, and we did. We were a bit concerned that a compensated subject might not be representative, but we hoped to get a big sample size to overcome that threat. We had good funding, so we were more concerned about Type II error than we were about sampling error. We scheduled more than 200 individuals for 20 different time slots over a 5-day period. We planned to accomplish the data collection in "stations," where the subject would progress from one spot to the next to provide all of the necessary data. With this process, we still needed five data collectors present at any given time. The assessment was pretty thorough and required the presence of a trained data collector, so it was quite the feat to choreograph.

On the day of the first planned data collection, it began to snow. It snowed so hard that the snowplows could not keep up, and businesses and schools were closing left and right. We managed to keep our data collectors around all day, but the subjects only started trickling in after lunch. We got a lot of cancellation calls. We talked about canceling the next day, but put off a decision until the morning. We figured if we could get there, then clients could get there, too.

Only about half of our data collectors made it in, and we were actually quite busy. It was clear, though, as the day progressed that we were not getting a representative population. We were obviously not collecting a baseline of risk-taking behavior in a public health population. Instead, we were collecting data from young adult males who owned four-wheel-drive vehicles and really needed 25 bucks. We were studying risk-taking behaviors in a population most likely to take risks.

The team had a quick consult and decided to stop the study, even though resources had already been expended. We decided that the flawed results were unlikely to warrant funding for Phase II and would not serve to inform the following study. It was a terrible disappointment to set it all up again—to back up and essentially start over. I thought, "What bad luck." It was a really well-designed study that was totally derailed by the weather.

Glenna Andrews, DrPH, RN

consideration of where bias might be expected to exert effects in the research process. Bias is introduced into research studies through five major areas:

1. Study design: When there is an incongruence between the aim of the study and its design, the likelihood of bias is increased. This disconnect may be due to the researcher's personal beliefs or greater familiarity with particular designs.
2. Selection and participation: The way the sample is selected and assigned to treatment groups can introduce sampling error into a study.

3. Data collection and measurement: Measurement bias can occur when assessment tools are not objective, valid, and reliable. Interviewing—a common means of qualitative data collection—can be influenced by bias in both question construction and the way the question is asked.
4. Analysis: It is a natural instinct to look for results that support a preconceived notion of effectiveness. Selective reporting of data can cause bias when data that are accurate but inconsistent with the researcher's beliefs are discarded.
5. Publication and dissemination: Studies are more likely to be published if they have statistically significant findings. Qualitative studies can suffer from publication bias when findings are not presented clearly and in depth (Smith & Noble, 2014).

Blinding can minimize bias, but it is not always possible in all studies. Using more than one observer or interventionist can help control for bias, but it can also produce experimenter or inter-rater reliability effects. This is a common problem that threatens the internal validity of research—protecting against one type of bias has the associated effect of creating another type of bias. Balancing the risk becomes a task for the researcher.

Self-selection bias can be a threat to a good design and can produce misleading results. Differences exist between subjects who volunteer to participate in a research study and those who are randomly selected, and these differences may not be immediately apparent (Knottnerus & Tugwell, 2014). For example, the results of a study to determine the effects of prayer on anxiety in presurgical patients might be skewed by individuals who pray regularly. A carefully constructed demographic questionnaire might help to reduce this threat.

A similar concern arises if subjects self-select into the control and intervention groups. For example, subjects who believe that massage will benefit their joint pain might choose to have the treatment, increasing the risk that a placebo effect might occur. Conversely, subjects who are skeptical of the effects of massage might elect to avoid the treatment, creating artificially negative results. Randomization into groups can greatly reduce this risk.

A broad range of potential methods and designs exists, and each option protects against some kind of bias (Savovic et al., 2012). Although randomized controlled trials are commonly held up as the strongest in terms of controlling bias, even they have potential sources of bias that must be accounted for. When threats to validity cannot be eliminated or controlled, then their effects must be quantified. Statistical analyses can help determine the amount of error and variability that is introduced by uncontrolled threats to validity.

Statistical Analysis

Statistical analyses can support the internal validity of a study by quantifying the probability of Type I and Type II error. The reader can then determine if the amount of error calculated for the study is acceptable, or whether the results should be used only cautiously in practice. The researcher can also support validity and clinical application of a study's results by calculating and reporting tests of effect size. Finally, valid conclusions are drawn when data meet the fundamental assumptions of the statistical tests used to analyze them.

Type I error:
Often called alpha (α) and referred to as the level of significance; the researcher erroneously draws a conclusion that the intervention had an effect.

Type II error:
Often called beta (β) and related to the power of a statistical test; the researcher erroneously draws a conclusion that the intervention had no effect.

Determining the Probability of Type I and Type II Error

Before accepting results as evidence for practice, the probability that an error was made should be evaluated. This assessment enables the researcher to quantify the role of error in the outcome. There are two types of error: Type I and Type II.

Type I error occurs when the researcher draws a conclusion that the intervention had an effect when, in fact, it did not. Type I error usually reflects weakness in the study design, because the cause of Type I error is usually an uncontrolled extraneous variable. Type I error is considered a serious flaw and threatens the overall internal validity of a study. An example of a Type I error is the following:

> Two groups of students were taught statistics using two different methods. The data indicate that Group A achieved significantly higher scores than Group B. However, Group A included subjects with higher math ability, and the teaching methods did not make a difference. Drawing a conclusion that the teaching method caused the result in this case is a Type I error. The differences in the scores were not based on the teaching methods, but rather were caused by extraneous variables (previous math ability).

A Type I error is called alpha (α). The term *level of significance* is simply the phrase used to indicate the probability of committing a Type I error. The maximum acceptable level for alpha in scientific research is generally 0.05; however, 0.01 may be chosen if the decision has important consequences for treatment. Alpha is set by the researcher *a priori*, meaning before the experiment begins. Its level is based on a thoughtful consideration of the stakes of being wrong. For example, an intervention that is intended to improve self-esteem might have an acceptable error rate of 5%; a test of a tumor-killing drug might more appropriately have a 1% error rate. Alpha is used as a standard of comparison for the *p* value, or the probability of a Type I error, that is yielded by most inferential statistical tests. When the calculated probability of a Type I error (the *p* value) is less than the acceptable level of a Type I error (alpha), then the test is considered to be statistically significant. Type I error is quantified, then, by the *p* value.

Type II error is the acceptance of a false null hypothesis or the statement that there are no differences in the outcome when, in fact, there are differences. An example of a Type II error is as follows:

> A study was conducted to determine whether breastfeeding or bottle feeding contributed to greater maternal fatigue in the first 30 days after birth. The researchers were able to recruit 30 breastfeeding mothers into the study, but only 6 bottle-feeding mothers consented to participate. No differences were found between the groups. The research reflects a Type II error in that a difference may have been present, but the small size of the sample did not enable the researchers to discover it.

A Type II error is called beta (β). The probability of obtaining a significant result is called the power of a statistical test; a more powerful test is one that is more likely to detect an outcome of interest. Type II error can occur when an experiment has insufficient power. It means that a treatment was effective, but the experiment did not reveal this condition. The best way to control Type II error is to ensure that the sample is large enough to provide sufficient power to the experiment to illuminate the findings. Type II error is calculated as 1-beta, or 1-power. For example, if the sample enables the researcher to document 90% power, then the probability of Type II error affecting the outcome is 10%.

The nurse may consider the question, "Which type of error is worse?" In health care, Type I error is generally considered more serious; such an error will lead the researcher to believe an intervention is effective when it is not. Focusing solely on tight controls of Type I error, however, means that significant findings may be overlooked. The relationship between Type I and Type II error is paradoxical: As one is controlled, the risk of the other increases. Both types of error should be avoided. Missing the opportunity to apply an effective treatment because its effects cannot be detected is unfortunate for patients and researchers alike. The best approach is to carefully consider and control sources of bias, set the alpha level appropriately, use an effective sampling strategy, and select a solid design for the question. Getting all these elements aligned requires a balancing of risks and benefits that is the task of the primary researcher. **Table 9.2** contrasts Type I and II errors and gives examples of each.

Calculating and Reporting Tests of Effect Size

Effect size must also be considered when evaluating the validity of a study. **Effect size** refers to how much impact the intervention or variable is expected to have on the outcome. Even though an experiment might yield statistically significant results, these may not translate into clinically important findings. An example of the impact of effect size is the following:

> Researchers want to determine the effects of aerobic exercise on heart rate in a sample of subjects with chronic supraventricular tachycardia (SVT). The researchers are specifically measuring the relationship between aerobic exercise and heart rate. If the relationship is strong, an effect will be detected even with a small sample size. Conversely, if it is determined that exercise has little effect on heart rate in patients with chronic SVT, a much larger sample would be needed to find any significant changes in heart rate in this study.

Large effect sizes enhance the confidence in findings. When a treatment exerts a dramatic effect, then the validity of the findings is not called into question. In contrast, when effect sizes are very small, the potential for effects from extraneous variables is more likely, and the results may have less validity (Diamond & Kaul, 2013).

Ensuring Fundamental Assumptions Are Met

Data analysis is based on many assumptions about the nature of the data, the statistical procedures that are used to conduct the analysis, and the match between the data and the procedures. Erroneous conclusions can be drawn about relationships if the assumptions of the statistical tests are violated. For instance, many statistical analyses assume that the data obtained are distributed normally—that is, that the population is distributed according to a normal or bell-shaped curve. If this assumption is violated, the result can be an inaccurate estimate of the real relationship. Inaccurate conclusions lead to error, which in turn affects the validity of a study.

Effect size: The size of the differences between experimental and control groups compared to variability; an indication of the clinical importance of a finding.

Table 9.2 Type I Versus Type II Errors

Example	Type I Error	Type II Error
A study is designed to test the effects of hydrotherapy on anxiety during the first stage of labor. All women who present to a single birthing center are invited to participate. Women are allowed to choose whether they use hydrotherapy.	Anxiety is reduced in the treatment group. BUT: All the women who choose hydrotherapy have a birth coach present. Is the reduction due to the hydrotherapy or to another cause (e.g., having a birth coach)?	Anxiety is not reduced in the treatment group. BUT: All the women who choose hydrotherapy have a higher level of anxiety prior to labor. Is the lack of response because the hydrotherapy does not work, or because the mothers had more anxiety to begin with?
A researcher tests the effects of a virtual preoperative tour of the surgical suite on postoperative length of stay in the postanesthesia care unit (PACU). During preadmission testing, patients are given an Internet access code that enables them to enter a virtual tour site. On admission, the subjects are assigned to a treatment group or a comparison group based on their self-report of completing the tour.	Length of stay in the PACU is shorter in the group whose members used the virtual preoperative tour. BUT: All the parents who took the virtual tour have personal computers and a higher level of socioeconomic resources than the control group. Is the shorter length of stay due to the virtual tour or to factors related to increased health because of socioeconomic advantage?	Length of stay in the PACU is no shorter in the group whose members used the virtual preoperative tour. BUT: All the patients who did not take the tour experienced previous surgery and so were already familiar with the surgical suite. Is the length of stay no shorter because the tour did not have an effect or because the control group did not really need it?
A nurse evaluates the effects of an evening backrub on the use of sleeping aids. Patients are randomly assigned to an experimental group or a control group. Patients in the experimental group are given a nightly backrub; patients in the control group are not.	Patients who receive the backrubs need fewer sleep medications. BUT: During the 10 minutes that the backrub is given, the nurses interact quietly with the patients about their concerns and treatment issues. Is the difference due to the backrub or the extra attention and counseling of the nurse?	Patients who receive the backrubs do not need fewer sleep medications. BUT: Only 10 patients assigned to the control group stayed more than one night, so the overall sample size was fewer than 25 subjects. Was the lack of a difference because the backrub had no effect or due to inadequate power to detect a difference?

Factors That Jeopardize Internal Validity

A good research design controls for factors that might potentially jeopardize the validity of the study results. A host of events and actions can threaten the researcher's ability to draw accurate conclusions about the effects of interventions. If these characteristics are measurable, they may be called extraneous variables. Many times, however, the effects of factors that affect the trustworthiness of results are not detected until after the experiment is complete, and they cannot be controlled or quantified.

The presence of factors that jeopardize internal validity does not necessarily mean the study is a weak one; almost all studies have some rival explanations for results. However, the rigorous researcher attempts to predict those factors that might logically be expected to affect the outcome of the study and takes action to prevent as many of their effects as possible.

GRAY MATTER

Threats to internal validity may include the following:
- History
- Maturation
- Testing
- Instrumentation
- Consent
- Treatment
- Multiple treatments
- Subject selection
- Attrition

Historical threats:
A threat to internal validity because of events or circumstances that occur during data collection.

Maturation:
A threat to internal validity because the changes that occur in subjects do not happen as a result of the intervention, but rather because time has passed.

Testing:
A threat to internal validity due to the familiarity of the subjects with the testing, particularly when retesting is used in a study.

Historical Effects

Historical threats refer to events or circumstances that occur around the time of the introduction of the intervention or that occur at any time during data collection. Although the event itself may be entirely unpredictable, it can be expected to exert an effect on the subjects and, as a result, the study conclusions.

Maturation Effects

Maturation in a research study is related to changes that occur in subjects over time but are not a result of the intervention or attribute being studied. Subjects can change for a variety of reasons, such as normal aging, physical growth, acquisition of knowledge and skills outside the study variables, or physical changes related to a disease process. For example, when studying the effects of relaxation techniques on the management of pain in patients with bone metastasis, the effects of the techniques will be minimized as the disease worsens.

Maturation is a particular concern in populations that are expected to change over time and in longitudinal studies. For example, populations that include children, individuals with chronic diseases, or the elderly are prone to the effects of maturation, particularly if measures are taken over an extended period of time.

Testing Effects

The threat of **testing** is related to the effects of taking a test and then retesting the subject. Subjects can become more proficient at test taking based on repeated experiences. For

Instrumentation:
A threat to internal validity that occurs because the instrument or data collection procedure has changed in some way.

Consent effect:
A threat to internal validity that occurs because the subjects who consent to the study may differ from those who do not in some way that affects the outcome of the study.

Treatment effect:
A threat to internal validity because subjects may perform differently when they are aware they are in a study or as a reaction to being treated.

example, the effects of different types of educational methods on the retention of skills necessary to manage central lines in the intensive care unit could be measured with a knowledge test. If the test were administered immediately following the instruction and then repeated within 2 weeks, results may indicate there is a large difference in the retention of knowledge and skills based on the educational method, so the conclusion is drawn that the methods made a difference. However, the results may be due to the subjects having seen the test before, rather than the effects of the teaching method. Methods to reduce the risk of this threat include scheduling the retesting at longer intervals and retesting subjects using a different test.

Instrumentation Effects

Instrumentation effects may occur because the instrument or data collection device has changed in some way. This can also be a threat when the data are collected by multiple individuals. In a study designed to determine if 3-year-old males exhibit aggressive behavior more frequently than 3-year-old females in a playgroup, for example, the observers may need to use specific criteria to score or count aggressive behaviors. If Observer 1 scores any physical contact as aggressive, but Observer 2 considers only hitting and kicking to qualify as aggressive, the resulting data will not be valid. Instrumentation-related threats can be reduced by training the observers carefully, using very specific protocols, and testing inter-rater reliability.

Consent Effects

Sometimes those subjects who consent to participate in a study may be different from those who do not consent in systematic ways, a factor known as the **consent effect**. The differences between participants and nonparticipants have been measured in multiple clinical trials and reported in at least two systematic reviews. El Emam, Jonker, Moher, and Arbuckle (2013) found as many as nine different demographic values that were different between those subjects who consented to participate in a study and those who did not; these variables clearly could introduce bias into a study. On average, in the systematic reviews, slightly more than half of the potential subjects consented to join the study (55.5%). This average dropped to 39% when subjects were asked if their responses could be audio-recorded—an important consideration in the design of qualitative studies, in which verbatim recording is often employed (Henry et al., 2015).

Treatment Effects

Subjects may react to the treatment itself, even if it does not exert a therapeutic effect. In this kind of **treatment effect**, the treatment itself may elicit a response that cannot be differentiated from a physiologic response. This threat to internal validity is the primary reason for the use of randomly assigned control groups and comparison groups.

Sometimes subjects in a study may perform differently because they know they are in a study. In such a case, changes occur in the subjects not because of the intervention, but rather because the subjects behave differently than they would normally—a phenomenon also referred to as the Hawthorne effect. The Hawthorne effect has been documented extensively, yet little is known about the conditions under which it occurs, the mechanisms and types of effects, or the magnitude of these effects (McCambridge, Witton, & Elbourne, 2014). It is so widely documented that it can be expected to exert some influence in nearly every interventional study that is accompanied by some level of informed consent.

As an example, consider an intervention designed to increase self-efficacy in patients who receive chemotherapy. All subjects were recruited into the study and randomized into either the intervention group or the control group. A pretest measure of self-efficacy was administered to all the subjects. All the subjects met with the researcher. However, the control group received written literature about chemotherapy, whereas the experimental group received a focused, structured intervention designed to increase self-efficacy. The posttest revealed that subjects in both the control and experimental groups demonstrated a statistically significant increase in self-efficacy, which could have simply been related to the subjects' awareness of being in a study.

The Hawthorne effect is of great concern if the researcher is in a position of perceived authority—as in leadership studies or when physicians lead research teams—so that subjects act in ways they perceive are desirable. Because of ethical concerns, however, it is difficult to control for this threat. Subjects need to be informed that they are in a study. Nevertheless, it is possible, with institutional review board (IRB) approval, to inform subjects that they are in a study but to be less explicit about what is being studied. The consent rate has been documented to be lower when explicitly worded consents are used (El Emam et al., 2013). In a study to determine the correlation among suffering, self-transcendence, and social support in women with breast cancer, for example, the instrument used to measure suffering was called the Life Experience Index rather than a measure of suffering. The concern was that calling it "suffering" might influence the responses.

Multiple-Treatment Effects

When multiple treatments are applied at the same time, it is difficult to determine how well each of the treatments works individually. Perhaps it is the combination of the treatments that is effective. Another concern is the effect of the order in which the treatments or interventions are administered. This concern about the sequence of events is particularly worrisome in interventional studies, where confirmation that the independent variable precedes the dependent one is important.

For example, a researcher might decide to study the effects of a skin cream applied manually to prevent skin breakdown. The cream is applied using circular massage. Patients receiving the cream treatment have a lower pressure-ulcer rate than patients who do not. However, this difference may be due to the act of massaging the area and not simply attributable to the application of the cream. Multiple-treatment effects threaten validity because they make it impossible to determine the unique contribution of each treatment to the outcome.

Selection Effects

Subject selection refers to the biases that may result in selection or assignment of subjects to groups in a way that is not objective and equitable. Selection effects can be exerted by the researcher through the sampling strategy or by subjects during the recruitment

Multiple-treatment effect:
An inability to isolate the effects of a treatment because multiple treatments are being used at the same time.

Subject selection:
A threat to internal validity due to the introduction of bias through selection or composition of comparison groups.

Attrition:
A threat to internal validity resulting from loss of subjects during a study.

Population validity:
The capacity to confidently generalize the results of a study from one group of subjects to another population group.

period. The more specialized the population under study, the more difficult it may be to recruit a representative pool of subjects. In a study to compare two smoking cessation treatment programs, for example, if Group A has 40 females and 10 males and Group B has 56 males and 4 females, there may be gender differences in response to the treatment programs. Randomization or random assignment to study groups counters this threat.

Attrition

Attrition refers to the loss of subjects during a study. For example, a longitudinal study to examine the effects of different types of exercise on weight loss began with 100 subjects but ended with only 44. Those who stayed in the study may have been more motivated to exercise, or they may have been more physically active before participating in the project. Other subjects could have moved, become ill or injured, or been unable to continue the study for a host of other reasons.

Some attrition is expected in any study. This type of risk becomes a concern when validity of the results is affected, such as when attrition is excessive or when the loss of subjects is systematic. Attrition risk can be avoided by taking the following steps:

- Advising subjects of the time commitment in advance
- Screening participants who might be likely to drop out of the study (e.g., those who have no computer)
- Making it convenient to continue participating
- Using technology-supported visit reminders
- Providing upfront scheduling (Page & Persch, 2013)

If and when subjects do leave the study, the researcher should determine the reason for their exit. An analysis and discussion of the reasons for attrition can help the researcher determine if the loss from the subject pool will result in systematic sampling error. For example, if all the individuals who leave the study do so because their illness worsens, then the study will be left with only those subjects who are less ill, so its internal validity will be compromised.

Factors That Jeopardize External Validity

External validity refers to the generalizability of the findings of the research to other settings or populations. The researcher should ask, "Can these findings be applied to other people or places?" For example, a study exploring the relationship of smoking to physical activity might not obtain the same results with a group of rural adolescents as it does with a group of adolescents from an urban setting.

Population validity refers to generalizing the findings from the sample to a larger group or population. For example, population validity is present if a study conducted on a group of 100 adults can be generalized to all adults with similar characteristics. If the sample is drawn from an accessible population, rather than the target population, however, generalizing the research results from the accessible population to the target population is risky. If the study is an experiment, then potentially different results might be found with subjects of different ages, ethnicities, or genders. A study of the effects of a support group on suffering in a population of women with lung cancer, for example, might reveal that subjects who attend support groups report lower levels of suffering—yet those findings might not be applicable to a population of males or even other females who are suffering due to causes other than lung cancer.

The extent to which the results of an experiment can be generalized from the set of environmental conditions created by the researcher to other environmental conditions is sometimes called ecological validity. This issue is a concern with experiments or interventional studies. Is the setting in which the study was conducted similar to or different from other settings? The setting may differ in terms of its geographic location, population characteristics, or level of care. For example, results from a study completed in an intensive care unit may not be generalizable to a rehabilitation unit.

Both population and ecological validity are important considerations when appraising research as evidence for nursing practice. The nurse must determine if the results are appropriate for application to a specific setting and group; this requires consideration of the effect of threats to external validity and the extent to which they were controlled.

GRAY MATTER

Threats to external validity may include the following:
- Selection effects
- Time and historical effects
- Novelty effect
- Experimenter effect

Selection Effects

As could be surmised, the selection of subjects is the process that will most strongly influence external validity. External validity is enhanced when subjects represent the population closely, so using a strong sampling strategy will enhance external validity. Sometimes, however, it may be impossible to gain access to a broad representation of the entire population. For example, suppose a researcher studying the effects of early ambulation on nausea can recruit subjects from only a limited geographic area. The effects of the location, setting, and types of patients who are accessible will subsequently affect the breadth of generalizability of the results from that study. The way the sample is selected, then, is a primary consideration in the evaluation of evidence for application to a specific practice.

The electronic health record has introduced a new source of potential threats to validity, particularly in regard to selection of subjects. Most studies have data sufficiency requirements; in other words, a subject's electronic record must be complete to be included. Rusanov et al. (2014) discovered significant bias toward sicker patients when sampling patients using a data sufficiency requirement. Although this requirement limits missing data, it affects both the type and the quantity of data that are subsequently collected.

Novelty effect:
A threat to external
validity that occurs
when subjects react
to something because
it is novel or new,
rather than to the
actual treatment or
intervention itself.

Experimenter effect:
A threat to external
validity due to
the interaction
with the researcher
conducting the study
or applying the
intervention.

Time and Historical Effects

Researchers should be cautious about transferring results obtained during one time period to a different time period. The conditions for the two time periods could be quite different. For example, the results of an intervention to teach new mothers how to feed a newborn in 1995 will not apply in 2014. The length of the hospital stay has been greatly reduced since the mid-1990s, and the amount of teaching time available may make the teaching method used in the older study ineffective.

Another threat to external validity is the amount of time it takes for an intervention or treatment to take effect. It is possible that the effects of the treatment or intervention might not become evident until weeks after the intervention is administered. In such a case, a posttest conducted immediately after an intervention might show no significant changes in the subjects. By comparison, if testing is done in 3 months, significant changes may be detected. For example, suppose an exercise intervention was introduced to a sample of older adults. Quality of life testing was conducted after 2 weeks of the exercise program but did not reveal any significant improvement in reported quality of life. However, when the same subjects were tested 60 days after continued participation in the exercise program, their self-reported quality of life might be significantly higher.

Novelty Effect

It is possible for subjects to react to something simply because it is unique or new. The treatment or intervention does not cause a change in such a case, but the subjects respond to the **novelty effect**. In a study to determine if online synchronous chat rooms were productive means to hold clinical postconferences, the initial response of the students was very positive; in only a few weeks, however, the attendance and response dropped dramatically. Conversely, it is possible that subjects will not change because the intervention is too new, but they will adjust to it over time. In the same project, using asynchronous discussion groups was unsuccessful at the start of the project, but as time passed, students adjusted to this method of conferencing and participation increased significantly in terms of both quantity and quality.

Experimenter Effect

It is also possible for subjects to react to the experimenter or researcher, such that the results could be very different if another individual conducts the study or applies the intervention. In a study of the sexual behavior of middle adolescents, for example, the response rate was approximately 25%. The researcher was a middle-aged Caucasian female, and the subjects were 15- to 17-year-old African American males in a high school in a major urban area. The surveys were incomplete, and the responses appeared to be random. When the same survey was administered by a 22-year-old African American male, the response rate was 88%, the surveys were completed, and the responses were appropriate. **Experimenter effects** pose a threat to external validity because the intervention may be effective only when applied by a particular kind of individual.

Balancing Internal and External Validity

It is the researcher's obligation to design and carry out studies in a way that maximizes both internal and external validity. However, just as the risks of Type I and II errors must be balanced, so the researcher is also challenged to find ways to control internal and external validity without compromising either one. The paradoxical relationship between the two types of validity makes this a formidable task.

Internal validity is supported by systematic, objective procedures carried out on randomly selected, large samples in tightly controlled settings. A review of the characteristics described in the previous sentence makes it clear that the more internal validity is controlled, the more artificial the study becomes. This artificiality limits external validity or generalizability. Nurse researchers function in applied settings with subjects who do not often behave in prescribed ways, and care is rarely delivered in laboratory settings. Finding a balance of control and usefulness is a constant challenge for creating research as evidence for nursing practice.

Trustworthiness in Qualitative Research

Many nursing research questions are best answered using a qualitative approach. The intent of qualitative research is to interpret, rather than to test, interventions. Qualitative research is sample specific and is not intended for generalization. The concern for internal and external validity, then, is not as paramount in the design of qualitative research.

Qualitative researchers are still concerned with representing reality accurately and in searching for truth, so creating confidence in the researcher's conclusions is still important. That is where the simple comparisons end, however. Qualitative researchers use different terminology, and there is disagreement among researchers about the concept of validity in qualitative research. Some believe validity is not compatible with the philosophy of qualitative research, whereas others argue that efforts to produce validity increase the credibility of the findings.

One set of authors found more than 100 sets of published criteria for the assessment of qualitative trustworthiness (Schou, Hostrup, Lyngson, Larsen, & Poulsen, 2012). They simplified the standards for evaluating a qualitative study so that only four categories of quality criteria were applied to assess the key elements of trustworthiness: credibility, transferability, dependability, and confirmability. Even so, 30 individual rating items were needed to draw conclusions about the usefulness of a study for application to practice, and nurses had difficulty applying some items reliably.

The controversy over the credibility of qualitative research focuses on the inherent bias in qualitative research and has led to a search for other means to ensure the results of such studies can be trusted. Pareira (2012) suggests that new standards for evaluating validity are needed in qualitative research. She suggests a combination of standards that address both the strength of the methods and the quality of the research experience. The terms "plausible," "believable," and "trustworthy" are generally used when discussing the validity of findings in qualitative studies; these terms reflect the premise that the findings can be defended when challenged.

Applicability and transferability:
The feasibility of applying qualitative research findings to other samples and other settings.

Replicability:
The likelihood that qualitative research outcomes or events will happen again given the same circumstances.

Some threats to the validity of quantitative studies jeopardize the validity of qualitative studies as well. For example, the Hawthorne effect, selection effects, and historical events may affect subjects in both types of studies. Nevertheless, some unique factors must be considered when judging the appropriateness of qualitative findings.

Although generalization is not a goal of qualitative research, the **applicability and transferability** of the findings is of great interest as evidence for practice. The researcher should provide an explicit description of the sample and setting so the reader can decide if this research can be applied to other samples. There is no test of significance in qualitative research. Instead, the in-depth description of the characteristics of the subject/sample being studied may allow one to conclude the extent to which it is comparable to other subjects/samples. If the subjects and sample are comparable, then one would be more comfortable transferring the results to other people or places. If it can be argued that what is being observed does not depend on the context or setting, then it might be transferred to other contexts. This conclusion enables the nurse to use the results as evidence in a dissimilar setting with more confidence.

Replicability enhances the trustworthiness of the results. The credibility of qualitative studies is supported if findings are confirmed by others, much like any other kind of research. However, this is not a simple process. Replicating a qualitative study is very difficult to accomplish because the original study is conducted in the natural setting, which will invariably change if the study is carried out with other populations or in other places. Any attempts at replication should be accompanied by a thorough discussion of the similarities and discrepancies between the two study settings and populations.

The qualitative researcher can take specific action to enhance the trustworthiness of the results and conclusions of such a study. A thoughtful consideration of potential threats to credibility can help the researcher plan reasonable methods to minimize their effects.

Strategies to Promote the Validity of Qualitative Research

Just as threats to validity must be considered and managed in quantitative design, so factors that may jeopardize the credibility of qualitative studies should be recognized and addressed. Qualitative research design is usually an emergent process, however, so many decisions are made as the study unfolds that will strengthen the reader's confidence in the findings. Certain characteristics are shared by all strong qualitative studies regardless of the specific type of qualitative design.

GRAY MATTER

The following methods promote the validity of qualitative research:
- Prolonged or varied field experience
- Use of verbatim accounts and triangulation
- Participant feedback
- Bracketing
- Audit trail

Prolonged or Varied Field Experience

Whenever possible, qualitative researchers should collect data over an extended period of time to allow the researcher to get an accurate picture of the phenomenon being studied. For example, a study examining the work environment in a critical care unit should account for the fact that the atmosphere may vary from day to day and over the course of a 24-hour period, as well as from nurse to nurse. Interviews to understand the experience of working in critical care should be done at many different times, on different days, and with different nurses to capture these variations.

Verbatim Accounts

Qualitative researchers should be careful to keep accurate field notes and to report results as direct quotes to avoid making inferences. Descriptions should be as close as possible to the participants' accounts. This fidelity in reporting ensures that the meaning that is captured is the respondents', not the researcher's interpretation of it.

Triangulation is the researcher's use of multiple sources to confirm a finding. In other words, isolated incidents and perceptions should not be the basis for drawing conclusions, but rather patterns of responses that appear frequently. To meet this criterion, the themes will be identified in the words of several respondents or identified in multiple ways (e.g., words, documents, and observations). Cross-checking information and conclusions using multiple data sources to increase understanding, use of multiple research methods to study a phenomenon, and the use of multiple researchers can increase the credibility of the results (Bekhet & Zauszniewski, 2012).

Participant Feedback or Member Checking

The procedure for obtaining participant feedback, which is also called member checking, involves discussing interpretations and conclusions with the participants. Checking the accuracy of the observations directly with subjects ensures that the researcher's interpretations and observations reflect what the participants actually meant. This step is essential to determine that the researcher has captured the real meaning of the data and has not interjected bias into the conclusions.

Bracketing the Researcher's Bias

Qualitative researchers are less concerned with bias than quantitative researchers are. Research conducted in an interpretive manner in a natural setting has inherent bias that is expected and accepted in qualitative research as long as it is not careless or excessive. Even so, the researcher should still critically examine personal biases and inclinations that might affect interpretation of the data.

Bracketing is a strategy used to control bias. A researcher who is aware of his or her own biases and makes them explicit is less likely to succumb to them—in other words, the effects of the bias are "put in brackets" so they can be set aside. The researcher must also bracket any presumed knowledge about a subject or topic during data collection and data analysis (Noble & Smith, 2015). The researcher needs to be open to ways in which gender, age, ethnicity, religion, politics, and other factors might affect the interview, observations, or participation in the project. A qualitative study by nature is unlikely to

Triangulation: A means of enhancing credibility by cross-checking information and conclusions, using multiple data sources, using multiple research methods or researchers to study the phenomenon, or using multiple theories and perspectives to help interpret the data.

Member checking: A method of ensuring validity by having participants review and comment on the accuracy of transcripts, interpretations, or conclusions.

Bracketing: A method of limiting the effects of researcher bias and setting them aside by demonstrating awareness of potential suppositions of the researcher.

Audit trail:
Detailed documentation of sources of information, data, and design decisions related to a qualitative research study.

be 100% objective; however, efforts should be made to convince readers that a high level of objectivity has been maintained.

Documentation of an Audit Trail

Documentation in qualitative research includes field notes and reports, interpretations, and thorough descriptions and reports of feedback. Careful records must be kept of each of these sources of information. In addition, the emergent nature of the design requires constant decision making, with a record of the rationale for each choice. This record of data and decisions constitutes an **audit trail** that allows the researcher to describe procedures and defend the results. A conscientious audit trail can also aid in replication of the research in other settings or populations. Records should be accurate, thorough, and complete. Strategies to ensure that these standards are met include writing early and often, including primary data in the final report, using rich descriptions, and getting frequent feedback on the documentation.

CHECKLIST FOR EVALUATING THE VALIDITY OF A RESEARCH STUDY

If the effects of an intervention are tested:
- ☐ Changes in the outcome are associated with changes in the intervention.
- ☐ The researchers clearly demonstrate that the intervention preceded the outcome.
- ☐ The researchers identified potential rival explanations and eliminated, controlled, or accounted for them.

To assess the role of bias:
- ☐ The researcher was blinded to group assignments.
- ☐ The primary researcher did not collect data.
- ☐ Subjects were selected using objective criteria and assigned to groups randomly.
- ☐ If the research took the form of a qualitative study, the author explicitly described a bracketing process.

Threats to internal validity/trustworthiness:
- ☐ Extraneous variables were identified and controlled.

- ☐ Historical events did not occur during the study that would affect the outcome.
- ☐ Maturation was not an alternative explanation for the results.
- ☐ If testing and retesting were involved, the time interval between tests was adequate to avoid a testing effect.
- ☐ Attrition from the study was not excessive or systematic.
- ☐ If a qualitative study, the author demonstrated:
  - Prolonged contact
  - Use of verbatim accounts
  - Triangulation
  - An audit trail

Threats to external validity/transferability:
- ☐ The sample was selected to maximize representativeness.
- ☐ The setting in which the study was done is adequately described to determine applicability.

Reading a Research Study to Determine Validity

Unfortunately, there is no section of a research report labeled "Validity." Instead, the reader must evaluate the validity of the design and determine whether the results obtained are believable. Nevertheless, it is possible to analyze a report in a systematic manner to determine which potential threats to validity exist, what the researcher did to control the threats, and whether these efforts were successful.

Two places where the reader can find information about the primary controls for validity are in the methods and procedures sections, where sampling, measurement, and analysis are described. The way samples are selected, responses are measured, and data are managed can all inhibit or enhance validity.

Most authors will describe the factors that jeopardized validity from their point of view. This description is usually found in the "Discussion" or "Conclusions" section, but it may appear in a separate section labeled "Strengths and Limitations." The list of factors may not be all-inclusive and is often subjective. Ultimately, it is the readers' obligation to determine whether the results apply to their patients and setting. Some studies will have very few threats that affect them; others will have multiple threats. There is no magic number of "acceptable threats." Some threats are also more important or have more damaging effects than others.

Replication of studies compensates for threats to internal validity. Studies that have been replicated many times, yielding similar results, have the highest level of validity and, therefore, constitute very strong evidence for practice. Studies that aggregate and review multiple studies, such as meta-analyses, systematic reviews, and integrative reviews, compensate for many threats to internal validity and provide the strongest evidence for practice.

Determining whether the researcher has controlled threats to validity can be a matter of judgment. Validity is an inexact concept that involves balancing controls with the risks of making errors. Achieving this balance is demanding, so weaknesses are inevitably discovered when a study is scrutinized. Because validity is one of the key characteristics of a study that determines whether it is strong evidence for practice, however, a critical eye is required. Internal validity instills confidence that an intervention will produce an effect; external validity means it can be used for the greater good; trustworthiness means findings can be applied to broader groups. All are critical as evidence for effective nursing practices.

Using Valid Studies as Evidence for Nursing Practice

Determining whether the results reported in a research study can, or should, be applied to nursing practice involves careful consideration of the validity of the study. If a study is not valid, then the results that were reported cannot reasonably be expected to occur in every setting. Many questions can be asked to determine if the independent variable actually caused or affected the desired outcome. Even when that answer is "yes," the nurse must still decide whether the results are applicable to a specific population.

The first order of critical analysis should be a systematic review of internal validity in a quantitative study or of credibility in a qualitative study. If a study has poor internal validity, then external validity cannot be achieved. Using a systematic approach, the study is reviewed for threats to internal validity and their effective controls. If a study is determined to have acceptable internal reliability, then a careful consideration of external validity should precede recommendations. The type of population and the setting should be carefully reviewed and applicability to a specific practice setting evaluated.

For example, suppose an intervention designed to reduce the incidence of falls is implemented in a long-term care facility. Fall data are carefully documented before and after the intervention. The data reveal a statistically significant decline in the number of falls on the study unit. However, the patient age and level of infirmity were reduced at the time and the number of unlicensed assistive personnel (UAP) was increased. The threat to the validity of the study is obvious: A multiple-treatment effect makes it impossible to determine which intervention had the result. Were patients less likely to fall because they were not as sick? Were more UAPs available to provide assistance? Or was the intervention alone responsible for the change? The threats to validity in this study mean its application to practice is limited until the study is replicated under more controlled circumstances.

If the study findings are, indeed, replicated several times, the nurse must still determine if the population and setting are similar enough to apply the findings to practice. The results of a fall study that was conducted in a long-term care facility may not apply to a medical–surgical unit. Results that were generated from a population of infirm elderly patients in a long-term care facility may not apply to outpatient surgical patients. Even studies that are internally valid and replicated may not be useful as evidence if the population and setting are so specific that the results have limited applicability.

Considering the internal and external validity of studies is a key step in appraising research for use as evidence in practice. Evaluation of threats to internal and external validity makes up a major component of the assessment process for determining the quality of a research study.

Creating a Valid Research Study

Designing a study that has strong validity or credibility is a challenge, even for experienced researchers. The nature of applied nursing research means human beings are involved, and humans' involvement introduces a level of unpredictability that makes it impossible to predict all threats to validity. Nevertheless, some threats to validity have the potential to affect almost any study. The conscientious research designer reflects on the most common threats to validity and creates design elements to ensure that an appropriate level of control is achieved. Table 9.3 describes common threats to validity and methods to ensure their control.

Blinding the researcher to specific elements of the study can help reduce the effects of bias. When the researcher is unaware of the group assignment of subjects and cannot link subjects to data, then the potential for influencing the outcome becomes much more remote. It may be necessary for the researcher to completely remove himself or herself from the setting during data collection to ensure that bias is controlled.

Selection effects are controlled almost exclusively through the way subjects are recruited, selected, and assigned to groups. Paying careful attention to the development of inclusion and exclusion criteria ensures that objective rationales are available for leaving some individuals out of a study. Random sampling and random assignment to treatment groups also have the effect of minimizing selection effects.

Table 9.3 Common Threats to Internal Validity and Associated Control Measures

Threat	What It Is	How It Is Controlled
History	Events occur during the study that have an influence on the outcome of the study	Random sampling to distribute effects across all groups
Maturation	Effects of the passage of time	Match subjects for age Use analysis of covariance (ANCOVA) to measure effects of time
Treatment effects	Subject reactions that are due to the effect of being observed	Unobtrusive measures Subject blinding Use of sham procedures or placebos
Instrumentation	Influence on the outcome from the measurement itself, not the intervention	Calibration of instruments Documentation of reliability Analysis of inter-rater reliability
Attrition	Subject attrition due to dropouts, loss of contact, or death	Project expected attrition and oversample Carefully screen subjects prior to recruitment Create thorough consent procedures so subjects are aware of what will be expected of them
Bias	Study is influenced by preconceived notions of the researcher or reactions of the subject	Blinding of researcher, data collectors, and subjects as to who is getting the experimental treatment
Selection effects	Subjects are assigned to groups in a way that does not distribute characteristics evenly across both groups	Random selection Random assignment Matching of subjects Stratified samples

Treatment effects are more difficult to control, particularly for ethical researchers interested in full disclosure. The Hawthorne or treatment effect may be present even in descriptive and correlation studies. The use of control groups or comparison groups can help ensure that any effects from participation in the study are spread evenly among subjects. Using sham procedures or comparing two interventions simultaneously can also control for changes brought about by treatment effects.

Other threats to validity will almost certainly occur during an experiment, no matter how well designed. The researcher has three basic ways to deal with these threats:

- *Eliminate the threat.* If a threat emerges that can be neutralized, removal of the threat can enhance the validity of the study results. For example, a researcher may ask research assistants to collect data if measures are subjective and bias is a concern. By removing himself or herself from data collection, the researcher has eliminated the effect he or she might have had on measuring a subjective trait.

- *Control the threat.* If a threat emerges that cannot be eliminated, the researcher can employ methods to control its effects or distribute its effects across all subjects or groups equally. For example, research to examine the effects of childhood developmental delays on school success may be affected by socioeconomic status. By matching all the groups on this variable through stratified sampling, the effects of limited resources will be distributed across all the groups equally, neutralizing its effect on the outcome.
- *Account for the threat.* If a threat occurs that cannot be eliminated or controlled, then the researcher must account for it in the write-up. All studies have weaknesses and threats to validity; it is up to the reader to determine if the weaknesses of a study outweigh its strengths. For example, a researcher was studying the attitudes of school nurses toward student violence when the Columbine High School shootings occurred. This historical event dramatically changed the responses of the school nurses. Although nothing could be done about the tragedy or its effects on the research study, the author reported the data as "before the incident" and "after the incident" and noted that it likely had an effect on the outcome.

When creating a study, the researcher must balance control of threats to internal validity with the need to maximize external validity. Generalizability is a key issue for research that is to be used as evidence. When a research study becomes too highly controlled, its artificial nature limits the applicability of its results to real-world populations. The researcher must balance each element that strengthens internal validity with a concern to maintain as much external validity as possible.

Summary of Key Concepts

- An internally valid research study is one in which there is sufficient evidence to support the claim that the intervention had an effect and that nothing else was responsible for the outcome.
- Specific conditions must be met to draw valid conclusions about causality: The intervention is related to the outcome; the intervention preceded the outcome; and rival explanations have been ruled out.
- Threats to internal validity can be minimized by collecting data, using an appropriate study design, and controlling bias.
- Statistical analyses can be used to rule out rival explanations for an outcome through the use of hypothesis testing, minimizing Type I and II error, considering effect size, and ensuring assumptions are met.
- When a researcher makes a Type I error, he or she has concluded that the independent variable exerted an effect when, in fact, it did not. Type I error is controlled by careful design and control.

- A Type II error has occurred when the intervention had an effect but that relationship went undetected. Type II error is primarily controlled with a strong sampling strategy and achieving an adequate sample size.
- Many factors can threaten internal validity, including history, maturation, testing, instrumentation, consent effects, treatment effects, selection effects, and attrition.
- External validity refers to the generalizability of the findings of the study to other populations or settings.
- Threats to external validity include selection effects, time and history, novelty, and experimenter effects.
- The researcher must make decisions that balance internal and external validity. As internal validity is more tightly controlled, it also becomes more artificial and has less applicability to broad populations.
- Qualitative research is judged by the trustworthiness and credibility of its results. The application of understanding from qualitative studies comes about through transferability and replication.
- Strategies to promote the credibility of qualitative research include prolonged contact, verbatim accounts and triangulation, member checking, bracketing, and audit trails.

For More Depth and Detail

For a more in-depth look at the concepts in this chapter, try these references:

Bleijenberge, I., & Verschuren, P. (2011). Methodological criteria for the internal validity and utility of practice oriented research. *Quality and Quantity: International Journal of Methodology, 45*(1), 145–156.

Craig, P., Dieppe, P., Macintyre, S., Michie, S., Nazareth, I., & Petticrew, M. (2013). Developing and evaluating complex interventions: The new Medical Research Council guidance. *International Journal of Nursing Studies, 50*(5), 587–592.

Crowder, S., & Broome, M. (2012). A framework to evaluate the cultural appropriateness of intervention research. *Western Journal of Nursing Research, 34*(8), 1002–1022.

Halbesleben, J., & Whitman, M. (2014). Evaluating survey quality in health services research: A decision framework for assessing nonresponse bias. *Health Services Research, 48*(3), 913–930.

Kumar, S. (2012). Conflicting research evidence in evidence-based practice: Whose bias do you seek? *Internet Journal of Allied Health Sciences and Practice, 10*(3), 10–13.

Malone, H., Nicholl, H., & Tracey, C. (2014). Awareness and minimization of systematic bias in research. *British Journal of Nursing, 23*(5), 279–282.

Moon, M., Wolf, L., Baker, K., Carman, M., Clark, P., . . . Zavogtsky, K. (2013). Evaluating qualitative research studies for use in the clinical setting. *Journal of Emergency Nursing, 39*(5), 508–510.

Rothstein, M., & Shoben, A. (2013). Does consent bias research? *American Journal of Bioethics, 13*(4), 27–37.

CRITICAL APPRAISAL EXERCISE

Retrieve the following full-text article from the Cumulative Index to Nursing and Allied Health Literature or similar search database:

Aurore, T., Deltombe, T., Wannez, S., Gosseries, O., Ziegler, E., Dieni, C., . . . Laureys, S. (2015). Impact of soft splints on upper limb spasticity in chronic patients with disorders of consciousness: A randomized, single-blind, controlled trial. *Brain Injury, 29,* 7–8, 830–836. doi: 10.3109/02699052.2015.1005132

Read the study carefully, searching for evidence of threats to internal or external validity. Pay particular attention to how the authors controlled these threats. Consider the following appraisal questions in your critical review of validity of this research article:

1. This study was a "single-blind" randomized trial. How does this differ from a double-blind study? Which kind of bias might it introduce into the study?
2. The sample was recruited from two different physical sites and levels of care. Which kind of bias might this introduce into the study?
3. There were considerable inclusion and exclusion criteria for sample selection. Which element of potential bias did each criterion address?
4. How did the protocol protect against researcher bias?
5. How did the researchers isolate the effects of each treatment? Which controls were in place to ensure any differences were attributable to a specific treatment?
6. Which other explanations can you think of for the differences between groups *exclusive of the treatment?*
7. Describe your level of comfort using these results as evidence for practice. How might these results be applied to nursing practice? What is the external validity— ecological and population—of this study?

References

Bekhet, A., & Zauszniewski, J. (2012). Methodological triangulation: An approach to understanding data. *Nurse Researcher, 20*(2), 40–43.

Diamond, G., & Kaul, S. (2013). On reporting of effect size in randomized clinical trials. *American Journal of Cardiology, 111,* 613–617.

El Emam, K., Jonker, E., Moher, E., & Arbuckle, L. (2013). A review of evidence on consent bias in research. *American Journal of Bioethics, 13*(4), 42–45.

Hartung, D., & Touchette, D. (2009). Overview of clinical research design. *American Journal of Health System Pharmacy, 66*(15), 398–408.

Henry, S., Jerant, A., Iosif, A., Feldman, M., Cipri, C., & Kravitz, R. (2015). Analysis of threats to research validity introduced by audio recording clinic visits: Selection bias, Hawthorne effect, both, or neither? *Patient Education and Counseling, 98*(7), 849–856.

Knottnerus, J., & Tugwell, P. (2014). Selection-related bias, an ongoing concern in doing and publishing research. *Journal of Clinical Epidemiology, 67*(10), 1057–1058.

McCambridge, J., Witton, J., & Elbourne, D. (2014). Systematic review of the Hawthorne effect: New concepts are needed to study research participation effects. *Journal of Clinical Epidemiology, 67,* 267–277.

Noble, H., & Smith, J. (2015). Issues of validity and reliability in qualitative research. *Evidence Based Nursing, 18*(2), 34–35.

Page, S., & Persch, A. (2013). Recruitment, retention, and blinding in clinical trials. *American Journal of Occupational Therapy, 67*(2), 154–161.

Pareira, H. (2012). Rigour in phenomenological research: Reflections of a novice nurse researcher. *Nurse Researcher, 19*(3), 16–19.

Rusanov, A., Weiskopf, N., Wang, S., & Weng, C. (2014). Hidden in plain sight: Bias towards sick patients when sampling patients with sufficient electronic health record data for research. *BMC Medical Informatics and Decision Making, 14*(1), 51. doi: 10.1186/1472-6947-14-51

Savovic, J., Jones, H., Altman, D., Harris, R., Juni, P., Pildal, J., . . . Gluud, L. (2012). Influence of reported study design characteristics on intervention effect estimates from randomized controlled trials. *Annals of Internal Medicine, 157*(6), 429–438.

Schou, L., Hostrup, H., Lyngson, E., Larsen, S., & Poulsen, I. (2012). Validation of a new assessment tool for qualitative research articles. *Journal of Advanced Nursing, 68*(9), 2086–2094.

Smith, J., & Noble, H. (2014). Bias in research. *Evidence-Based Nursing, 17*(4), 100–101.

Part IV

Research That Describes Populations

Chapter 10

Descriptive Research Questions and Procedures

CHAPTER OBJECTIVES

The study of this chapter will help the learner to

- Identify descriptive research designs and methods.
- Examine the importance of design decisions in descriptive studies.
- Compare the characteristics and applications of specific descriptive designs.
- Relate descriptive designs to evidence-based nursing practice.
- Appraise a descriptive study for strengths and weaknesses.
- Learn how to create a descriptive research design.
- Determine how to use descriptive research designs as evidence for nursing practice.

KEY TERMS

Case study	Longitudinal study	Spurious relationship
Correlation study	Prediction study	Suppressor variable
Cross-sectional design	Reversal designs	Tests of model fit
Epidemiology	Single-subject design	

Introduction

There is an old saying that goes, "You cannot know where you are going if you do not know where you have been." The descriptive researcher might more accurately say, "You cannot know where you are going if you do not know where you are." Experiments are the study of what may be; they are used to investigate interventions that may be effective or nursing actions that may prevent health problems. Descriptive research, in contrast, provides an understanding of what is. Understanding the potential that an intervention has for improving health must be based on an understanding of the conditions and the people that will be affected by it. Often, in-depth knowledge of the current state of affairs is necessary to hypothesize whether a change in practice is warranted or even desirable.

The purpose of descriptive research is the exploration and description of phenomena in real-life situations. In nursing practice, a descriptive design can be used to develop theory, identify problems, make decisions, or determine what others in similar situations are doing. Descriptive studies include a purpose and a question; these designs do not, however, have a treatment that is artificially introduced. Instead, descriptive research is the study of phenomena as they naturally occur. Such research helps nurses describe what exists, determine frequencies of occurrence, and categorize information so effective nursing interventions can be put into place (Grove, Gray, & Burns, 2014).

Descriptive studies are designed to provide in-depth information about the characteristics of subjects or a setting within a particular field of study. The researcher may collect data in the form of numbers or words, and data collection may be done via observation, measurement, surveys, or questionnaires. A wide variety of descriptive designs are available to the nurse researcher, but they all share one characteristic in common: No variables are manipulated in the study. When data are collected as numbers, the descriptive study is considered quantitative. Quantitative studies test theory by describing variables and examining relationships. In contrast, qualitative studies typically collect data in the form of words. This chapter focuses on quantitative descriptive designs; the use of qualitative methods to answer descriptive research questions is covered elsewhere in this text.

As the most basic research design, descriptive studies answer basic questions about what is happening in a defined population or situation. They may help the nurse identify existing health conditions, perceptions about an illness or treatment, emotional or psychological responses, or the current distribution of disease in a population. Descriptive studies can also help identify relationships between variables, such as the association between a risk factor and a disease. These studies are useful in determining the status of a population at risk of developing a condition (Polit & Beck, 2012).

Descriptive research plays an important role in nursing. Descriptive studies can be invaluable in documenting the prevalence, nature, and intensity of health-related conditions and behaviors. The results of these studies are critical in the development of effective interventions. In nursing, the only way to understand the beliefs and values of different individuals and groups is to describe them. This descriptive knowledge helps nurses develop interventions that will benefit individuals, families, or groups and enable them to obtain desirable and predictable outcomes.

SCENES FROM THE FIELD

The benefits of breastfeeding have been clearly established for both infant and mother in terms of reducing infections, obesity, allergies, diabetes, and some maternal cancers. Yet, in one international sample, only three-fourths of mothers initiated breastfeeding at birth, and more than half quit breastfeeding by 6 weeks postpartum. Of interest is the subgroup of mothers who intend to breastfeed but discontinue this practice in the first few days after birth. Understanding the reasons that mothers either avoid initiating this feeding method or intend to breastfeed but discontinue doing so is important in devising evidence-based nursing strategies aimed at improving mothers' success in starting and maintaining this ideal feeding method.

Brown and Jordan (2013) conducted a survey of more than 600 new mothers to examine breastfeeding cessation due to the birth experience and/or obstetric interventions. Their specific aim was to explore the differences in breastfeeding between mothers who had uncomplicated vaginal delivery and those who experienced labor and delivery complications. The authors used an exploratory cross-sectional survey design to answer the research question.

Mothers were asked to complete an Internet survey in relation to the birth and postpartum period of their youngest child. Babies who were low birth weight or premature were excluded, so the infants in this study were all of normal weight. The participants reported how long they breastfed their infants—even if only partially. Mothers also reported whether their birth experience was vaginal or surgical, and they responded to an open-ended item inquiring as to whether they experienced complications. Of the 602 women who responded to the survey, 101 did not breastfeed at all. Of the remaining mothers, 284 initiated but stopped breastfeeding. These mothers were asked to complete a 44-item questionnaire indicating their reasons for discontinuing. These Likert-style questions were developed based on a previous qualitative study and were piloted on a subsample of mothers for reliability and validity. Approximately half of these participants experienced a complication of labor—most frequently fetal distress, assisted birth, failure to progress, augmentation of labor, severe perineal tears, or postpartum hemorrhage.

The mothers were split into two groups—those who experienced a birth complication and those who did not—and differences between them were explored statistically. Mothers who experienced birth complications breastfed for a significantly shorter duration than those without complications. Specifically, surgical birth, fetal distress, failure to progress, and postpartum hemorrhage were all factors associated with shorter breastfeeding duration. The shortest time to discontinuation of breastfeeding was associated with maternal pain and the use of medications.

This study was a good example of a descriptive design in that it focused on a relatively small number of variables and explored relationships without attempting to determine cause and effect. Its results suggest that subsequent studies could focus on the causal nature of birth complications and ways that this effect could be mediated by nursing care. The Internet survey design enabled the researchers to access a broad sample of subjects, resulting in a large sample size. These exploratory descriptive data can be useful in designing interventions for new mothers, particularly those experiencing birth complications (Brown & Jordan, 2013).

GRAY MATTER

In nursing practice, a descriptive design can be used for the following purposes:
- Develop theory
- Identify problems
- Make decisions
- Determine what others in similar situations are doing

Descriptive Research Studies

As with any research study, the first step in descriptive research is to select a topic of interest, review relevant literature, and formulate a research question based on the identified problem. Descriptive research studies address two basic types of questions:

- Descriptive questions are designed to describe what is going on or what exists. An example of a descriptive question is "What percentage of school-age children are fully immunized in a school district?"
- Relational questions are designed to investigate the relationships between two or more variables or between subjects. An example of a relational question is "What is the relationship between the immunization rate and socioeconomic status in a school district?"

Table 10.1 Examples of Descriptive Research Questions and Designs

Type of Study	Typical Research Question
Descriptive	What is nurses' knowledge about best practices related to oral care?
Survey	How are nurses involved in decision making about patient care, the work environment, and organizational practices?
Cross-sectional	What are the differences in job satisfaction among nurses at different stages of their careers?
Longitudinal	What is the effect of urinary incontinence on the quality of life of long-term-care residents over time?
Case study	What are the appropriate assessments and interventions for a patient experiencing paraplegia after heart surgery?
Single-subject study	What were the responses of an individual with type 2 diabetes to culturally appropriate counseling from a nurse?
Correlation	What is the relationship between patient satisfaction and the timeliness and effectiveness of pain relief in a fast-track emergency unit?
Predictive	Can feeding performance in neonates be predicted by indicators of feeding readiness?

The descriptive research question includes some common elements. The population of interest is specified, as is the phenomenon of interest. If the question is relational, then two variables are identified. Because there is no intervention, there is no comparison group or expected outcome. In turn, descriptive research questions are relatively simple. It may be tempting to include several concepts in a single question, but the well-written descriptive research question focuses on a single concept. Multiple research questions may be called for when several concepts are of interest in a single study. Table 10.1 provides some examples of descriptive research questions.

A well-structured research question is the foundation for the determination of a specific design. As with any research study, it is worth the time and effort to consider the elements of the research question carefully because the details of the study design will be guided by this question.

Characteristics of a Descriptive Design

Drawing good conclusions in a descriptive study is completely dependent on the researcher's ability to collect data that are both credible and complete. The elements of a good descriptive design are intended to improve the probability of obtaining accurate data and/or responses to questions. A strong descriptive design should meet the following criteria:

- Include procedures that enhance the probability of generating trustworthy data
- Demonstrate appropriateness for the purpose of the study
- Be feasible given the resources available to the researcher and the existing constraints
- Incorporate steps that are effective in reducing threats to validity

The elements of a good design will help reassure the researcher that the results are valid and trustworthy. Even though descriptive designs are among the most basic studies, it is still important for the researcher to allow adequate time for planning prior to conducting the research. A typical descriptive study is used to acquire knowledge in an area where little research has been conducted or when little is known about the condition under study. The basic descriptive design examines a characteristic or group of characteristics in a sample, although many variations on this theme are possible. Such a design may be used for a pilot study or as the basis for designing more complex studies. It is useful in establishing the need for and the development of future, more intricate studies.

Fundamentally, descriptive designs can be classified as those that describe a phenomenon or population and those that describe relationships. There are, however, two additional ways to classify descriptive designs:

- *The number of subjects:* Descriptive designs may involve the study of an entire population, a sample, or multiple samples. They may also focus on single subjects or individual cases. A case is not necessarily a single individual, but rather a single subject. A *subject* may be defined any number of ways. For example, the study of an individual person, hospital, or city may all involve collection of data from a single entity.
- *The time dimension:* Some studies explore data collected from a sample at a single point in time, whereas others follow subjects or individual cases over time.

Within each of these classifications are explicit designs that enable the researcher to answer specific questions. The researcher will gain direction for making design decisions by considering the nature of the research question, the number of subjects that are appropriate and accessible, and the time span of interest.

Describing Groups Using Surveys

Of all the various types of descriptive studies possible, the survey design is the most commonly used. Surveys answer what, why, and where questions (Yin, 2013). Although the term *survey design* is commonly used to describe a study, it is more accurately considered a data collection method used in general descriptive designs. Surveys are used to collect data directly from respondents about their characteristics, opinions, perceptions, or attitudes. As part of this design, questionnaires or personal interviews are used to gather information about a population. A survey can be an important method for gathering data for both descriptive and relational studies. It can be used to answer questions about the prevalence, distribution, and interrelationship of variables within a population. Survey designs can be applied at a single point in time, or responses can be gathered over an extended time span. When this method is used, the researcher should obtain a survey sample large enough to represent the target population so the findings can be generalized. The generalizability of the study findings is a critical factor in ensuring their applicability in evidence-based practice (Schmidt & Brown, 2012).

The purpose of asking questions is to find out what is going on in the minds of the subjects: their perceptions, attitudes, beliefs, feelings, motives, and past events. Surveys are used to discover characteristics of people and learn what they believe and how they think, by collecting primary self-reported data.

Two types of questions may be included in surveys. The first type focuses on facts, allowing the researcher to obtain information about events or people. The second type focuses on words (rather than numbers) that express feelings and perceptions to give meaning to a phenomenon or event (Schmidt & Brown, 2012).

GRAY MATTER

The following are the four major steps in designing a general descriptive survey:
1. Select an appropriate sample.
2. Plan and develop instrumentation.
3. Administer the instrument and collect data.
4. Analyze the findings.

Survey Study Methods and Procedures

Designing a general descriptive survey proceeds through four major stages:

1. Selecting an appropriate sample
2. Planning and developing instrumentation
3. Administering the instrument and data collection
4. Analyzing the findings

The planning phase includes choosing a survey mode, which may be a questionnaire or an interview. During this phase, the instrument is selected or developed; in the latter case, it is also pilot tested for reliability and validity. The procedure for administering the instrument is described in a detailed protocol, thereby ensuring the subjects receive instructions that are consistent and unambiguous. Data are collected in an identical way from each subject so that differences in responses can be attributed to differences in the subjects, not variations in the administration method. Analysis of findings is accomplished through the application of descriptive statistics.

A survey is a widely used method of descriptive data collection. Its popularity reflects the fact that it is a relatively simple design that can be used to investigate a wide range of topics. Surveys offer a systematic method for standardizing questions and collecting data and can be an efficient means of gathering data from a large number of subjects. Survey research can take the form of an opinion poll, which can be completed on the Internet, by phone, or in person. Internet access is expected to increase the use of Internet-based research exponentially in the future (Tappen, 2011).

Strengths of Survey Studies

The use of a survey design offers many advantages for the researcher:

- Survey content is flexible and the scope is broad.
- Surveys are cost-effective methods for reaching large populations.
- Subjects have a greater sense of anonymity and so may respond with more honesty.

- Questions are predetermined and standardized for all subjects, minimizing researcher bias.
- Large sample sizes are possible.
- A large volume of data can be collected.

CASE IN POINT Survey Design

Lu et al. (2011), a group of bioengineers, wanted to build robots that could assist therapists in providing upper-body rehabilitation therapy after stroke. They wanted to find out the needs and preferences related to this intervention directly from therapists, so they developed an online survey. Their belief was that understanding the therapeutic requirements for the devices could help them design robotics that could be integrated more easily into clinical practice.

The researchers developed an 85-item questionnaire based on direct observation of therapists' practices. The survey queried respondents about movement patterns, level of assistance required, types of therapeutic activities, and accessibility. The survey was administered online internationally through professional organizations and email list services to physical therapists and physiotherapists. A total of 233 usable surveys were returned and analyzed.

The attributes that were deemed most desirable by the respondents included facilitating a wide range and variety of arm movements, being usable while seated, and giving real-time biofeedback to clients. In addition, support for patients' activities of daily living, which was thought to enhance the devices' usefulness in a home-based setting, was highly desirable. Low cost was also highly rated.

This survey was typical in that data were collected directly from respondents in an effort to understand their opinions about some subject. In this case, engineers were trying to understand the needs of therapists and patients so that they could build a useful robotic assistant. The sample was well selected for the purpose, and a sufficiently large group responded that these findings could confidently be applied as evidence for this project.

Limitations of Survey Studies

Although surveys offer many advantages, there are also some disadvantages associated with their use:

- The information obtained may be superficial and limited to standard responses.
- A survey cannot probe deeply into complexities of human behavior or explore contradictions.
- Content is often limited by subject recall, self-knowledge, and willingness to respond honestly.
- Questions may be misinterpreted by subjects, resulting in unreliable conclusions.
- Respondents may respond with socially acceptable responses to sensitive questions instead of honest answers.

The application of good design decisions can help maximize the advantages and minimize the disadvantages of survey designs. The use of reliable, valid instruments applied to large, randomly selected samples will result in the most credible results from a survey design.

Epidemiology:
The investigation of the distribution and determinants of disease within populations or cohorts.

Cross-sectional design:
Study conducted by examining a single phenomenon across multiple populations at a single point in time with no intent for follow-up in the design.

Describing Groups Relative to Time

Descriptive studies may focus on the characteristics of a population at a single point in time or on changes within a population over time. Prevalence and incidence studies are two types of descriptive studies from the field of epidemiology (Polit & Beck, 2012). Prevalence studies describe the occurrence of a disease in a population during a given time period. Incidence studies describe new cases of a disease or condition during an identified time period. Time-dimension designs are most closely associated with the discipline of **epidemiology**, which investigates the distribution and determinants of disease within populations. These populations are often referred to as cohorts in epidemiology. Cohort studies examine sequences, patterns of change, growth, or trends over time. By describing the characteristics of groups of people at specific time periods, the researcher attempts to identify risk factors for particular diseases, health conditions, or behaviors.

When the cohort is studied at a single point in time, it is called a cross-sectional study. If data are collected from the cohort at specific time periods over a span of months or years, it is called a longitudinal study.

Cross-Sectional Designs

The **cross-sectional design** is used to examine simultaneously groups of subjects who are in various stages of development; the intent is to describe differences among them. Studies of prevalence, for example, are commonly cross-sectional. A cross-sectional study is based on the assumption that the stages identified in different subjects at the single point in time are representative of a process that progresses over time. For example, a researcher may select subjects who have risk factors but have not yet developed a disease, subjects who have early-stage disease, and subjects who have the disease in chronic form. Other common ways to group subjects are by age or some demographic characteristic.

Cross-sectional designs are appropriate for describing the characteristics or status of a disease and the risk factors or exposures associated with the disease (Howlett, Rogo, & Shelton, 2014). They can also be used to infer the association between the characteristics of individuals and their health status. In addition, such studies are used to answer questions about the way a condition progresses over time when the researcher has access to a population consisting of individuals at various stages of disease or when longitudinal studies are not realistic. By definition, studies based on cross-sectional designs involve more than single subjects; that is, they are used for samples.

Cross-Sectional Study Methods and Procedures

In a cross-sectional design, the population of interest is carefully described. The phenomenon under study is captured during one period of data collection. Protocols guide the specific way in which data are collected to minimize bias and enhance the reliability of the data. Variables must be carefully defined and valid measures identified for each variable. Stratified random samples may be used to ensure that individuals who have specific characteristics or who are in various stages of disease are represented in proportion to their prevalence in the general population.

Strengths of Cross-Sectional Studies

The use of a cross-sectional design provides the researcher with many advantages, including the following:

- Cross-sectional designs are practical and economical.
- There is no waiting for the outcome of interest to occur.
- These studies enable the exploration of health conditions that are affected by human development.
- The procedures are reasonably simple to design and carry out.
- Data are collected at one point in time, so results can be timely and relevant.
- Large samples are relatively inexpensive to obtain.
- There is no loss of subjects due to study attrition.

Limitations of Cross-Sectional Studies

Although cross-sectional studies have many advantages, this design also has some drawbacks:

- The transitory nature of data collection makes causal association difficult.
- Cross-sectional studies do not capture changes that occur as a result of environmental factors or other events that occur over time.
- It may be difficult to locate individuals at varying stages of a disease or condition.
- Cross-sectional designs are impractical for the study of rare diseases or uncommon conditions.

Many of these limitations are overcome when a population is studied over time, rather than at a single point in time. Cross-sectional studies are often used as a starting point for a subsequent study carried out over time or as pilot studies for more complex longitudinal designs.

CASE IN POINT Cross-Sectional Design

It has been said that "sitting is the new smoking," in that the cardiovascular and other risks associated with sedentary behavior are becoming more apparent in the literature. Low levels of daily physical activity are of particular concern in patients who have experienced cardiovascular disease, as diminished activity has been shown to be predictive of mortality in this population.

Buijs et al. (2015) set out to assess the quantity and quality of daily physical activity among older patients who suffered from cardiac disease or who had experienced a cardiac event. They used a cross-sectional design to measure how physical activity changed over time and through the different stages of recovery.

A population of patients were recruited and sorted into three groups: an acute stage group, a rehabilitation group, and a maintenance group. The subjects used a physical activity monitoring device to record their data, which was measured continuously for 4 days. The researchers found that most of the patients—no matter their stage of illness—were not getting enough physical activity. The group in active rehabilitation engaged in the most exercise, but even they were sedentary 70% of the time. The acute and maintenance groups were statistically the same in terms of their level of physical activity. Their findings point to the need to continue support for physical activity in some way after cardiac rehabilitation is complete.

This research was a typical cross-sectional study, in that a population was selected that was experiencing various stages of a condition, and variables of interest were measured at a single point in time. This design enabled the researchers to describe a phenomenon at varying stages of illness without dealing with the limitations and attrition of measuring a group over time.

Longitudinal study:
Study conducted by following subjects over a period of time, with data collection occurring at prescribed intervals.

Longitudinal Designs

A longitudinal study follows one or more cohorts over an extended period of time. These designs are powerful ways to assess the effects of risk factors or the consequences of health behaviors. Longitudinal designs may answer questions about the way that characteristics of populations change over time, or they may quantify relationships between risk factors and disease. Longitudinal designs are often exploratory, seeking to answer questions about the nature of health conditions at various stages of human development. Such studies help determine trends and the benefits of treatments over both the short term and the long term. A cohort study tracks a group of people over time to determine if their outcomes or risks differ (Polit & Beck, 2012). This design is often called simply a cohort design, but it may also be known as a panel design. Longitudinal designs by definition involve repeated measures over time taken from the same group of subjects.

GRAY MATTER

Cohort studies examine the following variables:
- Sequences
- Patterns of change
- Growth or trends over time

Longitudinal Study Methods and Procedures

The first step in conducting a longitudinal study is to specify an appropriate population and the sampling procedures. A population is described in detail, and a sample that has adequate power is selected from the larger population. Power must be determined based not on the number of subjects who enter the study, but rather on the number required to complete it, because substantial attrition is expected over the extended time periods involved in longitudinal studies. The best longitudinal studies rely on random selection of participants to represent the population, although this is rarely a practical reality. Large samples represent the population best, provide the highest level of confidence in the findings, and compensate for the substantial attrition that is expected in longitudinal studies.

As part of the longitudinal design, variables must be clearly identified and valid measures identified for each. Reliable measures are extremely important in longitudinal studies because the data will be collected repeatedly. Both internal consistency and test–retest reliability are key considerations in the choice of instrumentation for longitudinal studies to ensure consistency over time.

Researchers can use two strategies to collect longitudinal data: retrospective or prospective. Retrospective studies are conducted to examine a potential causal relationship that may have already occurred. In a retrospective study, secondary data are used to obtain baseline measurements and information about periodic follow-ups and outcomes of interest. The stages of a retrospective longitudinal study are shown in **FIGURE 10.1**. The researcher performs the following steps:

1. Identify a suitable cohort that has been evaluated in the past.
2. Collect data on the expected causal variables from past records.
3. Obtain data about the hypothesized outcome from past or current measures.

The data are then analyzed to determine if there is a predictive relationship between the past event and the outcome of interest.

If a research question is written in the past tense, it is generally a retrospective study. Exploratory research questions about causal events can be answered using a retrospective study method. An effective retrospective study is dependent on access to accurate and complete data about a suitable cohort. These data can be collected from several past time points (Tappen, 2011).

In contrast, prospective studies answer research questions written in the future tense. Participants are enrolled at the beginning of the study and are studied over time (Polit & Beck, 2012). Interventions, data collection, and outcomes occur after the subjects are enrolled. The researcher recruits an appropriate cohort and measures characteristics or behaviors that might predict subsequent outcomes. As in retrospective studies, reliability of measures is critical, as are procedures to reduce attrition of subjects. Due to the time commitment required to complete longitudinal research, the researcher needs to encourage participants to complete the study (Schmidt & Brown, 2012). Loss of participants and inaccurate reporting of the losses may cause the study results to be misleading if these factors are not accounted for properly (Melnyk & Fineout-Overholt, 2011). The time periods at which data are collected are predetermined and based on a solid rationale.

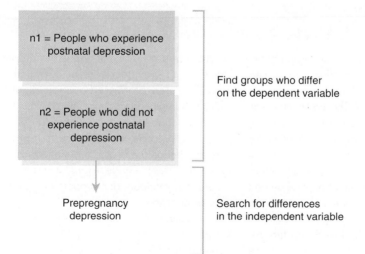

A retrospective longitudinal design

n1 = People who experience postnatal depression

n2 = People who did not experience postnatal depression

Prepregnancy depression

Find groups who differ on the dependent variable

Search for differences in the independent variable

FIGURE 10.1 Stages of a Retrospective Longitudinal Design

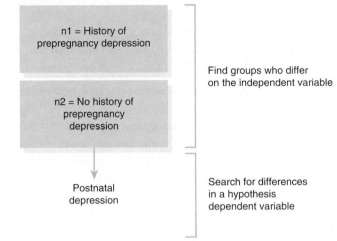

A prospective longitudinal design

n1 = History of prepregnancy depression

n2 = No history of prepregnancy depression

Find groups who differ on the independent variable

Postnatal depression

Search for differences in a hypothesis dependent variable

FIGURE 10.2 Stages of a Prospective Longitudinal Design

FIGURE 10.2 depicts the stages of a prospective cohort design. The researcher performs the following steps:

1. Recruit a sample from an identified population.
2. Measure the hypothesized predictor variables.
3. Measure outcomes at predetermined follow-up times.

The researcher can expect that a large volume of data will be collected over the life of the study, so procedures for data management should be considered in study planning.

CASE IN POINT Longitudinal Design

Mental health disorders are common during pregnancy and in the first postpartum year, affecting between 14% and 23% of women overall (Gordon, Henderson, Holmes, Wolters, & Bennett, 2016). The most common diagnoses during these periods are depression and anxiety, and these conditions increase the risk of complications for both mother and baby. Low-income women and minorities are at higher risk for these conditions—some sources estimate that the perinatal incidence of depression and anxiety is nearly 50% in these populations—yet they are also among the least likely to get appropriate treatment.

A group for researchers believed that the use of patient-centered eHealth tools could help these women avoid mental health issues during pregnancy. They recruited a group of low-income pregnant women through a clinic at a major medical center, all

of whom had a history of depression in pregnancy. The women's providers were included in the study as well. The researchers used a longitudinal design in which meetings occurred monthly, and the participants provided feedback in the design and use of eHealth tools. The outcome was an app that provided suicide prevention feedback, a patient decision aid for supporting treatment decisions, a screening tool for worsening symptoms, and support for high-risk women after discharge.

This study involved an unusual application of a longitudinal design, in that women's mental health was measured over time while they participated in the development of support tools. The highly engaging approach to data collection resulted in low attrition, which is usually the major weakness of this type of study.

Strengths of Longitudinal Studies

The use of a longitudinal design provides the researcher with many advantages, including the following:

- Longitudinal studies can capture historical trends and explore causal associations.
- Retrospective longitudinal studies are cost-effective and cost-efficient.
- Prospective longitudinal studies can document that a causal factor precedes an outcome, strengthening hypotheses about causality.
- Prospective studies provide the opportunity to measure characteristics and events accurately and do not rely on recall.

Limitations of Longitudinal Studies

Longitudinal studies also have some significant limitations:

- The principal disadvantages are attrition rates and the potential loss of subjects over time.
- Retrospective longitudinal studies are dependent on accurate, complete secondary data or the subject's ability to recall past events.
- Once a longitudinal study is begun, it cannot be changed without affecting the overall validity of the conclusions.
- Prospective longitudinal studies are expensive to conduct and require time and commitment from both subjects and researchers.
- Conclusions may be based on a limited number of observations.
- Large sample sizes are expensive to access.
- Systematic attrition of subjects is possible due to the long-term commitment required.

Substantial effort must go into the planning and execution of a longitudinal study—whether retrospective or prospective—if the researcher is to draw valid conclusions about the relationships between variables. Longitudinal studies are quite useful in assessing potential causal relationships, but their application is limited due to the difficulty of implementing them effectively.

Describing the Responses of Single Subjects

General descriptive designs involve evaluating the characteristics of groups of individuals or the way that whole populations respond to events. These designs allow researchers to draw conclusions about typical or average responses. Of course, typical responses do not tell the nurse how a single, unique individual may respond to a condition or a treatment. The study of a single subject, in contrast, can be an effective means for discovering the ways that individual people react to nursing practices and health conditions.

The purpose of studying single subjects is to assess individuals, with the expectation of generalizing the findings about that person to other individuals in similar situations or conditions. Single-subject designs may answer exploratory questions or serve as pilot tests for later experimental designs. Questions that focus on individual responses to treatments or health conditions over time are well served with

Case study:
The meticulous descriptive exploration of a single unit of study such as a person, family group, community, or other entity.

Single-subject design:
An investigation using a single case or subject in which baseline data are collected, an intervention is applied, and the responses are tracked over time.

single-subject designs. These designs attempt to explore real changes in the individual, which may be obscured in traditional analyses of group comparisons. Single-subject designs reflect what happens in clinical practice because nurses, as part of their plan of care, focus on an individual and not a group. In addition, a single-subject design may be the only approach possible for answering questions about patients with rare diseases. These designs usually involve data collected over time. Although they may actually include a small number of subjects, they are by definition not representative of entire populations.

Two methods are used to study individual subjects: case study and single-subject designs. A **case study** involves the meticulous exploration of a single unit of study such as a person, family, group, community, or other entity. It is purely descriptive, relying on a depth of detail and individual health data to reveal the characteristics and responses of the single case. By comparison, the **single-subject design** is essentially an experimental investigation using a single case or single subject. Baseline data are collected, an intervention is applied, and the responses of the individual are tracked over time. In essence, the individual subject serves as his or her own control.

Case Study Designs

A case study is the thorough assessment of an individual case over time in its real-life environment. This assessment may involve observation, interaction, or measurement of variables. When the data collection methods are limited to observation, interviews, documents, archived records, and artifacts, the resulting data are expressed in words and the design is qualitative. Often, however, the data that are collected are direct or indirect measures gathered via instrumentation or questionnaires; these numbers are then analyzed using quantitative methods. It is not unusual for a case study to involve a mixture of data collection methods that are both qualitative and quantitative. In fact, a characteristic of case study designs is that the number of subjects is small but the number of variables measured is large. It is important to examine all variables that may potentially have an effect on the situation (Burns & Grove, 2011).

Case study designs are effective for answering questions about how individuals respond to treatment or react to health conditions. Questions related to the effects of specific therapeutic measures can be addressed with a case study, and this design is often used to demonstrate the value of a therapy. The results of case study investigations are often applied as a teaching vehicle; for example, the "grand rounds" method is often used to introduce a practice via a demonstrated case. A case study approach can illustrate life-changing events by giving them meaning and creating understanding about the subject's experience. These strategies can result in a great depth of understanding about the phenomenon under study.

A case study is not intended to represent a population, but rather represents a means to test a theory or demonstrate the effectiveness of a practice from a unique and individual perspective. Often, the findings of a case study generate hypotheses that can subsequently be tested in subsequent studies that yield more widely generalizable results.

Case Study Methods and Procedures

The first step in a case study is obviously to identify an appropriate case. A "case" may be defined in a number of ways. The most common case is an individual, but a case also may be defined as a family, an organization, a county, a department, or any number of other delineations. Case study designs are often the result of opportunity—that is, a unique or unusual case presents itself to the nurse, who takes advantage of the opportunity to conduct an in-depth study over time. Case study designs may also come about through careful consideration of the criteria that should be present in a subject to test a theory, evaluate an intervention, or appraise responses to a condition over time. Case study designs require commitment on the part of both researcher and subject because these designs are longitudinal, and the subject is followed for a lengthy time period.

The key variables that are of interest are identified, defined, and captured through appropriate measures. It is important that these measures be stable and reliable over time, because they will be applied repeatedly over the life of the study. On initiating the study, the nurse researcher obtains a thorough history so that observations can be compared to previous behaviors and experiences. It is important to study as many variables in the situation as possible to determine which might have an effect on the subject's responses and actions. Because large amounts of data are generated, a conscientious data management plan is critical in the design of case study procedures. Analysis is time consuming; it requires meticulous effort and can be difficult. Measured changes must be quantified. In the most thorough case studies, the themes and responses of the individual are reported in a holistic context. This last element is one of the reasons why these studies often use a mix of methods.

CASE IN POINT Case Study Design

Individuals with visual impairments are among the people most likely to use a service dog, yet lack of experience or negative experiences with dogs may create fear barriers for these persons so that they do not get the full benefit of canine assistance. The authors of one research report used a case study design to examine a process of using a humane education course to improve the knowledge and skills of high school students who were blind but who had resisted use of a service dog (Bruce, Feinstein, Kennedy, & Liu, 2015). The researchers used a mixed method of measuring variables related to the participants over time as well as measuring variables for the entire group at a single point in time to determine effective ways of teaching young people with visual impairments about working with dogs.

The researchers used pre- and post-intervention interviews to obtain information about the students' personal experiences and perceptions about the dogs.

They also used pretests and posttests to measure knowledge; these tests were administered in the students' strongest reading formats. Video recordings were made that served as field notes; they were subsequently analyzed using qualitative thematic methods.

At the completion of the training, students were able to greet, feed, and play with the dogs. They learned about equipment and the roles of working dogs. The most effective instructional strategies were tactile, and involved practicing routines and repetition. Correcting misconceptions about dogs was also helpful, and all of the students gained knowledge about their service animal.

This case study was typical in that a very small number of subjects was studied in depth using mixed methods. Both quantitative and qualitative data were analyzed. The results, while not generalizable, could be used to generate hypotheses for future study, or to inform the care of individuals with similar conditions.

Strengths of Case Studies

Some of the advantages of using a case study design include the following:

- Case studies can provide in-depth information about the unique nature of individuals.
- Responses and changes that emerge over time can be captured and appraised.
- New insights can be obtained that can potentially generate additional studies.

Limitations of Case Studies

Disadvantages associated with using a case study approach include the following:

- There is no baseline measurement that can be compared with the intervention outcome.
- It is difficult to determine whether there is an improvement in outcome because causation cannot be inferred.
- Researcher objectivity is required when drawing conclusions, because interpretation may potentially be biased.
- Results cannot be generalized to larger populations.
- A lengthy time commitment is required.

Single-Subject Designs

Single-subject designs are the experimental version of a case study. These designs are used—as are case studies—to evaluate the unique responses of individuals to treatments or conditions. Single-subject designs differ from case studies, however, in that they are always quantitative in nature and involve distinct phases of data collection. Graphic analysis techniques are used to assess the data and draw conclusions. The organization of a single-subject design is also more structured than a case study in the sense that there is a specific sequence for measuring the baseline, introducing an intervention, and evaluating its effects.

While large randomized trials do have many notable advantages when used as evidence, many would argue that certain characteristics of single-subject designs make them an important addition and alternative to large-group designs. Single-subject studies may be more feasible, and more applicable to real-life conditions, particularly when the acceptability of treatments or the timing of responses is a primary question (Byiers, Reichie, & Sumons, 2012). This evidence is particularly helpful when compliance with a treatment program is important. Single-subject designs are effective means of answering questions about how a particular therapy will affect a single individual. The patient's response to a therapy or nursing practice can be evaluated without implementing large-scale experimental designs or recruiting big samples.

Single-Subject Study Methods and Procedures

A single-subject design has three basic requirements:

- Continuous assessment of the variable of interest
- Assessment during a baseline period before the intervention
- Continuing assessment of the responses of the individual after the intervention

The length of the baseline phase is unique to each subject; baseline measurements continue until the condition under study is stable. Because changes in the subject must be attributable to the intervention instead of random variability, stability in the measured variable is required during the baseline phase before the intervention is initiated (Polit & Beck, 2012).

Once the intervention is initiated, measurement continues over an extended period of time to capture trends or patterns that are assumed to represent a response to the intervention.

A number of different single-subject case designs are possible, most of which use a baseline phase and an intervention phase known as A and B, respectively. Measurements are captured repeatedly before and after the intervention. The most common single-subject design is referred to as the "AB" design. In the AB design, a baseline period of measures is captured (A) until the variable of interest stabilizes. An intervention (B) is then introduced, and measures are continued for a prescribed period of time. Changes in the subject during the B phase are considered attributable to the intervention; in other words, the subject serves as his or her own control.

Because single-subject designs suffer from many threats to internal validity, other designs can help mediate these threats. **Reversal designs** continue to measure the individual's responses as the intervention is withdrawn, or is withdrawn and then reinitiated. The design includes a reversal phase following the intervention. In the reversal phase, the intervention is withdrawn and conditions revert to what they were prior to the intervention. If a trend is identified in which a baseline is established, a change is noted after the intervention, and the change reverts to the baseline after the intervention is withdrawn, then the researcher's conclusions about the effects of the intervention are strengthened. These reversal designs may be identified as "ABA" or "ABAB."

The analysis of single-subject data occurs primarily through visualization and interpretation of the trends and patterns recognized in the subject's data over time. **FIGURE 10.3** depicts a single-subject graph that demonstrates an individual's response to treatment.

Reversal designs: Single-subject designs that continue to measure the response of the individual as the intervention is withdrawn or withdrawn and reinitiated.

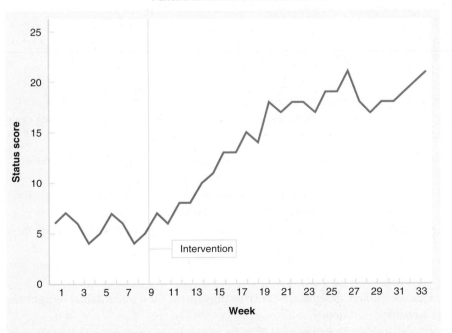

FIGURE 10.3 A Single-Subject Graph

GRAY MATTER

Single-subject designs include the following requirements:
- Continuous assessment of the variable of interest
- Assessment during a baseline period before the intervention
- Continuing assessment of the responses of the individual after the intervention

CASE IN POINT Single-Subject Design

Therapeutic horseback riding has been shown to have physical, social, learning, sensory, and psychological impacts in patients with a variety of disorders. Much of the research into this type of therapy has been conducted with programs that deliver the treatment to individuals with physical, social, or behavioral conditions. Holm et al. (2014) set out to determine whether therapeutic horseback riding could help achieve parent-identified improvement goals for children with autism spectrum disorder. These researchers used a single-subject design to determine if the therapy was effective, and to identify what "dosage," or frequency, was required to achieve a therapeutic effect.

Three boys with the identified disorder were recruited; their target behaviors were identified, and counts of these behaviors were collected in each phase of the study. The researchers measured the behaviors first for a baseline period, and then over several weeks with horseback riding "doses" of 1, 3, and 5 times a week. The treatment was then withdrawn, and measurements were continued. Compared to the baseline, 70% of the target behaviors were better during the intervention, and most of this improvement was retained after the treatment was withdrawn. Increasing frequency of therapeutic riding was associated with the percent improvement.

This study relied on a typical single-subject design, in that target behaviors were measured until a stable baseline was achieved, and then those behaviors were measured repeatedly as increasing "doses" of an intervention were applied. Continuing to measure after withdrawal of the treatment demonstrated the sustainability of the treatment effect. While not proof of cause and effect, the results of this study could be applied to similar subjects with this very specific condition in this age range. The study could also serve as a pilot for a larger randomized trial.

Strengths of Single-Subject Studies

Single-subject designs have some advantages over population-based studies when evaluating the effects of interventions:

- Single-subject designs are especially useful in exploring behavioral responses to treatment that might affect a patient's preferences and compliance.
- The unique responses of individuals can help the nurse determine whether a particular therapy will be effective for a specific kind of patient.
- Single-subject designs are flexible and involve multiple variations that may answer an assortment of questions.
- These designs explore real changes in the individual and can simultaneously serve as feedback about progress for the patient.
- Single-subject designs are easier to implement than longitudinal designs that require large samples.
- Single-subject designs provide intimate knowledge of a person's cognition, thoughts, actions, intentions, and environment (Polit & Beck, 2012).

Limitations of Single-Subject Studies

Although single-subject designs have many advantages, they also have some significant limitations:

- Single-subject designs are not generalizable to larger populations.
- Single-subject designs are not considered sufficient evidence for a practice change.
- Both researcher and subject must be committed to measures over time.

Even with these limitations, single-subject designs remain important in nursing research. Although nursing practice often affects the health of entire populations, it is also a profession that deals with people at their most vulnerable—people who need to be treated as the individuals they are. Understanding their distinctive responses, needs, and conditions can help the nurse identify evidence for practice that is relevant from both a scientific and a humanistic perspective.

Designs That Describe Relationships

By definition, descriptive research studies describe conditions as they exist. Many of these studies focus on a single characteristic, phenomenon, or group of variables. This emphasis does not, however, preclude describing the relationships between variables. Descriptive designs may be used to examine the relationships between variables in a single population or the relationship of a single variable among several populations. When these relationships are described in a quantitative way, the design is referred to as a **correlation study**.

Correlation studies may simply examine relationships among variables, or they may focus on the use of one variable to predict another. The latter type of study is called a **prediction study**. Likewise, tests of relationship or association may be used to determine whether a theoretical model fits reality. In other words, does a set of relationships exist in the real world in the way they are hypothesized in a researcher's model of reality? These studies involve the most complex descriptive designs, and often blur the line between descriptive and causal studies. In fact, these **tests of model fit** are often described as "causal models." Correlation and prediction studies are quite common in nursing research, and they are valuable approaches for generating evidence for practice. Tests of model fit are more rarely encountered due to their complex nature and the need for large samples.

Descriptive Correlation Designs

Correlation studies are used to answer questions about relationships or associations. They attempt to describe the strength and nature of the relationship between two variables without explaining the underlying causes of that relationship. These designs cannot lead to a conclusion of causality because they do not meet the requirement for temporality. In other words, the researcher cannot be sure which variable occurred first. Nevertheless, correlation studies can still be quite helpful in nursing practice. Specifically, such research can explain the strength and nature of relationships among variables or groups (Schmidt & Brown, 2012).

Most commonly, a correlation study is used to quantify the relationship between two variables in a single data set. For example, a correlation study might be used to determine whether there is a relationship between waiting room time and patient satisfaction. Correlation can also be used to determine if there is an association between a single variable

Correlation study:
A design that involves the analysis of two variables to describe the strength and direction of the relationship between them.

Prediction study:
Research designed to search for variables measured at one point in time that may forecast an outcome that is measured at a different point in time.

Tests of model fit:
Tests of association used to determine whether a set of relationships exists in the real world in the way the relationships are hypothesized in the researcher's model of reality.

in two populations; for example, a correlation study would be appropriate to determine whether satisfaction scores of patients and of their families are related. In either case, the design involves selection of an appropriate sample, measuring variables in a reliable and valid way, and analyzing the results using the correlation coefficient.

GRAY MATTER

Correlation designs are useful and realistic for clinical research studies for the following reasons:
- These methods can be used to study phenomena or clinical practices that cannot be manipulated, controlled, or randomized.
- Data can provide a solid base for further experimental testing.
- Results can serve as the foundation for designs about prediction.

Correlation Study Methods and Procedures

A correlation study is relatively simple to conduct. Criteria are developed that guide selection of the sample, and then the variables of interest are measured. In a correlation design, it is particularly important to have a representative sample, so random samples are superior to convenience samples. To obtain a true reflection of the variables being measured, large samples are needed. Relying on small samples may limit the size of the correlation coefficient, thereby underestimating the strength of the relationship.

Data collection in this type of study may be either prospective or retrospective. Prospective data collection gives the researcher greater control over the reliability and validity of measures, but it can be difficult and costly to implement. Conversely, retrospective data collection from secondary sources is efficient, but the data may not be reliable or may merely approximate the variables of interest. Determining whether to collect data prospectively or to gather data from secondary sources requires the researcher to consider the balance between validity and efficiency.

CASE IN POINT Correlation Design

The rate of cesarean delivery has increased dramatically in some industrialized countries. As many as half of high-income countries now have cesarean delivery rates exceeding 25% of all births. These types of births, when performed for unjustifiable reasons, may adversely affect the health and well-being of both mother and baby. Because a cesarean birth may result in a shorter gestation, babies may be born preterm. In addition, because the baby bypasses the normal birth canal and labor process, respiratory conditions may be more prevalent in the neonate. Cesarean births have also been associated with lower rates of breastfeeding and poorer quality of breastmilk.

Xie et al. (2015) took the high-level approach of studying birth data for 31 high-income industrialized countries to determine whether overall infant mortality was correlated with the cesarean birth rate. They found that both cesarean delivery and infant mortality rates varied widely among the countries. In some countries, as many as half of all births were surgical.

Cesarean delivery rates were positively correlated with infant mortality rates at a moderate level ($r = 0.41$), even after the data were adjusted for age and infant gender. There was a spurious relationship between cesarean delivery rates and preterm birth rates. Thus, it would appear that the mortality problem is related to prematurity as well as the mode of delivery.

This investigation was a typical correlation study in that the values of one variable were studied for the strength (moderate) and direction (positive) of the relationship with another variable. In this case, a clear spurious variable (prematurity) emerged that could explain some of the correlation. These results cannot be used as evidence that the mode of birth *caused* the infant mortality, but it could serve as the basis for a more rigorously designed study that could draw inferences about the results attributed to cesarean births.

Strengths of Correlation Studies

Correlation studies are common in nursing research because they have significant advantages:

- Correlation studies are relatively uncomplicated to plan and implement.
- The researcher has flexibility in exploring relationships among two or more variables.
- The outcomes of correlation studies often have practical application in nursing practice.
- Correlation studies provide a framework for examining relationships between variables that cannot be manipulated for practical or ethical reasons.

Limitations of Correlation Studies

Correlation studies have some distinct limitations that have implications for their use as evidence for practice:

- The researcher cannot manipulate variables of interest, so causality cannot be established.
- Correlation designs lack control and randomization between the variables, so rival explanations may be posed for relationships.
- The correlation that is measured may be the result of a **suppressor variable**—one that is not measured but is related to each variable in the relationship.

> **Suppressor variable:** A variable that is not measured but is related to each variable in the relationship and may affect the correlation of the data.

> **Spurious relationship:** A condition in which two variables have an appearance of causality where none exists. This link is found to be invalid when objectively examined.

This last limitation is one of the most significant: Demonstration of a correlation is not evidence of anything other than a linear association between two variables. Researchers often make the mistake of attempting to establish causality through a correlation study, reasoning that if two variables are related, one must have an effect on the other. In reality, correlation studies simply reveal whether a relationship exists between two variables; they cannot identify which variable occurred first and cannot isolate the effects of one variable on another—both conditions are required for causality. For example, there is a correlation between the malnutrition level of children and the time they spend in the Head Start program. Does this mean spending time in Head Start causes malnutrition? Of course not; this relationship is a reflection of a **spurious relationship**. In other words, some third variable—in this case, poverty—is the likely source of causality of both variables, giving the appearance of causality where none exists.

Despite their limitations, correlation designs are both common and quite useful for clinical research studies. They offer a realistic set of options for researchers because many of the phenomena encountered in clinical practice cannot be manipulated, controlled, or randomized. When applied and interpreted appropriately, correlation designs can provide a solid basis for further experimental testing. Although correlation cannot be used to determine causality, it can serve as the foundation for designs about prediction. In other words, if one variable is associated with an outcome in a consistent way, is it possible to predict the outcome for a given value of the variable? Answering this question is quite useful as evidence for practice and is the basis for a specific type of descriptive design—the predictive study.

Predictive Designs

Predictive designs attempt to explore which factors may influence an outcome. These studies may be used when a researcher is interested in determining whether knowing a previously documented characteristic (or set of characteristics) can lead to the prediction of a later characteristic (or set of characteristics). Predictive studies are sometimes called regression studies, based on the statistical test that is used for analysis.

Predictive studies are good choices for addressing questions that concern the ability to predict a given outcome with single or multiple predictor variables. They are tremendously useful as evidence in nursing practice because their results can be used to identify early indicators of complications, disease, or other negative outcomes so that preventive actions can be taken. Specific statistics that are generated from these studies can be used to predict an outcome for a single individual, given some specific data collected about that person. The tests used in predictive studies yield a statistic that enables the researcher to determine how well the predictive model works in explaining the outcome. Predictive studies can also be used to establish the predictive validity of measurement scales. In summary, predictive study methods are suitable for use with a variety of clinical questions.

Predictive Study Methods and Procedures

Predictive studies are very similar in design to correlation studies. The population is clearly identified, variables are defined, measures are captured with reliable and valid tools, and the data are analyzed and interpreted appropriately. The primary distinction between correlation and predictive designs is the type of analytic tool applied to the data and the interpretation of the outcome. Predictive designs are analyzed using regression analysis, which tests the predictive model for statistical significance and for explanatory capacity. Predictive studies are also distinct from correlation studies in that multiple predictors may be tested against a single numerical outcome, and these predictors may be a mix of ordinal- and interval-level measures. Even nominal data may be used if they are specially treated and coded in the analysis procedure. This makes the predictive study one of the most useful designs for clinical practice.

CASE IN POINT Predictive Design

Long-term glycemic control is a goal for young patients with type 1 diabetes mellitus. Jackson, Wernham, Elder, and Wright (2013) wanted to determine the predictors that best identified those young adults who would achieve and maintain long-term glycemic control. A cohort of 155 patients who had type 1 diabetes and were between the ages of 18 and 22 was recruited. This retrospective study used data recorded over a 14-year period to analyze the predictor variables associated with keeping HbA_{1c} levels within normal limits.

Healthcare practitioners seek interventions that can prevent the long-term effects of uncontrolled diabetes. The best indicator of long-term glycemic control in the study participants was early achievement of glycemic control, especially by the first year after diagnosis. The data from this study suggest that the efforts taken in the first year post diagnosis to control blood sugar pay off in the long run. As evidence, this study helps identify the effective timing of an intervention.

This study was a typical predictive model, in that a range of variables was measured for each subject and statistical techniques were used to determine the best predictors. The authors note that further study of these elements could lead to early detection and the development of effective interventions to achieve and maintain long-term control of type 1 diabetes (Jackson et al., 2013).

Strengths of Predictive Studies

Predictive studies are quite useful as evidence for nursing practice because they have significant advantages:

- A great deal of information is yielded from a single set of data.
- The results of the study can provide information about whole samples or can be applied to individual cases.
- A variety of levels of measurement may be used in the predictive model.
- The studies are relatively simple to design and implement, and they are cost-effective.
- The data that are used may be either prospective or retrospective.

Limitations of Predictive Studies

Despite their significant strengths, predictive studies have several drawbacks that researchers must consider when applying them as evidence for nursing practice:

- Although prediction can be quantified, there is no assurance of causality; suppressor variables may exist.
- The researcher may "go fishing," or explore large numbers of variables without a focused research question, resulting in an increased error rate.
- Regression analysis requires relatively large sample sizes, the need for which becomes amplified as the number of variables increases.

Predictive studies have the advantage of helping nurses identify patients at risk for subsequent health problems so that preventive strategies can be implemented. Because they can quantify the relationships between variables and outcomes, such studies are very useful as evidence for nursing practice. When multiple predictors and outcomes are suspected, the nurse researcher may hypothesize an overall model or a picture

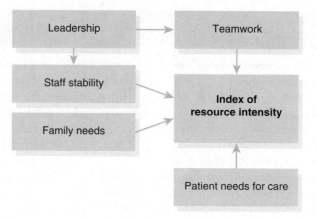

FIGURE 10.4 A Test of Model Fit

of relationships and interrelationships between variables. These models can then be evaluated using descriptive methods and procedures, which produces some of the most sophisticated descriptive studies used as evidence for practice.

Model-Testing Designs

An extension of predictive designs is the model-testing design. Although predictive designs quantify the relationship between a predictor and an outcome, model-testing designs quantify the accuracy of a hypothesized model of relationships and interrelationships. Model testing is the process of hypothesizing how various elements in the patient care environment interact, how these elements can be measured, and which paths of direct and indirect effects flow from variables to outcomes. The model-testing design requires that all variables relevant to the model be identified and measured. It also requires a large sample size and very precise measurement of variables. Notably, it requires that all variables of the model be measured (Burns & Grove, 2011). The analysis examines whether the data are consistent with the model. Model-testing designs represent the complexity of patient care realistically and thoroughly. **FIGURE 10.4** depicts such a model representing the environmental demands on the nurse.

Model-testing designs are quite complicated to plan and implement, and their analysis requires specialized software. The interpretation of model-testing designs requires substantial statistical expertise, with very large samples needed to achieve adequate power. For these reasons, they are not commonly used research methods for nursing evidence. Such complex designs are implemented to test hypotheses about complex relationships in the patient care environment, and are often used to develop nursing theory.

Reading Descriptive Research

The first step in the critique of the methods and procedures of a descriptive study is to determine the specific type of design used in the study. The design is usually specified generically as "descriptive" in the abstract and introduction of the study, and the specific type of descriptive design may appear there as well. If sufficient detail is not given in the early parts of the research report to determine the specifics of the descriptive design, the particulars should be included in the methods and procedures section. Enough detail should be provided that the reader can judge the researcher's decisions related to the specific design that was chosen. The type of design should answer the research question and meet the intent of the researchers. Information on the researcher's rationale for selecting the specific type of study for this question is helpful; a clear link between the purpose of the study and the type of design used to achieve it should be apparent.

If detail about the type of study is lacking, then the reader may need to closely examine the article for evidence of the type of design that was employed. Clues to the specific design may be found in the research question or objectives. Words such as *describe*, *explore*, *observe*, and *document* may indicate that a straightforward descriptive design was used. When individuals are referred to in the question, the study is likely a case study or single-subject design; such studies are always descriptive and are not considered experimental designs (regardless of how the author describes the design). If the research question uses words such as *relationship*, *association*, or *prediction*, then the study likely used a correlation design. No matter which design was used, it should have a clear link to the research question, and the specifics of the methods and procedures should match both the question and the stated design.

Other clues can be deduced from the description of the sources of data and the measurement procedures. If the only statistics that are reported are descriptive (e.g., mean, median, standard deviation), correlative (e.g., correlation coefficient, Pearson, rho), or for regression (e.g., *r*-squared, beta), then the study is descriptive, regardless of the author's designation. If the protocol for measurement involves record retrieval, abstraction of data from patient charts, or access to databases, then the design is almost certainly retrospective. If the protocol calls for recruiting subjects, then the study is prospective.

Scrutinize measures for documentation of the timing of data collection. Collecting data at a single point in time clearly means the study is a general descriptive, correlation, or cross-sectional study. In contrast, references to periodic data collection indicate that the study is a case study, a single-subject design, or a longitudinal study. Predictive studies may be of either type; it is not uncommon for researchers to collect predictor variables at a single point in time and outcome variables at some future point in time. The design of these studies, however, is revealed by their almost exclusive reliance on regression analytic techniques, so they should be identifiable from the type of statistics reported.

Although space restrictions in journals may limit the amount of information the author can provide about the study methods and procedures, a reasonably informed researcher should be able to replicate the study from the information provided. A descriptive study—although considered a basic design—should still demonstrate a systematic and rigorous approach to implementation. The population of interest should be defined, with inclusion and exclusion criteria specified for sample eligibility. Methods for recruiting and/or selecting subjects should be clear and unbiased; the reader needs to be watchful for signs of researcher bias or selection effects. Confidence in the conclusions drawn by the researcher and the capacity for generalizability are both dependent on a strong sampling strategy.

Scrutinize the measurement procedure to ensure that reliable and valid instruments were used to collect the data. The type of reliability that is documented should be specific to the descriptive design. For example, cross-sectional measures should have strong internal reliability because consistency across subjects is most important. Conversely, test–retest reliability is a bigger concern in longitudinal studies because stability over time is critical for drawing valid conclusions in these investigations. If data were collected retrospectively, look for operational definitions that ensure consistency in data retrieval. Mention should be made of training for data collectors and checks for inter-rater reliability if the study relied on multiple data collectors.

Finally, examine the conclusions section to ensure that the authors do not overinterpret or make inferences that go beyond what the results can support. Descriptive studies, at their most fundamental, can only describe. They may suggest or imply causal relationships, but no descriptive study can confirm a causal relationship. Making such a statement of causality is particularly tempting for the authors of correlation studies. This reasoning is understandable: If two variables are strongly related, then it is tempting to conclude that one affects or causes the other. In reality, without the controls that are inherent in an experimental design, and without a randomly chosen comparison group, it is impossible to confirm all the conditions necessary to establish true causality. The correlation documents the strength of a relationship but does not identify which variable came first. In addition, correlation studies do not allow the researcher to rule out rival explanations for the relationship through the control of internal validity. Ultimately, a correlation between two variables may represent the mutual effects of some completely different variable.

Descriptive studies are some of the most commonly undertaken types of research studies. With the preceding cautions in mind, they can be some of the most useful research studies for providing evidence for nursing practice. An understanding of the patient care situation as it exists can help the nurse plan strategies that meet existing needs and have a high likelihood of acceptance. Knowing what is can be a powerful means for creating innovative solutions to achieve what can be.

WHERE TO LOOK FOR INFORMATION ABOUT DESCRIPTIVE METHODS

- A descriptive study is usually explicitly identified as such in the abstract and early in the introduction of the article. It should be described early enough that the reader can evaluate the information that follows in the context of a descriptive study. If this information is not found in the introduction, then it should appear in the first paragraph of the methods and procedures section.
- The specification of the descriptive design should be easily identifiable and a major part of the research study write-up. The explanation may be concise, but it should provide enough detail that an informed reader could replicate the study.
- The specific type of descriptive design (e.g., cross-sectional, correlation, or single subject) should be detailed in the methods and procedures

section, even if the study has been identified generically as "descriptive" earlier in the study.
- Research reports may not explicitly portray a study as retrospective, even though these designs are very common in nursing research. Conversely, a researcher will generally state explicitly that a prospective study was conducted. The reader must scrutinize the data collection procedure to determine if any of the data were collected from secondary sources. Look for terms such as *ex post facto*, which is commonly used to describe retrospective designs.
- If the measurement process is complex, there may be a separate section for procedures, which may be labeled as such or called "protocols." This section may describe variables in detail as well as the measurement procedures.

CHECKLIST FOR EVALUATION OF DESCRIPTIVE METHODS AND PROCEDURES

❑ The design is identified as descriptive in the abstract and/or the introduction.

❑ The type of descriptive design is specified in the methods and procedures section.

❑ There is a clear and appropriate link between the research question and the descriptive design.

❑ The rationale for selection of a descriptive study is specific and appropriate.

❑ The primary variables of interest are clearly identified and defined.

❑ The interpretation and conclusions are congruent with description and do not imply causality.

❑ If the study is longitudinal, a rationale is provided for the timing of data collection.

Using Descriptive Research in Evidence-Based Nursing Practice

Descriptive research is not considered strong evidence for a change in nursing practice, but rather is more often used to assess current practice (Schmidt & Brown, 2012). Without the controls provided by experimental designs and control groups, these types of studies cannot provide strong conclusions about causality—a condition necessary for support of a nursing intervention. Nevertheless, evidence-based practice in nursing relies on expert judgment, clinical curiosity, and an understanding of patient preferences to design appropriate and acceptable interventions: This is precisely where descriptive research provides a great deal of value.

Descriptive evidence has many applications in nursing practice. Assessment, diagnosis, care planning, intervention, and evaluation of outcomes all rely on accurate description of phenomena, patient responses to care and conditions, and the acceptability of treatments.

GRAY MATTER

Though not considered the strongest evidence for a change in nursing practice, findings from descriptive studies can be used to support the following applications:
- Assessment of patients and patient care
- Identification of risk factors for disease
- Care planning
- Nursing interventions
- Evaluation of outcomes

Assessment of Patients and Patient Care

Descriptive studies can help the nurse determine the distribution of risk factors and disease in a population of interest. Of particular value is assessment of the signs and symptoms that patients exhibit as they react to treatments or respond to their health conditions. Predictive studies, for example, can help the nurse identify early signals that a patient may be at risk for a health condition or complication, so that preventive steps can be initiated. Case studies and single-subject designs aid the nurse in understanding how individual patients may respond to treatment and clarify the unique aspects of individuals that may affect their response to an intervention.

Diagnosis of Patient Care Conditions

Descriptive studies familiarize the nurse with the kinds of conditions that may present in a particular patient population, thereby supporting more accurate diagnoses of their nursing conditions. Cross-sectional and longitudinal studies help document the health needs of populations; model tests may also illuminate the relationship between conditions and nursing diagnoses.

Care Planning

Thorough description of the health needs of populations and the responses of individuals to care can help the nurse plan strategies to meet those patients' needs. Descriptive studies are particularly helpful in the design of effective patient teaching plans and health promotion activities. Individual compliance with a teaching plan depends on the patient's acceptance of the need for change and willingness to incorporate new behaviors into his or her life. Understanding the ways that individuals respond to health conditions can help the nurse design plans that meet each patient's goals more effectively.

Interventions

Descriptive studies facilitate interventions that are acceptable to patients and encourage compliance. A descriptive study can also detail the difficulties a nurse might have in implementing an intervention or the barriers that exist to changing a current practice. Case studies are particularly helpful in identifying which processes a nurse might use to implement a change in evidence-based practices or how a nurse was successful in helping an individual deal with his or her health conditions.

Evaluation of Outcomes

Descriptive studies help the nurse identify the outcomes that are reasonable and appropriate to evaluate after a treatment has been initiated or a health condition identified. Patient outcomes based solely on nursing actions and interventions are difficult to quantify because other care providers are also performing treatments and interventions that may factor into the outcome (Polit & Beck, 2012).

As part of their routine practice, nurses make decisions that have important implications for patient outcomes. Understanding the health problems of populations, the responses of individuals to health treatments and conditions, and the processes that nurses may use to initiate change are key considerations in evidence-based nursing practice. The diversity of descriptive research is matched only by its usefulness. The nurse is well served by reviewing descriptive research prior to planning interventions to maximize the probability that actions will be effective, efficient, and acceptable to those who are served by them. Descriptive research findings enhance both nursing practice and the patient experience.

A Note About Pilot Studies

A pilot study is an intentionally smaller version of a study, which utilizes a limited sample size or group of measures. Its primary purpose is to test the methods and procedures of a study prior to full implementation of that study. A pilot study can assess the planned study's costs, time, efficiency, and accuracy on a smaller scale. It may be used to test instrumentation for reliability and validity or data collection procedures for difficulties leading to inconsistencies. Grant-making agencies prefer to see studies that have been fully or partially tested on a pilot level before they dole out funding, because this step provides a level of assurance that the researcher can accomplish the research plan.

Although a pilot study is ideally a prospective part of the research plan, some researchers may wind up describing their study as a pilot because of an unacceptable response rate, use of a sample size with insufficient power, or inability to verify a measurement as reliable. In this case, the author may "live and learn" from the study by using it as a case study, in effect, to plan a more effective set of research processes.

Creating Descriptive Research

Descriptive designs are common in nursing research and are some of the most easily implemented studies. As such, they are appropriate for novice researchers in both academic and clinical settings. The information generated by a descriptive study can support evidence-based nursing practice—but only if the researcher performed a rigorous study that produced valid, credible results. "Descriptive" is not necessarily synonymous with "simple," and it is certainly not equivalent to "careless." Thoughtful consideration of the elements central to study design is needed before beginning a descriptive/correlation research study. A systematic series of decisions must be made to design a strong descriptive study:

- Clarify the purpose of the study and carefully construct a research question. It should be easy to provide a rationale for the selection of a descriptive study based on the purpose statement and the wording of the research question.
- Identify a design that will answer the question in the most efficient, effective way. The specifics of the design should be the result of careful consideration of both the strengths and the limitations of the design, as well as the skills and resources of the researcher.
- Describe the population of interest, and determine inclusion and exclusion criteria for the sample. Devise a sampling strategy that maximizes the representativeness of the population and supports the external validity of the findings.
- Clarify the variables of interest and write operational definitions for each before selecting measurement instruments. If multiple raters will be used in the study, create a data dictionary so that all the data collectors will understand what each variable represents. Use the operational definitions to identify the appropriate measurement tools, not the other way around.

- Identify a measurement procedure that will generate trustworthy data. If instruments or tools are to be used, ensure that they possess the appropriate psychometric properties for the specific study design that is proposed.
- Manage the data collection process carefully. Methods should be incorporated that will ensure reliability among raters, whether they are retrieving data from records or gathering data directly from subjects. This often includes training and observation for reliability before data collectors function independently.
- Design a process for maintaining the integrity of the data set. Specific measures should be planned for restricting access and ensuring confidentiality, such as use of password-protected files and locked file cabinets. Incorporate periodic quality checks into the data management process.
- Use the appropriate analytic tools for the question to be answered and the types of data being collected. Consider the level of measurement of each variable in selecting the specific statistical treatment.
- Report the analysis accurately and completely; report each test that was run, even if it did not contribute to the overall outcome of the study. This reduces the potential for selective retention of findings—a threat to validity of the study.
- Draw conclusions that are appropriate for the intent of the study and the results that were found. Although it is acceptable to note relationships that are suggested or implied by the data—and certainly to pose additional hypotheses that should be tested—descriptive studies can only describe.

Developing a design for a study will require careful attention to each of these elements. The fact that a descriptive design is common and basic should not lead the novice researcher to draw the conclusion that it can be accomplished without a great deal of forethought and planning. Considering these details will result in a stronger study.

Summary of Key Concepts

- The purpose of descriptive research is the exploration and description of phenomena in real-life situations.
- Descriptive research designs are used in studies that construct a picture or make an account of events as they naturally occur; the investigator does not manipulate variables.
- A descriptive design can be used to develop theory, identify problems, provide information for decision making, or determine what others in similar situations are doing.
- Two basic types of questions are addressed with descriptive designs: general descriptive questions and questions about relationships.
- Additional ways to classify descriptive studies are according to whether they involve groups of subjects or individuals and whether data are collected at a point in time or periodically over time.
- Retrospective studies rely on secondary data that have been collected in the past, often for other purposes; prospective studies involve data collection in the future for the express purpose of the study.

- Survey research involves collecting data directly from respondents about their characteristics, responses, attitudes, perceptions, or beliefs.
- Cross-sectional studies describe a population at a single point in time; longitudinal studies follow a cohort of subjects over an extended period of time.
- Descriptive designs can be used to measure the responses of unique individuals, either through case study or single-subject designs.
- Correlation studies examine relationships as they exist or may use variables to predict outcomes. These studies may also test models for their fit with reality.
- Although descriptive research does not enable the investigator to establish cause and effect between variables, these studies are still valuable as evidence for assessment, diagnosis, care planning, interventions, and evaluation.

CRITICAL APPRAISAL EXERCISE

Retrieve the following full-text article from the Cumulative Index to Nursing and Allied Health Literature or similar search database:

Codier, E., & Odell, E. (2014). Measured emotional intelligence ability and grade point average in nursing students. *Nurse Education Today, 34,* 608–612.

Review the article, focusing on the sections that report the question, design, methods, and procedures. Consider the following appraisal questions in your critical review of this research article:

1. Why did these authors select a descriptive design relating to the research purpose statement?
2. What is the specific descriptive design used by these authors?
3. Would you feel comfortable generalizing the results of this study to all nursing students? Why or why not?
4. Which efforts were made to ensure reliable, valid measures (e.g., operational definitions of variables, using instruments with low error)?
5. What are the strengths of the design, methods, and procedures of this study? Contrast them with its limitations.
6. Did the authors interpret the results correctly—that is, without any over-interpretation?

References

Brown, A., & Jordan, S. (2013). Impact of birth complications on breastfeeding duration: An Internet survey. *Journal of Advanced Nursing, 69*(4), 828–839.

Bruce, S., Feinstein, J., Kennedy, M., & Liu, M. (2015). Humane education for students with visual impairments: Learning about working dogs. *Journal of Visual Impairment & Blindness, 7,* 279–292.

Buijs, D., Ramadi, A., MacDonald, K., Lightfoot, R., Senaratne, M., & Haennel, R. (2015). Quantity and quality of daily physical activity in older cardiac patients. *Canadian Journal of Cardiovascular Nursing, 25*(3), 10–16.

Burns, N., & Grove, S. K. (2011). *Understanding nursing research: Building an evidence-based practice* (5th ed.). Maryland Heights, MO: Elsevier Saunders.

Byiers, B., Reichie, J., & Sumons, F. (2012). Single subject experimental design for evidence-based practice. *American Journal of Speech-Language Pathology, 21,* 392–414.

Gordon, M., Henderson, R., Holmes, J., Wolters, M., & Bennett, I. (2016). Participatory design of ehealth solutions for women from vulnerable populations with perinatal depression. *Journal of the American Medical Informatics Association, 23*(1), 105–109.

Grove, S., Gray, J., & Burns, N. (2014). *Understanding nursing research: Building an evidence-based practice* (6th ed.). St. Louis, MO: Elsevier, Saunders.

Holm, M., Baird, J., Kim, Y., Rajora, K., D'Silva, D., Podolinsky, L., . . . Minshew, N. (2014). Therapeutic horseback riding outcomes of parent-identified goals for children with autism spectrum disorder: An ABA multiple case design examining dosing and generalization to the home and community. *Journal of Autism and Developmental Disorders, 44,* 937–947.

Howlett, B., Rogo, E. J., & Shelton, T. (2014). *Evidence-based practice for health professionals: An interprofessional approach.* Burlington, MA: Jones & Bartlett Learning.

Jackson, C., Wernham, E., Elder, C., & Wright, N. (2013). Early glycaemic control is predictive of long-term control: A retrospective observational study. *Practical Diabetes, 30*(1), 16–18.

Lu, E., Wang, R., Hebert, D., Boger, J., Galea, M., & Mihailidis, A. A. (2011). The development of an upper limb stroke rehabilitation robot: Identification of clinical practices and design requirements through a survey of therapists. *Disability & Rehabilitation: Assistive Technology, 6*(5), 420–431.

Melnyk, B., & Fineout-Overholt, E. (2011). *Evidence-based practice in nursing and healthcare: A guide to best practice* (2nd ed.). Philadelphia, PA: Lippincott Williams & Wilkins.

Polit, D., & Beck, C. (2012). *Nursing research: Generating and assessing evidence for nursing practice* (9th ed.). Philadelphia, PA: Lippincott Williams & Wilkins.

Schmidt, N., & Brown, J. (2012). *Evidence-based practice for nurses: Appraisal and application of research* (2nd ed.). Burlington, MA: Jones & Bartlett Learning.

Tappen, R. (2011). *Advanced nursing research: From theory to practice.* Sudbury, MA: Jones and Bartlett.

Xie, R., Gaudet, L., Krewski, D., Graham, I., Walker, M., & Wen, S. (2015). Higher cesarean delivery rates are associated with higher infant mortality rates in industrialized countries. *Birth Issues in Perinatal Care, 42*(1), 62–69.

Yin, R. K. (2013). *Case study research: Design and methods* (5th ed.). Thousand Oaks, CA: Sage.

Chapter 11

Summarizing and Reporting Descriptive Data

CHAPTER OBJECTIVES

The study of this chapter will help the learner to

- Interpret descriptive data when summarized as measures of central tendency, variability, and correlation.
- Use graphical presentations of descriptive data to understand research findings.
- Critique the appropriateness of statistics used to summarize descriptive data.
- Select appropriate statistical techniques to summarize and present descriptive data.
- Evaluate the results section of descriptive studies as evidence for nursing practice.

KEY TERMS

Bar chart	Histogram	Scatter plot
Box plot	Line graph	Standard deviation
Coefficient of variation (CV)	Mean	Standardized score
Correlation analysis	Median	Standard normal distribution
Derived variable	Mode	Variance
Descriptive data	Range	
Frequency	Rate	

Introduction

Summarizing **descriptive data** is the first step in the analysis of quantitative research data. Because it is the first step, other steps depend on its careful completion. When descriptive data are summarized correctly, they provide useful information about participants in the sample, their answers to survey questions, and their responses to study inquiries.

Analysis of descriptive data entails the use of simple mathematical procedures or calculations, many of which are straightforward enough to be done with a calculator.

Descriptive data: Numbers in a data set that are collected to represent research variables.

Yet, these simple numerical techniques provide essential information in a research study. When it comes to descriptive analysis, those persons evaluating research as evidence have different needs than do those persons who conduct the research studies. The purposes of summarizing descriptive data for readers of research include the following:

- Giving the reader a quick grasp of the characteristics of the sample and the variables in the study to understand its appropriate application as evidence
- Providing basic information on how variables in a study are alike (measures of central tendency) and how they are different (measures of variability)
- Conveying information about the study through numerical and graphical methods to enhance understanding of the findings (Scott & Mazhindu, 2014)

The purposes of summarizing descriptive data for researchers include the following:

- Reviewing the data set using frequency tables to check for coding or data entry errors
- Visualizing the descriptive data—particularly the shape of distributions—to determine whether statistical assumptions are met for the selection of appropriate statistical analysis
- Understanding the characteristics of the participants in the study and their performance on variables of interest in the study
- Gaining an in-depth understanding of the data before inferential analysis

In quantitative research, a summary of descriptive data can be accomplished using statistical techniques such as measures of central tendency, variance, frequency distributions, and correlation. These statistics provide a method to summarize large amounts of data from a research study through meaningful numbers.

Care must be taken by researchers who create descriptive reports; correct statistical techniques must be selected for the data that have been collected. The level of measurement of a variable is a primary consideration when deciding which statistical technique to use to summarize descriptive data. In addition, the report of descriptive data needs to be presented in the most meaningful way—in other words, in a way that readers readily comprehend and cannot easily misunderstand. The same principles apply to nurses who use statistical techniques to summarize descriptive data in the clinical setting—descriptive data must be analyzed appropriately and reported in meaningful ways to others in the clinical setting. Of particular importance in evidence-based practice is using descriptive data before and after implementing the new practice; the questions of interest are "Does the evidence apply to the population of patients for whom the facility cares?" and "Is the change resulting in the desired outcomes?" (Melnyk, Fineout-Overholt, Stillwell, & Williamson, 2010).

When reading the analysis of descriptive data, the appropriateness of the statistical technique should be appraised. Even more critical, the summarization of the data and the nurse researcher's interpretation of the data must be critiqued by the reader to determine the level of confidence in the findings as evidence.

SCENES FROM THE FIELD

Treatments that are planned but not delivered are a serious source of adverse events for patients in an acute care unit. Missed nursing care may be even more serious in the neonatal intensive care unit (NICU), where even small departures from the plan of care can lead to serious complications. Tubbs-Cooley and colleagues (2015) conducted a descriptive study to determine the frequency and type of missed care as reported by NICU nurses and the factors that may have contributed to these omissions.

These researchers surveyed a random sample of certified NICU nurses in seven states who provided direct care. They used an existing survey—the MISSCARE Survey—that consists of three sections: questions related to the characteristics of the nurses, questions about the frequency and type of missed nursing care activities, and questions about the possible reasons for the missed care. The data, which were collected via a web-based survey, comprised both ordinal and nominal (classification) data.

Tubbs-Cooley et al. (2015) reported the findings in tables with sufficient information to determine both the typical values and the ranges of responses. The ordinal data were represented in tables that allowed the reader to see the actual counts and percentages for responses by item. This helped support the credibility of the analytics and the interpretation of the results.

A range of care activities was found to be missed. Most frequently missed were routine rounds, oral care for ventilated infants, parent education, and parental involvement in care and oral feedings. The activities missed least often were reassuring—these NICU nurses were particularly attentive to hand washing, safety, physical assessment, and medication administration. The nurses reported the most common reasons for missed care were the frequent interruptions and urgent patient situations that arise in an intensive care environment. As would be expected, unexpected upturns in patient volume and care intensity were also reported as issues leading to missed treatments.

This evidence was presented well and the variables were measured and analyzed appropriately. NICU nurses can use this information as evidence in developing care plans and practice guidelines that enable nurses to ensure that every patient gets every treatment needed, at the time it is needed.

An Overview of Descriptive Data Analysis

Statistical analysis of descriptive data is conducted to provide a summary of data in published research reports. These data serve as the starting point for the reader to begin making decisions regarding the strength and applicability of the research as evidence for practice in specific populations. Descriptive data are derived from a data set to represent research variables for the purpose of summarizing information about the sample and do not involve generalization to a larger set of data such as the population. For example, a data set could contain variables including ages of participants, years of experience as a nurse, and scores on a job satisfaction instrument. Simply put, descriptive statistics use numbers narratively, in tables, or in graphic displays to organize and describe the characteristics of a sample (Polit, 2010).

Descriptive statistics involve a range of complexity, from simple counts of data to analyses of relationships. The most commonly encountered descriptive statistics are classified in the following ways:

- Counts of data, expressed as frequencies, frequency tables, and frequency distributions
- Measures of central tendency, expressed as the mean, median, and mode

- Measures of variability, including the range, variance, and standard deviation
- Measures of position, such as percentile ranks and standardized scores
- Measures of relationship such as correlation coefficients
- Graphical presentations in bar charts, line graphs, and scatter plots

The specific types of summary statistics that are applied to descriptive data are driven by the nature of the data and the level of measurement of the variable. It is important to apply as many descriptive techniques as necessary to provide an accurate picture of the variable, rather than giving only a single measure that may mislead a reader. For example, providing a percentage of 100% hand-washing compliance for a month may look very good, but if the frequency count is omitted—especially if that count is $n = 1$—a complete picture is not provided.

Understanding Levels of Measurement

The initial, and perhaps most vital, step in descriptive analysis is to identify the level of measurement for each variable so as to choose the appropriate statistical analysis. This decision is the responsibility of the researchers who create descriptive studies and is an important point for critique by nurses who read research reports. Data can be collected in one of four possible levels of measurement: nominal, ordinal, interval, or ratio. Each level has characteristics that make it unique, and each requires a particular type of statistical technique. Table 11.1 shows descriptive statistical techniques that are appropriate for each level of measurement.

Nominal-level data are those that denote categories and have no rank order; numbers given to these data are strictly for showing membership in a category and are not subject to mathematical calculations. Nominal data can be counted, but are not measured, so they can be summarized using statistics that represent counts. Fall precautions is an example of nominal data: Either a patient is on fall precautions or the patient is not. Summary statistics appropriate for this level of measurement are frequency, percentage, rates, ratios, and mode.

Table 11.1 Levels of Measurement and Appropriate Summary Statistics

Level of Measurement	Distributions	Central Tendency Mode	Variability	Shape
Nominal	Frequency Percentage	Mode		
Ordinal	Frequency Percentage	Mode Median	Range Minimum/maximum	
Interval/ratio		Mode Median Mean	Range Minimum/maximum Standard deviation Variance	Skew Kurtosis

Ordinal data are also categories but have an added characteristic of rank order. These data differ from nominal data in that the categories for a variable can be identified as being less than or greater than one another. However, because the level of measure is still categorical, the exact level of difference cannot be identified. A pain scale, in spite of its representation as a series of numbers, is an example of ordinal data. For example, while we know a score of 7 on this scale is greater than a 5, the difference cannot be quantified. For example, we cannot conclude that the difference between a 7 and a 5 on the pain scale is the same as the difference between a 4 and a 2 on the same scale; we simply know that one number is higher than the other. Further, we do not know that a score of 5 for one patient is the same as a score of 5 for another patient. The fact that the pain scale is represented by numbers also does not necessarily mean the characteristic under study has been quantified. In our example, we do not know exactly how much pain exists; it is just rated against other experiences of pain for that patient. The patient's score has simply been ranked against all other values of the variable. Statistical techniques appropriate for ordinal data include those appropriate for nominal data plus range, median, minimum, and maximum.

> **Frequency:**
> A count of the instances that an event occurs in a data set.

Interval and ratio data are recorded on a continuous scale that has equal intervals between all entries; length of stay is an example. Data collected on interval or ratio levels result in numbers that can be subjected to many mathematical procedures, including mean, standard deviation, variance, and evaluation of the distribution (skew and kurtosis).

Identifying Shape and Distribution

Initial analyses of data are meant to help the researcher identify the distribution, and therefore the shape, of the variable's data. The outcome of this analysis, coupled with the level of measurement, guides the researcher in selecting the appropriate statistics to represent the variable's center and spread.

Summarizing Data Using Frequencies

Frequency is a statistical term that means a count of the instances in which a number or category occurs in a data set. Frequencies are commonly used in clinical settings; for example, a frequency might be used to document the number of infections by surgery type, the number of patient falls by nursing unit, or the number of nurses who leave in the first 18 months of employment. In research, frequencies are used to count the number of times that a variable has a particular value or score. A researcher may collect data on nominal-level variables or ordinal-level variables and then generate a frequency count per category to summarize the data. For example, if information about gender were desired, two values (male and female) would be collected; the number of participants in the study who were male and the number who were female would be tallied.

Frequency data can also be used to calculate percentages, rates, and derived variables. A percentage is a useful summary technique that shows the relative frequency of a variable. For example, if gender was measured as a variable and there were 180 female participants in a sample of 400, the percentage of female participants would be 45%. The number 45% is more meaningful as a summary value than the frequency count because readers can tell quickly that slightly less than half of the sample was female. To calculate

Rate:
A calculated count derived from dividing the frequency of an event in a given time period by all possible occurrences of the event during the same time period.

Derived variable:
A new variable produced when data from other variables are combined using a simple formula.

the percentage in this example, the number of female participants is divided by the number of participants in the entire sample (180/400 = 0.45 or 45%).

Rates that are clinically important can be calculated to provide information about data trends over time. Like a percentage, a **rate** is calculated by dividing the frequency of an event in a given time period by all possible occurrences of the event during the same time period. The difference is that percentages by definition are "per 100," whereas rates can have a different denominator, such as per 1000 patient-days. Monthly fall rates are an example; the number of falls in a month is divided by the total number of patient-days in that month and then multiplied by 1000 to give the number of falls per 1000 patient-days. This allows for comparison between units based on opportunities for falls (each day) instead of the raw count (number of falls). When calculated periodically, patient outcomes expressed as rates can be monitored as a basis for action planning to improve care (Altman, 2006).

Derived variables are created when data from other variables are put into a simple formula to produce a new piece of information—a new variable. An example of a derived variable is the hospital length of stay. It is calculated by summing the number of inpatient days on a nursing unit (a frequency) in a month and then dividing this sum by the number of patients in the unit. Rates and derived variables may be used to represent the effects of extraneous variables or to describe baseline performance. Operational definitions of these variables are important to include to facilitate consistency in the method of calculation.

Summarizing Data Using Frequency Tables

Interval-level data can be summarized in a frequency table as well, but they must be grouped into categories first, which requires converting the data into ordinal data. Because interval-level data can fall anywhere on a continuous scale, each data point could theoretically be a unique number; as a result, there can be many different values in the data set, which makes interpreting the data difficult. As an example, **Table 11.2** contains

Table 11.2 Unordered Data Set of Years as a Nurse

Years as a Nurse

13	5	23	5	3
7	5	30	20	5
8	6	17	21	11
7	6	27	5	18
2	1	9	9	16
2	1	3	5	9
1	5	30	1	28
2	2	16	3	12
5	5	20	15	17
23	20	17	9	24

Table 11.3 Frequency Table for Years as a Nurse

Years as a Nurse	Frequency	Percentage
1–3	11	22
4–9	18	36
10–17	9	18
18–30	12	24
Total	50	100

Bar chart:
A graphic presentation for nominal or ordinal data that represents the categories on the horizontal axis and frequency on the vertical axis.

Histogram:
A type of frequency distribution in which variables with different values are plotted as a graph on x-axes and y-axes, and the shape can be visualized.

a data set that could benefit from summary as a frequency table. To create a frequency table for interval-level data, the data are sorted from lowest value to highest value, categories are created for the data, and the number of occurrences in each category is counted. Collapsing several years together provides an even clearer picture. Table 11.3 represents the same data in a frequency table that includes both counts and relative frequency (percentage). Representing complex data in this way enhances interpretation and understanding of the values. Although no patterns were readily apparent in the data in the original table, review of the frequency table makes it clear that most participants in the study had few years of nursing experience; in fact, the majority of participants had nine or fewer years of experience.

Summarizing Data Using Frequency Distributions

In many ways, graphical presentation of data is easier to understand because the data are presented in summary fashion with colors, lines, and shapes that show differences and similarities in the data set. An easy chart to create is a bar chart for nominal or ordinal data. The most common way to design a bar chart is to have categories of the variable on the x-axis (horizontal) of the chart and the frequency for each category on the y-axis (vertical). Bar charts provide the reader with a quick assessment of which category has the most occurrences in a data set. For example, a bar chart of patient safety occurrences (nominal data) can show which occurrences happen the most, thereby providing information on which areas should be the focus of improvement efforts.

A bar chart showing the frequency per category for ordinal data enables evaluation of the shape of the distribution of values. Such graphs are called frequency distributions or histograms. For example, the values of subjects' pain ratings can be represented in a graph with the value (pain rating) placed on the x-axis and the number of cases with that pain rating on the y-axis. **FIGURE 11.1** depicts a histogram of pain rating data. It shows categories for values of the variable across the horizontal dimension, with frequencies being displayed on the vertical dimension. In this histogram, the reader can see that most of the values of the variable "postop pain" were between 4 and 6.

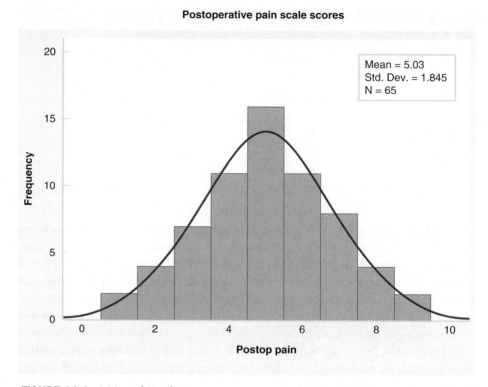

FIGURE 11.1 A Normal Distribution

Another useful feature of the histogram is that it shows the curve of the data. The researcher can see whether the data in the study are normal, are skewed, or have an abnormal kurtosis. Based on the distribution of the data, the researcher will then select the statistic for describing the center and spread of the data. Figure 11.1 depicted an approximately normal distribution. A normal distribution, often called a bell curve, has a large proportion of values of the variable in the middle of the distribution and smaller proportions on the ends (tails). The shape of the distribution is symmetrical, meaning that the right and left sides of the distribution are mirror images. The shape of the distribution of a variable in a research study is important because many statistical procedures require the assumption of a normal distribution to yield reliable results (Field, 2013).

Some variables are not symmetric, so they do not have a normal distribution. Asymmetric distributions may be described as demonstrating skew or kurtosis. A skewed distribution has a disproportionate number of occurrences in either the right or left tail of the distribution. Describing the type of distribution is counterintuitive: The skew is described by the direction of the tail. For example, distributions with more values in the positive end of the distribution trail out to the negative end and so are described as negative skew; those with more values on the lower end of the scale

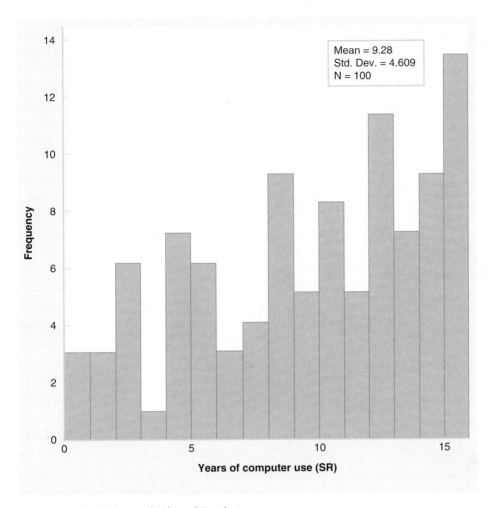

FIGURE 11.2 A Negatively Skewed Distribution

will trail out to the positive end and so are called positive skew. **FIGURES 11.2** and **11.3** demonstrate skewed distributions. Kurtosis refers to an unusual accumulation of values in some part of the distribution, particularly in the size of the tails. Those distributions with large tails are called leptokurtic; those with small tails are called platykurtic. A leptokurtic distribution is depicted by the histogram in **FIGURE 11.4**.

Researchers who create data have a responsibility to check the descriptive data for compliance with the underlying assumptions of the statistical techniques selected for use. These assumptions often include a requirement for variables to have a normal distribution (not skewed or kurtotic) and to have equal variances (similar spread of scores around the mean). A visual inspection of the graphical display of values of a variable via a histogram can give a researcher a quick indication of whether the variable meets the requirements of the statistical test.

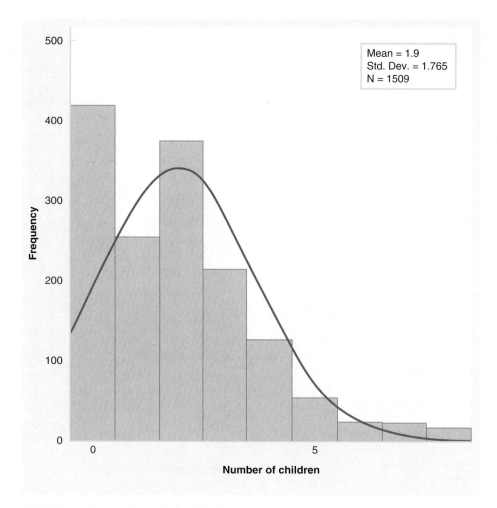

FIGURE 11.3 A Positively Skewed Distribution

Describing the Center and Spread

By first checking the shape of the distribution of data for a variable, the researcher becomes able to select the most appropriate statistics to describe the variable's center and spread. Measures of central tendency are used to describe the variable's center; they include the mean, median, and mode. The spread, or variability, of the variable's data is calculated via standard deviation, range, and percentiles.

Summarizing Data Using Measures of Central Tendency

A measure of central tendency is a single number that summarizes values for a variable. These measures represent the way the data tend toward the center; they comprise a single number used to reflect what may be a typical response in the data set. For example, when researching care of a geriatric population, the ages of the participants in a sample will be an important variable to evaluate in the study. Instead of listing all the ages of participants,

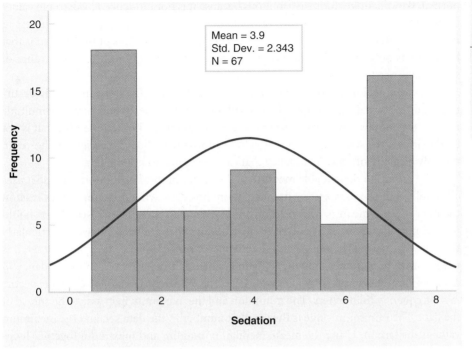

Number of sedating medications

Mean = 3.9
Std. Dev. = 2.343
N = 67

Mean:
The average; a measure of central tendency.

Median:
A measure of central tendency that is the exact midpoint of the numbers of the data set.

FIGURE 11.4 A Distribution with Kurtosis

a researcher can summarize the data using a measure of central tendency such as the average (mean) age of participants in the sample. If, for example, the mean age were 25 rather than 75, the reader would know that participants were young adults rather than elderly participants. Other measures of central tendency include the median and the mode.

The **mean** is commonly called the average. This number is calculated by adding all scores in the data set and dividing the sum by the number of scores in the data set. Therefore, only data measured at the interval and ratio levels are appropriate for calculating a mean score. The mean is an easily recognized and interpreted measure of central tendency. It is familiar to most readers and easy to calculate. The mean, however, is disproportionately affected by extreme values. For example, the mean length of stay of joint replacements would be 3 days if five patients each stayed in the hospital for 3 days—but it would also be 3 days if four patients each stayed 2 days and one patient stayed 7 days. This sensitivity to extreme scores is a weakness of the mean; thus data that are normally distributed are most appropriate to submit to the calculation of a mean score.

The **median** is another measure of central tendency, but it is not a calculation; it is a location. To find the median, the values of a data set are arranged in sequence from smallest to largest, and the center of the data set is determined by finding the exact midpoint of the data. Using the example from the previous paragraph, patients who underwent joint replacements and had hospital lengths of stay of 3, 3, 3, 3, and 7 days would have a median length of stay of 3. When there is an even number of values in the data set, the

Mode:
A measure of central tendency that is the most frequently occurring value in the data set.

Range:
A measure of variability that is the distance between the two most extreme values in the data set.

Variance:
A measure of variability that gives information about the spread of scores around the mean.

two most central values are averaged to obtain the median. The median can be used with normal, skewed, or kurtotic distributions because it is not influenced by extreme values in the data set. It can be used with ordinal, interval, or ratio data, but its usefulness in inferential statistical procedures is limited. The primary weakness of the median is that it represents only the middle of the data set and can be used in only a narrow range of statistical procedures.

An additional measure of central tendency is the **mode**, the most frequently occurring value in the data set. Some data sets will not have a mode; others may have multiple modes. The mode is an easy statistic to determine, but it has limited usefulness. It is not used in inferential statistics and provides little information about a data set. It is, however, the only measure of central tendency that can be applied to nominal data.

The mean is a dependable measure of the center of the distribution because it uses all numbers in the data set for its calculation; however, when extreme values exist in the data set, the mean is drawn toward that extreme score. Thus researchers should use the mean statistic with caution in distributions that are badly skewed, particularly those involving small sample sizes. The median is the middle point of the data set; it is not sensitive to extremes, making it a good choice as a measure of central tendency in distributions that are skewed. The mode helps the reader understand if any value occurs more frequently than others. The minimum and the maximum help assess the spread of the data. The minimum value is the smallest number in the data set, and the maximum value is the largest. Using the mean, median, minimum, and maximum together helps the reader of the data used in research obtain a fuller, more accurate picture of the study findings. How these numbers come together to characterize a data set is demonstrated in **Table 11.4**. Such numbers give an indication of the breadth of variability in the data set, but more sensitive statistics are needed to evaluate the way individual values vary from the typical case.

Summarizing the Variability of a Data Set

Although a typical case can be described statistically, values for individual subjects will differ, sometimes substantially. Statistical techniques can demonstrate variability in ways that enhance understanding of the nature of the individual values represented by the variable scores. With skewed data, a researcher can use a variable's **range** as well as percentiles to appropriately represent the variability of the data. To calculate the range, the analyst would first identify the minimum and maximum values in the data set. The range, which is determined by subtracting the minimum value from the maximum value of the variable, is the simplest way to represent the spread of the data. This single number provides an indication of the distance between the two most extreme values in the data set. The range is easy to calculate, which makes it useful for getting a quick understanding of the spread of scores. However, more powerful measures use every number in the data set to show the spread of the individual values.

Variance and standard deviation are the most commonly used statistics for measuring the dispersion of values from the mean. Just as the mean is used to represent the center of normally distributed data, so the standard deviation and variance are representations of the variability of data. The variance and standard deviation provide information about

Table 11.4 Interpreting Measures of Central Tendency

The variable of length of inpatient stay for adult community-acquired pneumonia has values of:

- Mean: 1.4 days
- Median: 0.78 day
- Minimum: 0.5 day
- Maximum: 12.3 days

Meaning

The median is smaller than the mean; this indicates a positively skewed distribution, because more scores will be in the lower half of the distribution. Thus most people stay in the hospital for shorter periods than this mean value, and some extreme values are likely artificially inflating the mean length of stay. The broad range between minimum and maximum reflects that the scores are spread out.

The variable of length of inpatient stay for pediatric community-acquired pneumonia has values of:

- Mean: 2.2 days
- Median: 2.4 days
- Minimum: 0.5 day
- Maximum: 4.6 days

Meaning

The median and the mean are roughly equal; this indicates the distribution is likely a normal one. The range between minimum and maximum is not large, and the similarity between the measures of central tendency is a sign that extreme values are unlikely to have an effect on these statistics.

The variable of length of inpatient stay for aspiration pneumonia has values of:

- Mean: 4.3 days
- Median: 5.6 days
- Minimum: 0.8 day
- Maximum: 8.9 days

Meaning

The median is larger than the mean; this indicates a negatively skewed distribution because more scores are in the upper half of the distribution. Thus more of these patients stay in the hospital longer than the average length of stay. There is a moderate range between the minimum and the maximum, and a moderate difference between the measures of central tendency, indicating there may be only a few extreme values in the data set.

the average distance of values from the mean of a variable. Variance can be calculated using a calculator, a spreadsheet, or statistical software. The calculation of variance and standard deviation is explained in the box on page 305; it is illustrated here to provide an understanding of the concept.

The calculation results in a single score that provides information about the spread of scores around the mean. When the variance increases, the distance of scores from the

Standard deviation:
The most easily interpreted measure of variability of scores around the mean; represents the average amount of variation of data points about the mean.

mean is larger and the distribution is spread farther away from the mean. The distribution will appear flat and spread out, as illustrated in **FIGURE 11.5**. Conversely, when the variance decreases, the distance of scores from the mean is smaller, meaning more scores are clustered around the mean, and the distribution is taller, as depicted in **FIGURE 11.6**. The distribution will appear tall and thin. The variance is based on a squared value, so it may be difficult to interpret.

The square root of the variance, the **standard deviation**, is a more easily interpreted measure of the distance (spread) of scores around the mean because its scale is proportional to the original set of numbers and represents data in the same way as the variance. Large standard deviation scores relative to the mean indicate that values in the data set are spread out from the mean, and small standard deviation scores relative to the mean indicate that values are close to the mean. The standard deviation is more frequently reported in research reports than is variance because it is more easily interpreted (Szafran, 2012). Variance, however, is more commonly used in the calculation of other statistics, such as those used to determine standard error and the differences between groups. It is helpful to calculate at least one standard deviation value manually to understand its underlying conceptual meaning.

Variance and standard deviation are subject to the same limitations as the mean because all scores in the data set are used in the calculation, and the mean is used in

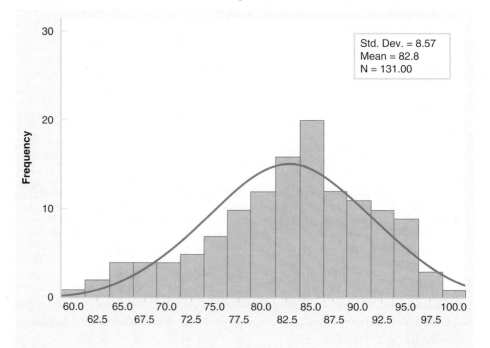

FIGURE 11.5 Distribution with a Large Variance

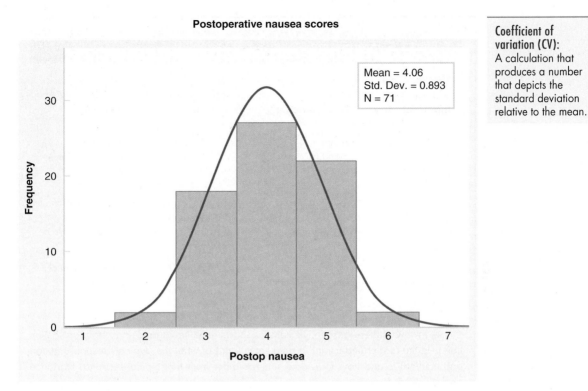

FIGURE 11.6 Distribution with a Small Variance

Coefficient of variation (CV): A calculation that produces a number that depicts the standard deviation relative to the mean.

the calculation. Thus extreme scores in the data set will affect both the variance and the standard deviation. When it is appropriate to use a mean to describe the data set (i.e., with a fairly normal distribution without extreme skew), it will be appropriate to use variance and standard deviation.

Calculating the Variance and Standard Deviation

The mean and standard deviation are powerful building blocks for other statistical techniques because they can be manipulated algebraically. In some cases, readers of research reports want to compare the variability of scores across different groups or even different studies. The **coefficient of variation (CV)** is a calculation that produces a number that depicts the standard deviation relative to the mean, allowing for the comparison of the variability of different variables measured with different scales; the comparison of standard deviations alone does not allow for an accurate comparison. The formula for the coefficient of variation is $CV = 100(SD/\bar{x})$. **Table 11.5** depicts data with their associated measures of variability and an interpretation of these statistics. The larger the CV, the greater the variation; conversely, the smaller the CV, the smaller the variation.

Table 11.5 Interpreting Measures of Variability

The Variable of Length of Inpatient Stay:	Has Values of:	Resulting in a Coefficient of Variation:	Meaning:
Adult community-acquired pneumonia	Mean: 1.4 days Standard deviation: 0.8 day	$(0.8 / 1.4) \times 100$ $= 0.571 \times 100$ $= 57.1$	A moderately large amount of variability
Pediatric community-acquired pneumonia	Mean: 2.2 days Standard deviation: 0.2 day	$(0.2/2.2) \times 100$ $= 0.090 \times 100$ $= 9.0$	A very small amount of variability
Aspiration pneumonia	Mean: 4.3 days Standard deviation: 1.1 days	$(1.1/4.3) \times 100$ $= 0.256 \times 100$ $= 25.6$	A small amount of variability

A review of these descriptive statistics shows how the variance and standard deviation help the reader understand a data set in terms of what the "typical" response (mean and median) is and how individual subjects differ from that typical response (variance and standard deviation).

Summarizing Data Using Measures of Position

Values from a data set can be divided into parts so that readers can understand where a particular value lies in relation to all other values in the data set. The percentile rank is the most commonly used statistical technique for this purpose. A percentile is not synonymous with a percentage; rather, a percentile represents the percentage of values that lie below the particular value of interest. For example, a score of 92% on an exam may be at the 100th percentile if it is the highest score in the class. Conversely, it may be at the 0 percentile if it is the lowest score in the class. The minimum score in a data set is always at the 0 percentile, the maximum score is always at the 100th percentile, and the median is always the 50th percentile (given that 50% of the scores are always below the median). Percentiles are common ways to represent healthcare data such as patient satisfaction and scores on standardized tests, when a fairly narrow range of scores is expected.

Quartiles are identified by dividing the data set into four equal parts. The first quartile contains the 0 to 25th percentile rank (that is, the lowest 25% of the scores), the second quartile contains scores in the 26th to 50th percentile rank, the third quartile contains scores in the 51st to 75th percentile rank, and the fourth quartile contains all scores greater than the 76th percentile rank. This technique is particularly helpful when the researcher is examining achievement or when performance of some subjects relative to performance of others in the study is important. It is also a useful technique for dividing scores on interval-level variables into logical groups to study differences between them.

Sometimes a researcher may want to transform scores gathered in a research study into **standardized scores**, which express the distance from the mean for a single score. Just as the standard deviation represents the spread of scores around the mean for an entire data set, so a standardized score represents the distance of a single point from the mean. This distance is represented by the standard deviation so that standardized scores can be compared across variables, even if the scale of measurement is radically different. The most commonly used standardized score is the z-score. The z-score is calculated by finding the difference between the individual value and the mean, then dividing that number by the standard deviation. The resulting score depicts the variable in terms of its relative position in the overall data set.

When all of the scores in a data set have been converted to a z-score and depicted as a histogram, the result is called a standard normal distribution. A **standard normal distribution** has a mean of 0 and a standard deviation of 1. This transformed distribution retains its original shape, and the z-scores can be used to determine in which percentile a given score would fall. This kind of analysis is helpful in determining the probability that an individual score would fall in a specific place in the distribution. Distributions with a bell shape have approximately 68% of scores between +1 or −1 standard deviation and 95% of scores between +2 or −2 standard deviations, as shown in **FIGURE 11.7**. These characteristics of a standard normal distribution are very useful as a basis for determining the probability that a specific statistical finding is due to standard error and become the basis for judging random chance in inferential analyses.

Standardized scores:
A measure of position that expresses the distance from the mean of a single score in standard terms.

Standard normal distribution:
A bell-shaped distribution in which the mean is set at 0 and a standard deviation at 1.

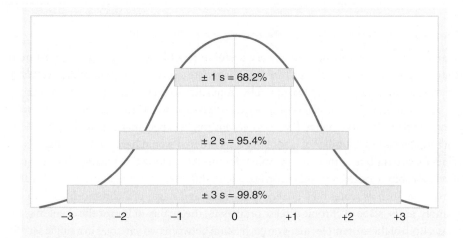

FIGURE 11.7 The Standard Normal Distribution

Correlation analysis:
A measure that depicts the strength and nature of the relationship between two variables.

All of the descriptive statistics presented thus far are considered univariate, meaning they are used to study a single variable at a time. Such statistics are appropriate for analysis of data collected for general descriptive studies. Descriptive statistics can also be applied to describe bivariate relationships, or the study of two variables at a time.

A Note About Scale

The word *scale* is used frequently when talking about descriptive data. Scale refers to the units of measurement of the variable. For example, height is commonly measured with a scale of inches, and weight is commonly measured with a scale of pounds. Scale is also used with respect to the potential range of the data. Height has limitations of scale in that people are not taller than 7.5 feet; thus, if height were measured in inches, its scale would be restricted to the range of 0 to 90 inches. Weight in people, by comparison, has been measured as high as 1000 pounds. Thus height will never have as many possible "units" as weight. If we try to compare these two scales—if we wanted to compare their means, for example, to see if a person of average height is also of average weight—the scale size means the average number of units of weight will always be several times as big as the average number of units of height.

Is an individual who is 15 pounds above average in weight and 2.5 inches above average in height an overweight person? It is hard to tell using the raw values. Using percentiles or standardized scores to represent numbers eliminates this problem. Instead of expressing a value in terms of its absolute number of units, the value is expressed by its relative position on the scale. This enables us to compare where each value falls relative to its specific scale, in a standard way, so that unit-to-unit comparisons are possible. Thus, if an individual is 1 standard deviation above the mean in weight and also 1 standard deviation above the mean in height, he or she is not overweight. Measures of relative position enable the comparison of values across variables, regardless of the scale with which they are originally represented.

Summarizing Scores Using Measures of Relationship

Bivariate descriptive statistics can be very useful in describing the strength and nature of relationships between variables and are the appropriate tests in correlation studies. **Correlation analysis** examines the values of two variables in relation to each other. This type of analysis can be used to examine the relationship between two variables in a single sample or between a single variable in two samples. For example, one might expect that the number of patients in a hospital and the number of laboratory tests ordered would have a relationship: As the values for patient census increase, the values for number of tests ordered increase. This type of relationship is called a positive correlation. A different example may show a negative correlation, such as scores on a quality-of-life scale and stages of a chronic disease. In this example, as the stage of chronic disease progresses, the quality of life for the client may decrease. Both of these examples focus on correlation between two variables in a single sample. Alternatively, the values of a single variable may be appraised for its relationship between two samples; for example, there may be a positive correlation between the adult weights of mothers and their daughters. It is important to note that correlation does not imply causation.

Correlation statistics can be shown both numerically and in graphic forms. The notation of rho or *r* is used to represent a bivariate correlation in a sample. The most common correlation coefficients are the Pearson product moment correlation and the Spearman's rank order correlation. The former is used for interval- or ratio-level data, and the latter for ranked or ordinal data. In either form, the correlation can be positive or negative, with values between −1 and +1, inclusive. Values of exactly −1 or +1 are known as perfect correlations, reflecting a perfect linear relationship in which a change of one unit in a variable is accompanied by a change of exactly one unit in the other variable. A correlation coefficient with a value of 0 has no correlation. The direction of the relationship is interpreted from the sign; a negative correlation coefficient reflects an inverse relationship (as one variable increases, the other decreases), whereas a positive correlation coefficient reflects a positive relationship (as one variable increases, the other variable increases as well). The strength of the relationship is interpreted based on the absolute value of the coefficient itself, regardless of its sign (Kremelberg, 2010). An example of interpretation of correlation coefficients for a set of variables appears in **Table 11.6**.

Table 11.6 Interpreting Measures of Correlation

Variable 1	Variable 2	Correlation Coefficient	What the Sign Means	What the Number Means
Pneumonia length of stay in days	Results of pulmonary function tests	−0.850	The negative sign indicates an inverse relationship; as results of pulmonary function tests improve, length of stay in days decreases.	0.8 to 1.0 absolute value indicates a strong relationship.
Pneumonia length of stay in days	Number of comorbid conditions	+0.678	The positive sign indicates a positive relationship; as the number of comorbid conditions increases, the length of stay also increases.	0.6 to 0.8 absolute value indicates a moderately strong relationship.
Pneumonia length of stay in days	Nutritional status	−0.488	The negative sign indicates an inverse relationship; as the quality of nutritional status improves, the length of stay in days decreases.	0.4 to 0.6 absolute value indicates a moderate relationship.
Pneumonia length of stay in days	Annual days absent from work	+0.213	The positive sign indicates a positive relationship; as the annual days absent from work increase, the length of stay in days increases.	0.2 to 0.4 absolute value indicates a weak relationship; less than 0.2 indicates no relationship.

Line graphs:
A graphic presentation that plots means for a variable over a period of time.

Box plot:
A graphic presentation that marks the median of the values in the middle of the box and the 25th and 75th percentiles as the lower and upper edges of the box, respectively. It indicates the relative position of the data for each group and the spread of the data for comparison.

An advantage of the correlation coefficient is that it can be an efficient way to determine both the strength and the direction of a relationship with a single statistic. Nevertheless, a correlation coefficient reflects only a linear relationship; in other words, the relationship has to be proportional at all levels of each variable before it will be depicted accurately with a correlation coefficient (Motulsky, 2010). Some important relationships in health care are curved, rather than linear, and are not represented well by a correlation coefficient. For example, a dose–response curve will follow a curvilinear trajectory, but it is still a very important relationship in nursing care.

A note is in order about correlation coefficients and statistical significance. Often, a *p* value, indicating the probability of chance, is reported with the correlation coefficient. It is sometimes erroneously interpreted as evidence that the relationship is a significant one. In reality, the *p* value indicates the probability that the measured relationship is due to standard error. Even very weak correlation coefficients can be statistically significant, and strong correlations can result in no statistical significance. The strength and direction of the correlation coefficient are the characteristics that must be interpreted to determine whether the correlation is clinically significant, and this can be determined only by the application of the clinician's expert judgment (Privitera, 2012).

A correlation coefficient is an efficient and easily interpretable way to describe the degree and direction of a linear relationship between variables. These relationships can also be represented graphically using a scatter plot. Scatter plots are effective means for evaluating relationships and determining if those relationships are linear. They are one of a group of graphical presentations that can illustrate statistical results in a visual way, which are often more easily interpreted and understood by readers.

Summarizing Data in Graphical Presentations

It is just as important to use the correct graphical technique as it is to use the correct statistical technique to summarize descriptive data. In some ways, graphical presentation of data is easier to understand because the data are presented in summary fashion, with the colors, lines, and shapes of the graph highlighting differences and similarities in the data set. Earlier in this chapter, bar charts and histograms were shown as graphs commonly used in identifying the distribution of data. **Line graphs**, by comparison, are used to show change over time. Values for the variable are summarized by period of time using a mean, and then each period of time is followed for a defined time frame, such as monthly for a year. Line graphs are used in time-series designs, in single-subject designs, or to determine the effectiveness of a new intervention or research protocol. Line graphs are easy to read and quickly show results over time.

Sometimes the best way to display the data is to illustrate where the majority of the scores lie in the data set. A **box plot** provides a good method to show this, particularly when a variable is measured in different groups. The box plot is a visual representation of measures of position. The median of the values for a variable in all groups of participants is marked in the middle of the box. The 25th and 75th percentiles for each group form the lower and upper edges of the box, respectively. Scores contained within the box are those between the 25th and 75th percentiles and represent the middle 50% of the values for each group. The minimum and maximum values are marked with an X or connected by a line to the box. The resulting chart is sometimes called a "box and whiskers plot," referring to the box with lines extending from the top and bottom; it shows a side-by-side comparison of the relative position of data for each group. This representation gives the reader a picture of the spread of the data (minimum and maximum values) and where 50% of the values lie (within the box), as well as the middle point, or median (line in the middle of the box). **FIGURE 11.8** depicts a box-and-whiskers plot for a measure of postoperative pain in the hours after surgery. Inspection of the graph shows the reader that hour 4 is the point at which pain reaches its peak, after which it gradually declines.

Scatter plots require graphing two variables measured from the same subject at the same time and show the nature of the relationship between those two variables. When all data in the set have been plotted, the graph shows whether the points are closely grouped (associated) or scattered (no association). The closer the dots are to forming a discernible, straight line, the more tightly associated the variables are to one another. **FIGURE 11.9** depicts three data sets containing two variables as scatter plots. The scatter plot on the left shows two variables that have a positive relationship to each other, the center scatter plot shows two variables that have a negative association, and the scatter plot on the right shows no association between the two variables.

Charts and graphs provide useful information to readers when used appropriately. Bar graphs are easy to create for nominal and ordinal data. Frequency data from different groups can be compared using bar graphs so a reader can quickly see which group has the highest number of instances of a particular variable. Histograms are used in a similar

Scatter plot:
A graphic presentation that indicates the nature of the relationship between two variables.

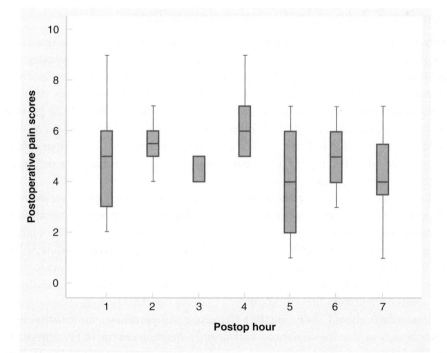

FIGURE 11.8   A Box-and-Whiskers Plot

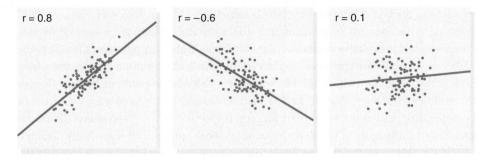

FIGURE 11.9 Scatter Plots

manner for interval-level or ratio-level data. The bars in histograms are connected, which denotes a variable that has continuous numbers. Histograms have the added feature of showing the shape of the distribution of a variable. Line graphs are usually created to show the mean value of a variable over some period of time. This type of graph is particularly helpful when a change in the mean (either higher or lower) might signal the need to change a nursing practice. Whereas the line graph typically shows the mean over time, the box plot shows the distribution over time. Each box contains the 25th to 75th percentiles of the distribution. Watching trends over time using a box plot is helpful if the median point or the middle 50% of the distribution is important. Finally, a scatter plot is an effective way to visually represent the strength and direction of a relationship between two variables.

Common Errors in Summarizing Data

The most elementary error is made when an inappropriate statistic is used to summarize data. For example, a mean should never be calculated for race, gender, or other categorical data. However, those researchers who are new to statistical analysis may forget these levels of measurement and, seeing numbers on the screen, run descriptive analysis. Although the statistical analysis computer package will certainly calculate a mean when provided the correct commands, the resulting number is meaningless. What would a mean of 5.6 on the variable race indicate? An error! Other problems may occur when data are entered incorrectly; this type of mistake is addressed later in the chapter in the section on creating descriptive data.

Erroneous conclusions can be drawn about variables when some data are presented without the benefit of seeing all appropriate descriptive data. Descriptive data analysis of a variable should always include measures of central tendency and variability. For example, a variable measured for two different groups can have approximately the same mean but a different spread of scores around the mean. The interpretation of the performance of the groups depends on knowing both the values for a typical case and how far individual data points deviate from the typical case.

Researchers should always disclose frequency and percentage information in research reports so that the reader can understand whether a change in percentage over time is a function of sample size or a change in the values of the variable. For example, a researcher studying the development of pressure ulcers within the first month of admission to a nursing home over a 3-month period of time reported the following percentages: 8%, 7.5%, and 0%. The reader might logically believe that the last month signaled a breakthrough in preventing new ulcers. In fact, the percentage is calculated by taking number of ulcers and dividing by total admissions for the month. When these data are also presented as 6/75, 6/80, and 0/20, a different conclusion can be drawn: The number of admissions has declined.

A common error in the interpretation of descriptive data is overinterpretation of the results. In other words, the researcher interprets the data in a way that goes beyond what the statistics were intended to reflect. This problem is most common with the correlation coefficient. Although the correlation coefficient is an excellent way to represent the strength and direction of a relationship between two variables, it is limited to description of that relationship. Because the variables are measured simultaneously, the researcher cannot draw conclusions about causality. It is not uncommon, however, for a researcher to interpret a strong correlation as evidence that one variable has an effect on, causes, or in some way influences the other. In fact, correlation is evidence only of a relationship, not of causation, and overstating the relationship should be avoided (Rosner, 2010).

When a researcher has a good command of statistical techniques, it can be tempting to present data in complicated ways that are sophisticated enough to amaze fellow researchers. However, the point of reporting descriptive analyses is to inform, not to impress. The readers of research that is intended as evidence for nursing practice are generally practitioners, not statisticians. If the write-up requires the help of a statistician to interpret its results section, then the author has not presented the findings well. Descriptive data should be provided in the most uncomplicated fashion that accurately and completely represents the findings so that understanding and application to practice are maximized.

A final pitfall to avoid is presenting data graphically in a way that hides important aspects of the data set. This type of error is generally unintentional, but it can limit the reader's understanding of the research results. For example, showing only the mean values will hide the distribution of the variable. The researcher needs to create different types of charts to determine which one best displays the meaning of the data. The best way to report descriptive analysis is in the most accurate, complete, and understandable way that is not easily misinterpreted.

GRAY MATTER

The following are common errors in summarizing descriptive data:
- Inappropriate statistics
- Incorrectly entered data
- Selected data presented without the context of the whole data set
- Lack of disclosure of frequency and percentage information
- Overinterpretation of results
- Inconsistent presentation of data
- Graphic representation that hides important aspects of the data set

Reading the Descriptive Data Section in a Research Study

Descriptive statistics are the statistics that the reader of nursing research will most commonly encounter. Even studies that have more sophisticated and complex intentions will still present descriptive data about the sample and the individual variables. A thorough understanding of descriptive statistical concepts will assist the reader in determining the fundamental characteristics of the subjects and variables in a study, thereby helping the reader to determine whether the results of the study can be applied in a particular setting (Garden & Kabacoff, 2010). Reading the descriptive statistics can be confusing, however, because of the technical jargon associated with statistical analysis and the Greek letters that are used as symbols. Table 11.7 summarizes the notations that are used to represent descriptive statistics for populations and samples. The most commonly used symbols represent statistics within a sample; they include n, x, s, and s^2, which represent data set size, mean, standard deviation, and variance, respectively.

In evidence-based practice, the ability to discern the applicability of research findings to an area of practice is vital to the success of the modified practice. While newly discovered research may be sound and well designed, it is important to review the descriptive statistics of the study to decide whether the outcomes of the research can be achieved in another setting. Descriptive statistics enable the reader to paint a picture of the sample to whom the research outcomes apply, thereby allowing the reader to compare his or her own patient population with the sample used in the research. For example, if the study sample is composed of subjects with an average age of 36 with a relatively small standard deviation, then a facility that treats primarily Medicare patients would be well advised to avoid application of the results of that research (Craig & Rosalind, 2012).

The report of descriptive data analysis usually follows the methods section, although descriptive statistics may appear in the description of the sample and research variables. The report of descriptive data is typically the third or fourth major heading in a research report and is often called "Results" or "Findings." Readers of research reports will often see the sample described first. Following the description of the sample, descriptive data for

Table 11.7 Summary of Symbols Used for Descriptive Statistics

	Symbol for Population	Symbol for Sample
Data set size	N	n
Mean	μ (mu)	$\bar{x}$
Standard deviation	σ (sigma)	s
Variance	σ^2 (sigma squared)	s^2
Correlation	ρ (rho)	r

Table 11.8 Means of Test Anxiety Score by Group and Time

Group	N	Mean	SD
Pretest			
Control	38	25	8.38
Cognitive-behavioral	38	27.33	10.21
Hypnosis	38	23.63	8.52
Posttest			
Control	36	24.58	10.12
Cognitive-behavioral	34	19.25	10.44
Hypnosis	35	18.20	7.05

variables used in the study are presented. Some authors use narrative descriptions of the scores for variables, whereas others use tables to display data. Likewise, research reports are more likely to present descriptive data about variables relative to group membership.

An example of descriptive statistics by group membership appears in Table 11.8. These data represent a study of three groups—two intervention groups and a control—that had their level of test anxiety measured in the pretest and posttest periods. The reader can see that test anxiety scores decreased in both the cognitive-behavioral and hypnosis intervention groups, whereas the control group stayed essentially unchanged.

Readers of research reports should not accept the results without an appraisal of the appropriateness of data analyses. The reader can systematically evaluate whether appropriate decisions have been made for data analysis and reporting by asking a series of guiding questions:

- Which variables were included in the study?
- What was the level of measurement for each variable?
- Were the descriptive statistics appropriate for the level of measurement of each variable?
- Were the descriptive statistics appropriate for the research question (that is, descriptive or correlation)?
- Were the descriptive results presented in the appropriate form for maximum understanding?

With patience and persistence, most readers should be able to comprehend the meaning of the findings from a descriptive research study. Descriptive data provide the reader with an understanding of the sample and variables through measures of central tendency and variability. This information lays the foundation for more complex statistical analysis such as inferential statistics.

WHERE TO LOOK

Where to look for descriptive results:

- The report of descriptive data is typically the third or fourth major heading in a research report and may be called "Results" or "Findings."
- Statistics that describe the size, composition, and characteristics of the sample are often presented

first in this section, or they may appear with the description of the sampling procedure.

- The report typically includes descriptive reports for each individual variable and each scale or summary score; these may be presented in tables, figures, graphs, or narrative form.

CHECKLIST FOR EVALUATING DESCRIPTIVE RESULTS

- ❏ The descriptive report of the sample provides enough details to judge the adequacy and characteristics of the sample.
- ❏ The presentation of descriptive statistics is understandable and clear.
- ❏ Complete descriptive statistics are presented for each variable (e.g., measures of both central tendency and variability).
- ❏ The tables, graphs, or charts complement the text and enhance understanding.

- ❏ Graphical representations are consistent in scale and orientation.
- ❏ The descriptive statistics are not misleading, open to misinterpretation, or confusing.
- ❏ The descriptive results give a full and clear picture of the variables under study.
- ❏ The data have not been overinterpreted and conclusions do not go beyond what the statistics can support.

Using Descriptive Data Analysis in Practice

Nurses use descriptive data in clinical practice every day. Descriptive analysis is used when nurses check trends in vital signs (minimum and maximum values, line graphs), when they review infection rates for a clinical unit (number of patients with infections divided by all patients), and when they calculate average length of stay for clients with certain diagnoses (sum of inpatient days in a month divided by number of patients in the unit). Descriptive data can inform nursing practice in relation to the way diseases, complications, and health issues are distributed in the population of patients. Moreover, nurses who conduct quality improvement studies use descriptive data to develop evidence about the outcomes of those efforts. Even though this type of evidence is positioned lower on the hierarchy of evidence, it provides data that can guide clinical nurses in improving nursing practice and clinical outcomes. Descriptive analyses are often the first step in designing an intervention study that will provide conclusive evidence for a practice change. When searching externally for practice change, the evidence needs to be reviewed to determine its validity, reliability, and applicability—all of which begin with the descriptive statistics of the research.

In the coming years, nursing practice will be impacted as increasingly more data become available through what is being referred to as "big data" or "data science." The emergence of big data has occurred in tandem with the move to electronic health records (EHRs) from paper-based record keeping. Because incredible amounts of patient data are now available in digital form, the opportunity exists for large-scale analysis of those data for purposes of population health analysis, environmental health impacts, and other large-scale studies. Nurses, for example, will be able to utilize these data to analyze and construct optimal clinical practices. Standardization of EHR input is the linchpin necessary for wide usage of these available data, and utilization of descriptive statistics to summarize the available information will be key to understanding their implications (Sensmeier, 2015).

When considering the types of descriptive data that would be useful in practice, nurses might ask the following questions:

- Which type of data would be useful to track clinical outcomes?
- What are the operational definitions for data to be collected when tracking clinical outcomes?
- What is the appropriate level of measurement for the data?
- Which types of descriptive statistics could summarize the data best?
- Which graphs, charts, and tables might best illuminate the trends in clinical outcomes?

Asking these questions can lead nurses to develop systems to collect descriptive data and create reports that can inform their own practice as well as communicate the need for practice change to others.

Creating Descriptive Data Summaries for a Research Study

Researchers who report descriptive data from a research study must create and follow a data analysis plan, paying careful attention to detail. It is only through systematic attention to the data analysis process that appropriate results are generated and errors are detected and corrected before final analysis.

The first order of business is to review the research design and research questions/hypotheses. This review helps to orient the researcher to the major aims of the study and the specific types of analyses that should be used to describe the sample and to answer research questions.

After completing this review, the researcher should follow a step-by-step process of preparing the data for analysis. It is likely that preparing the data for analysis will take more time and effort than the actual analysis itself. It is not unusual to take several days to enter, inspect, and clean the data, but only minutes to run descriptive statistics. This process may feel laborious, but it is imperative to ensure accurate, complete results.

In the initial stages of data collection, the researcher labels all surveys or tools with a unique number so that data from different participants can be retrieved later, if necessary, without confusion. A codebook is developed with numerical codes substituted for words that describe nominal variables. For example, the researcher may collect data on gender, race, and marital status. The researcher may label males as 1 and females as 2. These numbers lack mathematical meaning; they simply serve as categories that enable a statistical analysis computer program to count instances of data in those categories. The codebook should be stored as an electronic or paper record with the data file so the codes can be easily retrieved and referred to during analysis.

Regardless of the way the data are collected, an organized system of maintaining data integrity must be established. Data from each participant should be filed in such a way that retrieval of the data is easy. A notebook, file folder, or computer file is commonly used for this purpose. Because the security of the data is the responsibility of the researcher, the data should be password protected if stored on a computer, or locked in a filing cabinet if a paper system is used. As data are generated in the research study, they should be reviewed for completeness and accuracy before storing.

Once the data collection phase is over, the data entry phase begins. Data must be meticulously entered into statistical software using the codes that were developed earlier. Verification of the data quality is completed by having a second person compare the raw data with the data that were entered for each participant in the study; these should match. The researcher next runs some initial descriptive statistics to catch any outliers or errors in coding. The minimum and maximum values are particularly helpful in finding data outliers and errors. For example, in a study on resuscitation events, a participant who reports being involved in 100 events in the past year when the next highest value is 25 would be considered an outlier on that variable. This number may be correct or it may be an error. The researcher should inspect the raw data for that participant to determine the veracity of the data. Another common mistake is simple miscoding that is not caught in the earlier verification; entering a 3 as a code when the only options are 1 or 2 will be found in this initial analysis. An easy way to find this type of coding error is to run frequencies on the data set. Once outliers and errors have been found, the data are cleaned by returning to the raw data set to correct the data entry errors. The file is then saved with a name that denotes it is the cleaned data file.

The early analysis phase begins with inspection of the cleaned data file for missing values—that is, data that were not recorded by a participant. Several options are available to the researcher in such cases, including deleting participants with missing data, deleting the variable with missing data, or substituting a value (mean or estimate) for the missing data (Marshall & Jonker, 2010). The early analysis phase also entails looking at sample characteristics of participants compared to those who started the study but did not complete it. The researcher should inspect the characteristics of the sample to see if those participants who persisted in the study differed in some way from those who withdrew. This comparison can help identify any attrition bias.

Next, the researcher may need to change (transform) the data in preparation for making summative scales. Often items on research instruments are worded in reverse to reduce response set bias. Once the data are collected, the researcher needs to change the scoring of the reversed items so he or she can add them to positively worded items. This transformation is done using the statistical analysis computer program. When all transformations have been completed, items can be combined into subscales or scale scores by following the scoring directions. Finally, the researcher is ready to perform the descriptive analysis for the purpose of reporting results from the study.

To begin the descriptive analysis, the researcher should develop a list of variables in the study. For example, the researcher might collect data on variables including gender, race, marital status, age, medical diagnosis, conditions, length of stay in the hospital, and other characteristics. The researcher should list each variable, the level of measurement, and appropriate descriptive statistics for that level of measurement. If data have been numerically coded—for example, if "male" is coded as "1" and "female" as "2"—then a permanent codebook should be created for later reference during interpretation of the results.

Once the researcher has developed the list of appropriate descriptive statistics for variables, then the data analysis procedures can be run. Descriptive analysis can be completed using a variety of methods. Simple descriptive analyses can be calculated by hand, using an electronic calculator. Although the process is laborious and subject to error, it is possible to compute most descriptive statistics without complex software. Spreadsheet programs can also be used to calculate descriptive statistics, including measures of central tendency, variability, relative position, and correlation. Advantages of spreadsheet software include its wide availability and its capacity to produce both graphical and numerical representations of data. Specific statistical software is the fastest and most efficient way to complete a descriptive analysis. It can yield both numerical and graphical summaries of data and can be used to analyze and compare measures for subgroups as well as the entire sample. The key advantage of using statistical software for descriptive analysis is that the data are prepared and ready for more complex analyses if needed.

Reporting Descriptive Results

Although descriptive results are reported in myriad ways, there are standards for the way in which descriptive results are reported. The goal of descriptive reporting is to convey the most complete information in the most straightforward and concise way. Thebane and Akhtar-Danesh (2008) developed a set of standards for reporting descriptive results for nursing research, and these can serve as a guide when writing this section of a report. The appropriate report for each type of data includes:

- *Interval*: Report the mean, followed by the standard deviation in parentheses—for example, mean age was 38.6 (s = 2.4).
- *Ordinal*: Report the median, with the minimum and maximum scores following in parentheses—for example, median pain score was 4 (min = 1, max = 7).
- *Nominal*: Report the number for each category followed by the percentage in parentheses—for example, number of females was 25 (51%).

When the data set includes outliers, a box plot should also be provided for reference. Any methods used to deal with missing data should be described in enough detail that the reader can determine how these procedures might have affected the results.

A common question is how accurately to depict the data—that is, how many decimal places should be reported. Guidelines developed by Lang and Secic (2006) set the seminal standard for reporting precision:

- *The mean:* To, at most, one decimal place more than the original data.
- *Standard deviation:* To, at most, two decimal places more than the original data.
- *Percentages:* For sample size greater than 100, report to one decimal place. For between 20 and 100 subjects, report percentages as whole numbers. For fewer than 20 subjects, report the actual raw number.

Tables and graphs are helpful in visually understanding the data and condensing large amounts of information into smaller sections.

Summary of Key Concepts

- Summarizing descriptive data is the first step in the analysis of quantitative research data.
- Descriptive data are numbers in a data set that are calculated to represent research variables and do not involve generalization to larger populations.
- Nominal and ordinal data are best represented by frequencies, percentages, and rates.
- Interval- and ratio-level data can be represented by measures of central tendency, variability, and relative position.
- Measures of central tendency include the mean, median, and mode. The mean is easily calculated and interpreted but is influenced by extreme scores. The median represents the midpoint of the data but does not reflect extremes well. The mode is the most frequently occurring value; it is of limited usefulness in descriptive analysis.
- Measures of variability include the variance, standard deviation, and CV, all of which represent how spread out the data values are in relation to the mean.
- Measures of relative position include percentiles and standardized scores, which enable the comparison of values when the scales of measurement are different.
- The relationship between two variables in a sample is represented by the correlation coefficient.
- A frequency distribution enables the researcher to determine the shape of the variable's distribution, which may be normal, skewed, or kurtotic.
- Data must be analyzed using the correct statistical procedure for the level of measurement of a variable.
- The data may be presented numerically and graphically in a way that conveys the most accurate information about the variables in the study.
- Errors in reporting descriptive data include using the wrong statistics for the level of measurement; presenting incomplete, overly complicated, or misleading data; and drawing conclusions that go beyond what the data will support.
- Data must be meticulously collected, entered, checked for quality, and cleaned prior to analysis.

CRITICAL APPRAISAL EXERCISE

Retrieve the following full-text article from the Cumulative Index to Nursing and Allied Health Literature or similar search database:

Klainin-Yobas, P., He, H., & Lau, Y. (2015). Physical fitness, health behavior and health among nursing students: A descriptive correlational study. *Nurse Education Today, 35*(12), 1199–1205.

Review the article, focusing on the sections that report the results of the descriptive analyses. Think about the following appraisal questions in your critical review of this research article:

1. List all of the variables that are measured in this study. For each, determine whether the variable consists of nominal-, ordinal-, or interval-level data.
2. Which level of measurement is yielded by the Overall Physical Health Scale? Which information in the article leads you to this conclusion?
3. Which level of measurement is yielded by the individual items in the Health Behaviour Questionnaire? Which information in the article leads you to this conclusion?
4. Did the authors use the correct descriptive statistics for the level of measurement of the variables?
5. Are the statistics represented in the most understandable way? Discuss the use of tables relative to the type of information being reported. Are there graphical representations that could simplify the report?
6. Do the authors provide the right descriptive numbers about the sample, measurement instruments, and results?

References

Altman, D. (2006). *Practical statistics for medical research.* London, UK: Chapman and Hall.

Craig, J., & Rosalind, S. (2012). *The evidence-based practice manual for nurses.* New York, NY: Churchill Livingstone/Elsevier.

Field, A. (2013). *Discovering statistics using IBM SPSS statistics* (4th ed.). London, UK: Sage.

Garden, E., & Kabacoff, R. (2010). *Evaluating research articles from start to finish.* Thousand Oaks, CA: Sage.

Kremelberg, D. (2010). *Practical statistics.* Thousand Oaks, CA: Sage.

Lang, T., & Secic, M. (2006). *How to report statistics in medicine* (2nd ed.). Philadelphia, PA: American College of Physicians.

Marshall, G., & Jonker, L. (2010). An introduction to descriptive statistics: A review and practical guide. *Radiography, 16,* e1–e7.

Melnyk, B., Fineout-Overholt, E., Stillwell, S., & Williamson, K. (2010). The seven steps of evidence-based practice. *American Journal of Nursing, 110*(1), 51–53.

Motulsky, H. (2010). *Intuitive biostatistics: A nonmathematical guide to statistical thinking.* New York, NY: Oxford University Press.

Polit, D. (2010). *Statistics and data analysis for nursing research* (2nd ed.). Upper Saddle River, NJ: Pearson.

Privitera, G. (2012). *Statistics for the behavioral sciences.* Thousand Oaks, CA: Sage.

Rosner, B. (2010). *Fundamentals of biostatistics* (7th ed.). Pacific Grove, CA: Duxbury Press.

Scott, I., & Mazhindu, D. (2014). *Statistics for healthcare professionals, an introduction* (2nd ed.). London, UK: Sage.

Sensmeier, J. (2015). Big data and the future of nursing knowledge. *Nursing Management, 46*(4), 22–27.

Szafran, R. (2012). *Answering questions with statistics.* Thousand Oaks, CA: Sage.

Thebane, L., & Akhtar-Danesh, N. (2008). Guidelines for reporting descriptive statistics in health research. *Nurse Researcher, 15*(2), 72–81.

Tubbs-Cooley, H., Pickler, R., Younger, J., & Mark, B. (2015). A descriptive study of nurse-reported missed care in neonatal intensive care units. *Journal of Advanced Nursing, 71*(4), 813–824.

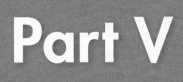

Part V

Studies That Measure Effectiveness

Chapter 12

Quantitative Questions and Procedures

CHAPTER OBJECTIVES

The study of this chapter will help the learner to

- Examine quantitative research designs and methods.
- Describe the importance of design decisions in quantitative studies.
- Compare the characteristics and applications of specific quantitative designs.
- Relate quantitative designs to evidence-based nursing practice.
- Appraise a quantitative study for strengths and weaknesses.
- Learn how to create a quantitative research design.

KEY TERMS

Case-control study

Causal-comparative study

Comparison group

Control group

Experimental designs

Ex post facto research

Nonequivalent comparison group before/after design

Nonequivalent comparison group posttest only

Quasi-experimental designs

Time-series designs

Introduction

Evidence for nursing practice means that nurses are able to practice based on what they know, rather than what they think. Quantitative research enables the nurse researcher to determine what is known. The purpose of quantitative research is to use measurement to determine the effectiveness of interventions and to report these effects with an identified level of confidence. Quantitative research is generally reported using numbers, which is helpful because mathematics and statistics are universal languages. Nurse researchers focus on detecting truth; quantitative methods and procedures allow the nurse to describe what is known in a standard, universally understandable way.

Pain is the so-called fifth vital sign, and its management is an important part of the critical care nurse's job. Intubated patients, in particular, are prone to high levels of pain both because of the number of procedures they must undergo and because they cannot communicate. Optimal pain management minimizes stress and discomfort to enhance the effectiveness of mechanical ventilation. Oftentimes, pharmacologic pain management is indicated, but it brings both benefits and harms. Analgesics are not free from adverse effects, and their prolonged use may increase healthcare costs. A group of critical care nurses in a Tehran, Iran, hospital tested the effects of a nonpharmacologic intervention—listening to natural sounds through headphones—to see if this alternative treatment might reduce the level of self-reported pain among patients on mechanical ventilation (Saadatmand et al., 2015).

The researchers used a randomized, double-blind, placebo-controlled trial to test the listening intervention. They randomized 60 patients into an experimental group, which listened to nature sounds through headphones, and a control group, which listened to no sound through identical headphones. The patients were asked to self-rate their pain on a standard pain scale at baseline and again at 30-minute intervals during the intervention and for 30 minutes after the headphones were removed. Although the patients' pain levels were similar at baseline, pain scores in the intervention group fell significantly, and they were lower than the scores in the control group at every measurement point.

This study involved a purely quantitative design that controlled a number of potential extraneous variables. Measuring the variables over time allowed each patient to function as a control, so improvements could be evaluated over time as well as at each time period. These positive effects were sustained throughout each time period. Studies on effective, nonpharmacologic ways to control pain in this critically ill population are needed as evidence for nursing practice; testing these innovative approaches rigorously for effectiveness is essential.

Quantitative research involves the measurement of variables of interest and subsequent statistical analysis of the data. Quantitative analysis can be used for the following purposes:

- Determine the effects of an intervention
- Measure the relationships between variables
- Detect changes over time

Quantitative studies provide some of the strongest evidence for nursing practice because they enable the researcher to draw conclusions about the effectiveness of interventions. These studies are designed to provide high levels of control so that confidence in the results is enhanced. If all conditions are controlled so that the effects of a variable or intervention can be isolated, then the probability is low that the outcome is due to something other than the intervention. Quantitative methods allow the researcher to measure the probability that some other factor caused the outcome—specifically, extraneous variables, measurement error, and sampling error, among others. Quantitative designs are intended to isolate and evaluate the effects of an intervention, treatment, or characteristic (which are referred to as independent variables) on a specific outcome (referred to as the dependent variable).

Quantitative studies can also answer questions about relationships between a cause and an effect, although sometimes causality must be inferred. For example, the relationship between risk factors and disease cannot be tested with a true experimental design, because it is not ethical to expose healthy individuals to risk factors they would otherwise not experience. As a result, researchers must study these variables as they naturally occur. Because such studies do not allow researchers to control many extraneous variables, other explanations for the outcome may arise. Subjecting these kinds of study data to quantitative analysis allows the researcher to determine the probability that a relationship was caused by something else and to express risk relationships in quantifiable ways (Sanz, Matesanz, Nieri, & Pagliaro, 2012).

Quantitative studies may be undertaken to determine changes over time in a single group of individuals. In essence, subjects serve as their own controls in these studies. Time-series analysis can provide substantial information about the effectiveness of interventions because these kinds of studies yield measures of both how much difference the intervention made and how long it took for that effect to become detectable.

These kinds of studies are useful as evidence for nursing practice in multiple ways. The focus on scientific studies as a basis for evaluating the effectiveness of interventions is a cornerstone of evidence-based nursing practice. Quantitative studies can help the nurse appraise the effectiveness of an intervention, determine the relationship between actions and patient responses, and measure changes over time. Overall, such studies play an important role in establishing evidence-based practices and testing new or improved interventions.

Quantitative Research Questions

Quantitative studies address a considerable number of research questions, though these questions are usually focused on the effects of interventions, actions, risk factors, or events. These questions often begin with words such as *what* and *when*, and they use active verbs such as *affect*, *influence*, or *change*. Overall, quantitative research studies focus on establishing a statistical relationship between variables and measuring the probability that error was responsible for the outcome (McCusker & Gunaydin, 2015). The research questions they address, then, will have variables that can be operationally defined and measured in a numerical way.

The quantitative research question includes some common elements. It is most amenable to the PICO approach, which focuses on the following elements:

- Population of interest
- Intervention under study
- Comparison that makes up the control
- Outcome of interest

In cases where the intervention is a naturally occurring "cause," such as a risk factor, some researchers—particularly epidemiologists—prefer the PECO approach. It includes the following four elements:

- Population of interest
- Exposure to a factor of interest
- Control or comparison group
- Outcome of interest

Table 12.1 Examples of Quantitative Research Questions and the Study Designs Used to Answer Them

Research Question	Design Used to Answer It
What are the effects of early ambulation (within 24 hours) and later ambulation (after 24 hours) on the rate of postoperative nausea in patients undergoing bariatric surgery?	Experimental designs
What is the effect of focused imagery on the pain associated with chest tube removal after coronary artery bypass graft surgery as compared to receiving no focused imagery for chest tube removal?	Experimental designs
Does the presence of an alarm on biomedical equipment result in faster nursing response times than when biomedical equipment has no alarms?	Quasi-experimental designs
Does the implementation of an evidence-based practice council in a hospital result in better patient outcomes than when there is no evidence-based practice council?	Quasi-experimental designs
Are symptoms of myocardial infarction recognized in a shorter period of time in men than they are in women after presentation to an emergency department?	Causal-comparative designs
Do women who conceive via in vitro fertilization have higher levels of parenting anxiety than women who have naturally occurring pregnancies?	Causal-comparative designs
Do women who have more than three children have higher rates of chronic urinary tract infections than women who have two or fewer children?	Case-control designs
Do men with abdominal hernias have a higher rate of abdominal aneurysms than men who have not been diagnosed with abdominal hernias?	Case-control designs
Is aggressive, early pulmonary rehabilitation effective in preventing long-term complications of community-acquired pneumonia?	Time-series designs
Does participation in a nursing residency result in increased retention of new graduate nurses?	Time-series designs

It is clear that the PECO question mirrors the PICO approach closely, except that the "intervention" is not manipulated or artificially introduced into the experiment (McKeon & McKeon, 2015).

A carefully constructed research question gives the researcher guidance in research design and communicates a great deal about the study in a single statement. It is a key tool for ensuring a quantitative study has all the elements needed for a controlled trial. Table 12.1 provides some examples of quantitative research questions that are appropriate for quantitative study.

Characteristics of a Quantitative Design

Several different types of studies are classified as quantitative designs, but they all have some basic characteristics in common. In particular, they all rely on numbers to measure effects and to quantify error. These designs are best suited to study objective characteristics and human responses that can be quantified. Such studies involve comparing groups of subjects in some way—either between groups or within a single group over time. Quantitative designs are intended to be used with representative samples so that the findings can be generalized to larger groups of people with a high level of confidence that the study's outcome will be the same. Most quantitative studies are aimed at determining effects, whether they are directly attributed to a cause or inferred because of a measured relationship (Fain, 2013). It is the establishment of the relationship between an independent variable and a dependent one that requires the controls that are built into quantitative studies.

GRAY MATTER

Characteristics of all quantitative design studies include:
- Relying on numbers to measure and quantify variables
- Studying objective characteristics and responses that can be measured
- Comparing groups of subjects in some way
- Applying interventions to samples to generalize the study results to broader populations
- Aiming to determine effects of an intervention through a high level of control

An Interest in Variables

Quantitative studies focus on measuring relationships among variables. These variables may be classified as either independent (an intervention) or dependent (an outcome). In this case, the researcher is interested in the effect of the independent variable on the dependent variable. Quantitative studies require quantifying the variables of interest, so these variables are usually objective characteristics or responses that can be reported as numbers. For example, the objective characteristics of heart health can be measured in the form of blood pressure, heart rate, serum cholesterol, and other indicators of cardiac risk. In contrast, the responses of pain, anxiety, and nausea have to be reported by the affected individual, rather than measured by the researcher, so they are often recorded on scales or other instruments.

Quantitative researchers are also interested in a third type of variable: the extraneous variable. Extraneous variables are not part of the central study, but still exert an effect on the outcome. Many of the design elements in quantitative studies are intended to mitigate these effects through controls.

Control over Variables

Quantitative studies exhibit a high level of control over the variables of interest. An independent variable is controlled by the researcher; it is introduced into a patient care situation and manipulated to determine its effects. The researcher then puts measures in place to identify when the dependent variable has occurred and to quantify that response. The requirement for control over variables is not limited to those variables internal to the study. Indeed, a key focus of quantitative designs is to control variables that are extraneous to the study but that may exert an effect. The quantitative researcher attempts to eliminate these variables through strong design, if possible. If the effects of the variables cannot be avoided, then the researcher must control them through the sampling strategy, intervention protocols, or statistical analysis. On occasion, some variables cannot be eliminated or controlled, or the variables may arise during the experiment, such as an external event. In such a case, the researcher accounts for the variables' effects in the research report.

This level of control lets the researcher rule out alternative explanations for the outcome in a systematic way. It increases the reader's confidence that the intervention—and nothing else—caused a given effect reported in the study write-up.

The Use of Measurement

Quantitative analysis is, at its most fundamental level, based on quantifying something. It is clear, then, that variables in quantitative studies will be measured. Measurements may be direct or indirect, and values may be collected prospectively or retrospectively. Data may be gathered from primary or secondary sources. The measures themselves must be reliable and valid to rule out measurement error as an extraneous effect. Quantitative studies are characterized by data collection using instrumentation that yields numerical data. Data may be collected at a single point in time, at a baseline and again after an intervention, or over time periods. Given the use of measurement in quantitative studies, the reliability of the instruments, raters, and measures is a central concern.

Comparisons of Groups

Most quantitative studies focus on a comparison of groups of some kind. Comparisons may be made between the following groups:

- An intervention group and a control group
- A group with a risk factor and a matched group without that risk factor
- The same group at baseline and after treatment

Comparisons between groups are usually applied to test the effects of an intervention. With sufficient control and a strong sampling strategy, if differences between groups are detected, then it can be assumed that the intervention was the cause. When control groups are not possible, the researcher can study the effects of a risk factor by comparing outcomes for groups with and without the risk factor. Comparisons within groups, such as studies utilizing a time-series design, can reveal both whether a treatment has an effect and when it is likely to occur. Regardless of the question and intent, some comparison between or within groups is characteristic of all quantitative designs.

A Priori Selection of a Design

Quantitative designs are selected after the research question is clarified and the literature review is complete, and then they are not changed. Although some aspects of the study may necessarily need to adapt to changing conditions, the bulk of the decisions about quantitative designs are made before the study begins. This minimizes the potential for introducing researcher bias or changing the study after it has begun, both of which might alter the results. Thus the *a priori* selection of design, protocol, and analytic method is characteristic of good quantitative designs.

The details of the design are determined by the nature of the research question and the resources of the researcher. Fundamentally, quantitative designs can be classified in the following ways:

- Experimental designs answer questions about the effectiveness of interventions.
- Quasi-experimental designs answer questions about the relationships among variables.
- Comparisons of intact groups answer questions about differences in the characteristics of groups.
- Time-series designs answer questions about the effectiveness of interventions over time.

A general design is selected early in the research planning stage. All of these designs represent variations on the central theme, but each has distinctive applications and characteristics. These properties provide the researcher with guidance in the development of the specific research protocol and plan.

The Gold Standard: Experimental Design

Experimental designs answer questions about the effectiveness of interventions. These studies are considered the "gold standard" for evidence-based practice because they provide convincing support for the value of a treatment (Hall & Roussel, 2012). Experimental designs are often referred to as randomized controlled trials because these designs have in common the random assignment of subjects and a high level of control. Because subjects are randomly assigned to groups, the researcher can assume the groups are basically similar in most ways. Sometimes such studies are referred to simply as "clinical trials." Design elements of the experiment enable the researcher to control extraneous variables so the effect of an intervention can be isolated and quantified. An experimental design also enables the researcher to measure the effects of error and calculate the probability that the results were due to random events rather than the intervention. Overall, experimental designs—particularly when such studies are conducted in multiple sites or when multiple studies are reviewed in aggregate—are considered the strongest evidence for practice and are at the top of the evidence pyramid.

In experimental designs, the researcher shifts from being a passive observer and data collector to taking an active role in the intervention. In other words, the researcher is not looking for relationships, but hoping to cause them. A clinical trial is the typical experiment: Subjects are randomly assigned to either an experimental group or a **control group**, the intervention is applied to the experimental group but withheld from the control group, and differences in a specified outcome are measured. If differences are found, then they can be assumed to be attributable to the intervention because all other differences between the groups are controlled.

Experimental designs: Highly structured studies of cause and effect applied to determine the effectiveness of an intervention.

Control group: A subgroup of the sample of an experimental study from which the intervention is withheld.

Characteristics of Experimental Designs

Experiments have some fundamental characteristics that enable researchers to draw conclusions about cause and effect. Recall that three conditions must be met to draw a conclusion about cause and effect:

1. The cause must precede the effect in time.
2. Rival explanations for the outcome must be ruled out.
3. The influence of the cause on the effect must be demonstrated.

Experimental designs are structured to demonstrate these characteristics and allow the researcher to draw conclusions about causality.

The Independent Variable Is Artificially Introduced

The independent variable (the "cause" in cause and effect) is introduced and manipulated in an experiment. Although much can be deduced from studying naturally occurring phenomena, extraneous variables make it difficult, if not impossible, to isolate the effect of a single intervention (Hall & Roussel, 2012). In an experimental design, the only difference between groups is the intervention, so its effects can be isolated and quantified. Manipulating the independent variable also enables the researcher to sequence the treatment so that a subsequent outcome can be revealed, which is one of the conditions necessary to infer causality.

Subjects Are Randomly Assigned to Groups

A hallmark of the experimental design is random assignment of study participants to groups. When subjects are randomly assigned to groups, then it can be assumed that all their other characteristics are randomly (and equally) distributed in both groups. This feature enables the researcher to draw a conclusion that the only difference between the two groups is the intervention. Randomization means the researcher can rule out rival explanations, which is a second condition for determining causality.

Experimental Conditions Are Highly Controlled

In experimental designs, the researcher builds in controls for extraneous effects of variables or subject characteristics. Controls may be incorporated into sampling strategies, methodology, data collection, or analysis, but the most common approach is the use of a control group. These controls also help the researcher rule out rival explanations for the outcome—the second condition necessary to establish causality.

Results Are Quantitatively Analyzed

In an experimental design, the differences between groups are measured quantitatively and analyzed using inferential statistics. Inferential statistics yield numbers that are helpful in two ways: They allow the researcher to determine the probability that random error is responsible for the outcome, and they give the reader of the study write-up information about the size of the effect. Statistical analysis enables the researcher to draw a conclusion that the independent variable had an influence on the outcome, which is a third condition for concluding a cause-and-effect relationship exists. Statistical analysis also enables the calculation of the magnitude of the effect.

Questions That Are Best Answered with Experimental Design

Experimental designs are best applied to answer questions about the effectiveness of interventions. The ability to introduce a treatment in a highly controlled situation enables the researcher to draw conclusions about causality, influence, and relationships. Questions that focus on the sequence between a cause and an effect are also answered with experimental designs. Some words that appear in questions addressed by experimental designs include *affect, cause, relate, influence,* and *change.* Examples of questions include the following:

- What is the effect of continuous, low-level zinc ingestion on the occurrence of the common cold among college students?
- Does a video game orientation to the surgical suite change the level of anxiety preoperatively for children as compared to children who receive a traditional orientation?
- Does access to a clinical consultant influence the level of use of evidence-based practice on a patient care unit as compared to a unit that has no clinical consultant?

Experimental Design Methods and Procedures

Conducting experimental studies requires that the researcher make decisions about how the study will be carried out to demonstrate the key characteristics. Design of the methods and procedures involves a series of systematic steps based on carefully considered choices.

- *What is the population of interest?* Objective inclusion and exclusion criteria help the researcher consider and describe the specific population of interest.
- *How will subjects be assigned to groups?* Experimental designs all require random assignment to groups, but multiple methods for randomization may be employed.
- *How will the intervention be applied?* Carefully considered, detailed directions for applying the intervention will minimize error associated with inconsistent application of the treatment.
- *What will be the comparison?* For some studies, the comparison is "no treatment"—that is, a true control group. However, it is usually not ethical to withhold treatment from a patient in the name of science. Thus the comparison is made to a standard treatment, or in some cases, to a sham treatment (to control treatment effects).
- *How will the outcome be measured?* Reliable, valid measures are required to minimize measurement error, ensure accuracy, and measure with precision.
- *How will differences between the groups be quantified?* The choice of statistical tests is part of the planning process.

Strengths of Experimental Designs

Experimental designs are the gold standard for evidence-based practice. Studies with such designs are considered some of the best scientific evidence available for support of nursing practice. The use of an experimental design offers many advantages for the nurse:

- Studies based on experimental designs are considered the strongest evidence for practice.
- These designs are the only ones that allow a definitive conclusion about cause and effect, so they are ideal for testing the effectiveness of interventions.

- Experimental designs are recognized and valued by other disciplines.
- Experimental designs are generally understood by the public and patients.

Limitations of Experimental Designs

Despite their clear strengths, only a small percentage of healthcare research studies is based on experimental designs. Additionally, of those experiments reported in the literature, many have serious flaws—for example, groups may be assigned in ways other than randomly, or serious errors may affect the outcome (Melnyk & Fineout-Overholt, 2014). Although experiments offer many advantages, some of the disadvantages associated with the use of this method include the following:

- Experimental designs are complex and difficult to carry out.
- These designs require substantial resources in terms of time, researcher skill, and access to subjects.
- Many aspects of health care cannot be manipulated (for example, the presence of a risk factor, the worsening of a disease).
- Increasing control means the experiment becomes more artificial, so that generalizability of the findings may be limited as a result.

CASE IN POINT Experimental Design

Preterm infants manifest pain and stress during traumatic procedures such as the heel stick for blood samples. A number of individual nonpharmacologic methods have been found to be effective in reducing pain in this population, including non-nutritive sucking, administration of oral sucrose, and facilitated tucking. While evidence shows a modest effect for each of these interventions, researchers wanted to test combinations of them as means to reduce pain in preterm infants. In the study carried out for this purpose (Yin et al., 2015), controlling for interactions between treatments was complex, requiring five randomly selected comparison groups, each of which was provided with a different combination of interventions. This in turn required a large sample—110 infants—to adequately test each group of interventions. All were compared to a control group that received routine nursing care during the procedure.

All of the procedures were effective alone and in some combination with other interventions, but the magnitude of effect of all three combined was the largest. Observable signs of pain decreased by more than 32% in this group. The results clearly support the use of all three interventions simultaneously to achieve the greatest benefit for the infant. The authors were also able to determine that heel stick procedures can, indeed, be atraumatic when conducted while infants are stable, quiet, appropriately positioned, and soothed with nonpharmacologic methods before gently sticking the heel and squeezing blood.

This randomized trial was a complex and well-executed example of isolating the effects of both individual interventions and groups of them. Randomization minimized a host of threats to the study's validity and made the results stronger as evidence for practice in the neonatal unit.

More Common: Quasi-Experimental Designs

Experimental designs provide clear evidence of the effectiveness of interventions, yet they are uncommon in nursing and health care in general. This rarity reflects the difficulty in achieving the high levels of control that are characteristic of experiments in an applied setting. In addition, it is not always desirable—or ethical—to manipulate an independent variable or to withhold treatment, so alternative designs must often be selected. **Quasi-experimental designs** have many of the characteristics of experimental designs except for one key feature: These studies do not randomize subjects to groups, but rather work with intact groups or convenience samples. Because of this single feature, control and generalizability are limited.

Characteristics of Quasi-Experimental Designs

Quasi-experimental designs have many characteristics in common with experimental designs. Specifically, the researcher identifies independent and dependent variables of interest and strives to control as many extraneous variables as possible. Subjects are separated into groups, and differences between the groups are measured. Data are collected numerically and analyzed statistically.

The primary difference between experimental and quasi-experimental designs is the lack of random assignment to treatment groups. This characteristic weakens quasi-experimental studies when compared to experimental ones because, without randomization, it cannot be assumed that the intervention and comparison groups are equivalent at the beginning of the study. This leaves room for other explanations for the outcome, so a clear conclusion about cause and effect cannot be drawn.

Quasi-experimental designs often involve studying intact groups. Such an approach may be employed because it is impractical or impossible to deliver the intervention to some members of a group and not others. For example, a nurse educator may be interested in the effectiveness of a patient education intervention used on one patient care unit and compare outcomes to another patient care unit that does not use the educational intervention. In this study, a **comparison group** exists, but it is not a true control group because the subjects are not assigned to groups randomly.

Quasi-experimental studies can still provide strong evidence because they meet two of the three conditions for inferring causality: The independent variable precedes the dependent variable, and the influence of the independent variable can be measured. They cannot, however, completely eliminate the possibility that rival explanations are responsible for the outcome, because those explanations are not controlled by randomization.

Questions That Are Best Answered with Quasi-Experimental Designs

Quasi-experimental designs can be used to answer many of the same types of questions as their experimental counterparts. For example, questions about the effectiveness of interventions are often addressed with quasi-experimental designs. The questions often begin with *what* or *how* and use action verbs to indicate an expected effect. The variables are measurable and can be quantified using numbers.

The primary difference between quasi-experimental and experimental designs lies in the way results are interpreted, rather than the way the questions are worded. Quasi-experimental designs are not as strong as experimental designs because they are not controlled, and it cannot be assumed the sample truly represents the population. If the researcher is careful not to over-interpret the results, then quasi-experimental studies have a great deal to contribute to the body of nursing knowledge.

Quasi-experimental designs: Studies of cause and effect similar to experimental designs but using convenience samples or existing groups to test interventions.

Comparison group: A subgroup of the sample of a quasi-experimental design from which the intervention is withheld. Subjects are similar to and compared with the experimental group, but they are not randomly assigned.

Quasi-Experimental Design Methods and Procedures

Quasi-experimental design decisions are made *a priori*, as are experimental ones. Although there are many similarities between experimental and quasi-experimental methods, there are some key differences between the two types of designs:

- *Identify the population of interest.* In quasi-experimental studies, identifying the population is heavily dependent on the accessible population and the way that subjects are naturally divided into groups.
- *Identify group assignments.* Quasi-experimental studies often rely on convenience samples made up of intact groups. As such, group membership is not *assigned* so much as it is *identified*. The criteria for membership in a group are clearly identified, however, so the researcher controls selection effects.
- *Apply an intervention.* The independent variable is identified and applied to the treatment group using standardized, detailed procedures.
- *Measure the outcome.* Quasi-experimental studies have dependent variables, which are measured in both groups to determine if the intervention affected an outcome.
- *Perform quantitative analysis of differences in groups.* Statistics are applied to determine the magnitude of any effects that are identified and the probability that sampling error is responsible for the outcome. Different statistics may need to be applied, however, because many inferential tests assume randomness, and adjustments in calculations are called for with convenience samples.

CASE IN POINT Quasi-Experimental Design

Suctioning is a key nursing intervention for postoperative patients undergoing open heart surgery. Physician preferences for open- or closed-suctioning systems drive the choice of a suctioning method. Two nurse researchers studied the effects of each type of system on hemodynamic parameters using a quasi-experimental design (Ozden & Gorgulu, 2015). The study sample consisted of 120 patients who met inclusion criteria. Half of these patients were suctioned using the open-suctioning method; the other half were suctioned with the closed-suction method. The outcomes measured were heart rate, mean blood pressure, PaO_2, $PaCO_2$, SaO_2, and pH. These values were measured before, immediately after, and at 5 and 15 minutes after suctioning.

The researchers found that heart rate, arterial blood pressure, and arterial blood gases of the patients were negatively affected by the open-suctioning system, and these indicators took some time to return to the baseline level. These outcomes were not adversely affected by the closed-suctioning system.

The researchers concluded that closed-suctioning systems can be used more safely than open-suctioning systems in patients who have experienced open heart surgery.

This study is a good example of a quasi-experimental design, in which all the elements of a pure experiment are present except randomization. In this case, the choice of a treatment was affected by the physicians' preferred procedures. The lack of random selection means that there are still concerns about potential selection bias and sampling error. Otherwise, the detailed procedures described and the large effect sizes noted would indicate these conclusions are supported and could be applied to practice. These findings would be even stronger evidence if they were replicated in subsequent trials.

Quasi-experimental studies are not as strong as pure randomized trials in testing interventions, but they are often more realistic to implement and provide moderately strong evidence for practice.

The most common quasi-experimental design is the **nonequivalent comparison group before/after design**. In this design, subject responses in two or more groups are measured before and after an intervention. The only difference between this design and a true experiment is the lack of randomization. The strongest of the quasi-experimental designs, the nonequivalent comparison group before/after design provides good evidence for nursing practice.

On occasion, researchers are unable to collect pretest data before the intervention is introduced. In this case, serious flaws are introduced into this design, which is classified as **nonequivalent comparison group posttest only**. In these studies, it is impossible to determine which subject characteristics were present when the experiment began. Because there is no basis for determining the baseline equivalence of the groups, a multitude of extraneous variables may potentially be introduced. In addition, temporality of the independent variable cannot be established because a baseline was not measured.

Strengths of Quasi-Experimental Designs

The use of a quasi-experimental design offers many advantages for the researcher, including the following:

- Quasi-experimental studies are more feasible than true experiments in an applied setting.
- True experiments may not be feasible or ethical; it may be impossible to deliver an intervention to some people in a group and not others.
- Quasi-experimental studies introduce a level of control that reduces the effect of extraneous variables.
- Accessible subjects can be used for the study so that larger samples may be obtained.

Limitations of Quasi-Experimental Designs

Although quasi-experimental designs offer many advantages, some of the disadvantages associated with the use of this method include the following:

- It is inappropriate to draw firm conclusions about cause and effect without random assignment to groups.
- Groups may not be equivalent in characteristics, such that extraneous variables are introduced.
- Rival explanations for the outcome exist and may weaken confidence in the results.

Designs That Focus on Intact Groups

All the designs considered thus far in this chapter have focused on studies in which the independent variable is introduced, manipulated, or added to the situation in some way. In some cases, though, the independent variable is not *introduced* so much as it is *located*. In other words, the researcher must find subjects in which the independent variable is a natural occurrence and compare these individuals to those in whom the variable is naturally absent. The researcher then measures an outcome of interest—the dependent variable—in both groups to infer causality.

Nonequivalent comparison group before/after design: The strongest type of quasi-experimental design in which subject responses in two or more groups are measured before and after an intervention.

Nonequivalent comparison group posttest only: A type of quasi-experimental design in which data are collected after the intervention is introduced. Lack of baseline data may introduce extraneous variables in the results.

Ex post facto research: An intact-group design that relies on observation of the relationships between naturally occurring differences in the intervention and outcome.

The studies that rely on this approach are sometimes called nonexperimental designs because the independent variable is not manipulated. Indeed, technically it should not be called an independent variable at all because this factor is not changed or introduced. It is, however, very common to use the independent/dependent terminology when referring to the variables in this group of studies.

Intact-group studies can take on one of several forms. **Ex post facto research** (based on a Latin phrase meaning "operating retroactively") relies on the observation of relationships between naturally occurring differences in the presumed independent and dependent variables. It is so named because the data are usually collected after the fact, meaning that both the independent and dependent variables have already occurred. This design weakens the capacity of these studies to support cause-and-effect conclusions because the researcher cannot prove temporality. In other words, the researcher depends on the subject's recall to determine if the independent variable preceded the dependent one.

CASE IN POINT Ex Post Facto Design

Attention-deficit/hyperactivity disorder (ADHD) has been studied extensively in children, but little is known about how this condition affects individuals and their families as they move into adulthood. Montejo et al. (2015) studied 100 adult participants—half of whom were formally diagnosed with adult ADHD and half of whom were not—to determine their family functioning, parental bonding, and adult relationships. The participants were identified from the patients treated by a single Spanish hospital in its Department of Psychiatry. Outcomes were measured with two reliable and valid tools: one that measured family function and another that measured parental bonding.

The results showed that emotional connections were different in those families with at least one adult who was diagnosed with ADHD. Parental bonding,

however, did not appear associated with ADHD except for the "care" dimension. This dimension represents bonding based on control rather than affection. The authors concluded that families with adults who suffer ADHD demonstrate some dysfunctional characteristics, and their parental caring behaviors may be affected by the presence of the ADHD-diagnosed member.

The ex post facto design used in this study compared a group with a naturally occurring condition to a group that did not have the characteristic. Statistical tests were used to identify relationships between these two groups. Findings from ex post facto studies can be used as evidence for practice, albeit with caution. These studies represent the measurement of relationships, not causal models.

Causal-comparative study: An intact-group design that involves categorization of subjects into groups. An outcome of interest is measured and differences are attributed to the differences in classification of subjects.

Studies of intact groups may also be classified as **causal-comparative**. These nonexperimental investigations seek to identify cause-and-effect relationships by forming groups based on a categorical classification. In other words, groups are determined based on certain characteristics that the individuals inherently possess. Groups are then assessed relative to an outcome of interest. Subjects may be assigned to groups based on any categorical classification, such as gender, ethnicity, or geographic region. An outcome of interest is then measured to determine if the groups differ. If they do, it is assumed that the differences in the outcome are due to the differences in the classification of the subject. For example, a researcher may be interested in determining if men and women express the same amount of anxiety prior to cardiovascular angiography. In this case, the independent variable is loosely interpreted as "gender" and the dependent variable is "anxiety."

A third type of intact-group design is the **case-control study**. These studies are common in epidemiology and public health because they enable researchers to study the links between causative agents and disease (Dawson & Trapp, 2016). Case-control studies are often used to judge the relationships between risk factors and disease states or between an event and an outcome (Conway, Rolley, Fulbrook, Page, & Thompson, 2013). For example, an infection control nurse might be interested in determining the source of infections on a given patient care unit. Patients who developed an infection would be matched carefully with patients who did not, and both groups would be appraised for exposures to potential infectious agents. In this case, the independent variable is interpreted as "exposure" and the dependent variable is "infection." Case-control studies are always performed by looking backward in time. For this reason, they are sometimes referred to simply as retrospective studies, in contrast to longitudinal studies, which must be prospective (Dawson & Trapp, 2016).

> **Case-control study:** An intact-group design that involves observation of subjects who exhibit a characteristic matched with subjects who do not. Differences between the subjects allow study of relationships between risk and disease without subjecting healthy individuals to illness.

CASE IN POINT Causal-Comparative Design

Some data indicate that the presence of *Helicobacter pylori* bacteria may accompany an altered immune system. It has been hypothesized that multiple sclerosis (MS) is also linked to defects in the immune system. A team of researchers set out to determine if patients with MS had a higher incidence of *H. pylori* infection than patients who did not suffer from MS (Gavalas et al., 2015). The authors identified 44 patients with relapsing MS and 20 controls who did not have the disease. The presence of *H. pylori* was confirmed by quantitative histological survey.

The overall prevalence of active *H. pylori* infection in the MS patients was more than 86%, compared with 50% in the 20 matched control participants. During the study, the researchers discovered that two other autoimmune disorders—hypothyroidism and ulcerative colitis—were also exclusively present in the MS group. Other conditions diagnosed during the histological examination also demonstrated greater incidence in the MS group, including esophageal and duodenal ulcers and Barrett's esophagus.

This study is typical of causal-comparative research in that no intervention was manipulated, and data about the independent variable were collected retrospectively. A group was identified whose members experienced a condition—in this case, MS—and was compared to a group whose members had no such experience. Comparable outcomes—in this case, histological diagnoses—were measured in the two groups. Although not definitive for identifying a cause-and-effect relationship, causal-comparative studies such as this one still provide evidence that can be applied to practice. For example, Gavalas et al.'s (2015) study would support examining patients with MS for other autoimmune and gastrointestinal disorders. When a chronic disease is the subject of study, such that introduction of a diagnosis is not ethically possible, causal-comparative studies may be the strongest design available to answer the research questions.

The Kinds of Questions That Studies of Intact Groups Answer

Ex post facto research is useful for studying the effects of events that occur for some individuals but not for others. For example, the nurse may want to investigate whether patients who experience medication errors have longer lengths of stay in the hospital than patients who do not. In such a case, the nurse would select records from patients with medication errors and compare them to the records from patients without errors, thereby determining if there is a difference in their length of stay.

Causal-comparative studies are useful for understanding the relationship between causal variables and their potential effects, particularly when the intervention is of a group nature. It is difficult, for example, to provide an innovative educational technique to some students in a classroom and not to others. Likewise, it is nearly impossible to study changes in the way patient care units are organized or managed without using causal-comparative studies. Without huge, unwieldy samples, the researcher cannot apply the intervention randomly. These designs are useful for addressing questions that involve the way groups react to interventions or to study the effectiveness of management strategies, educational efforts, or developmental work.

CASE IN POINT Case-Control Design

Ventilator-associated pneumonia (VAP) rates are high among trauma patients, particularly those with brain injury. Finding no definitive research that compared the risk factors for VAP specific to patients with these conditions, Gianakis, McNett, Belle, Moran, and Grimm (2015) conducted a case-control study to attempt to pinpoint these risk factors. Their retrospective study examined data abstracted from the records of 157 trauma patients with and without brain injury, and sought to identify predictive risk factors.

Demographic and clinical characteristics were evaluated, as well as injury severity scores, coma indicators, intubation type and location, documented aspiration, in-hospital mortality, and number of ventilator, intensive care unit (ICU), and hospital days. The primary outcome variable was diagnosed VPA.

Many clinical and demographic characteristics were comparable between the groups, including severity of injury and the number of ventilator days. Both groups were at high risk for VAP, mostly due to characteristics that are not controllable, such as patient age, severity of injury, and location of initial intubation. Of these variables, age was the strongest predictor of VAP in trauma patients with head injuries, and the overall incidence of the condition was higher in this group. The best predictor of VAP for the trauma patients without head injury was the number of ventilator days, which is a prevalent predictor among the general population. It is clear that risk of VAP is related to a host of factors, and most of these are present in trauma patients both with and without head injury.

This study is a typical case-control design in that Gianakis et al. (2015) found subjects with and without the dependent variable (head injury) and explored differences in the measured variables in each group. Although they cannot definitively identify causal agents, case-control studies can guide the nurse to identify and minimize potential risk factors.

Investigating the differences between intact groups gives the nurse valuable information about the relationships between actions and responses. Such designs are helpful for the study of relationships between risk factors and disease because it is not ethical to subject a healthy individual to a risk factor just to study its effects. In this case, it is necessary to find individuals with risk factors and then compare their outcomes to those of individuals without the risk factors (Sathian, Sreedharan, & Mittal, 2012). For example, the nurse may wish to determine if patients who are unable to ambulate until the second postoperative day have a higher risk of thromboemboli than patients who are able to ambulate on the first postoperative day.

The research questions explored in intact-group investigations often begin with "What is the difference... ?" or "What is the relationship between... ?" to reflect an expectation that the independent variable will have a demonstrable effect. Good questions for these studies will have an identified population, a variable of interest, some comparison group, and an outcome.

Methods and Procedures for Studies of Intact Groups

Studies of intact groups require a systematic approach and efforts to exert as much control as possible. Because these studies have neither random assignment nor a manipulated intervention, the evidence they provide is much weaker than that produced by experimental or quasi-experimental designs. The researcher, then, should make an effort to control as much as possible to strengthen the conclusions. A systematic approach includes the following steps:

- *Identify the population of interest.* As in quasi-experimental studies, identifying the population is heavily dependent on the existence of an accessible population and the way subjects are naturally divided into groups. Inclusion and exclusion criteria are particularly important in these studies to minimize selection effects.
- *Identify group characteristics.* The independent variable of interest is operationally defined so the researcher will be certain that a subject possesses it; the comparison group is carefully matched on all other characteristics. This process of carefully matching subjects with the independent variable and those without it is critical for case-control studies. Matching helps to control extraneous variables such as gender, age, and diagnosis.
- *Define the outcome of interest.* The dependent variable is operationally defined so it can be quantified and measured.
- *Measure the variables.* The variables are measured either directly or indirectly, from either primary or secondary sources. In the case of ex post facto research, record retrieval is often necessary. Reliability and validity of measures are important considerations to minimize measurement error.
- *Perform quantitative analysis of differences in groups.* Statistics are applied to determine the magnitude of any effects that are identified and the probability that sampling error is responsible for the outcome.

As can be seen, many procedures in studies of intact groups are intended to minimize error associated with measures, sampling, and analysis because it is impossible to control the extraneous variables with these designs. Minimizing other sources of error through adequate controls strengthens the ability to use the results as evidence for practice.

Strengths of Studies of Intact Groups

The use of studies of intact groups offers many advantages for the researcher:

- These designs are a practical way to study interventions that are of a group nature or that cannot ethically be withheld or manipulated.
- Studies of intact groups are helpful in applied settings because they provide direction for educators, managers, and group leaders.
- These designs are relatively easy to carry out and are often implemented using secondary data.

Time-series designs:
A type of
quasi-experimental
design in which only
one group receives
the intervention; an
outcome is measured
repeatedly over time.

Limitations of Studies of Intact Groups

Although studies of intact groups offer many advantages, some of the disadvantages associated with the use of these methods include the following:

- The researcher cannot draw definitive conclusions about cause and effect using these studies.
- Because data collection often relies on secondary sources, the researcher must depend on the accuracy and completeness of existing records.
- Because the researcher forfeits control of the independent variable, he or she cannot ensure that extraneous variables did not affect the outcome.

Time-Series Designs

A final type of experimental design has a dual focus: The researcher is interested in both the effects of an intervention and the timing of its effects. Time-series designs are sometimes categorized as quasi-experimental because they do not have randomly assigned groups. Indeed, time-series designs have only one group: the group receiving the intervention. A baseline is measured and an intervention applied, and then measures are taken periodically over a specified time period. In these studies, subsequent measures are compared to the baseline measure, and any changes that emerge are assumed to be due to the intervention. In such designs, subjects actually serve as their own comparison group, with subsequent responses being compared to data for the same subjects in the preintervention period.

The Kinds of Questions That Time-Series Designs Answer

Time-series designs answer questions about the effectiveness of interventions and the timing of responses. In some cases, the effects of an intervention may have a delayed onset or may take time to fully develop. For example, a study of functionality after total knee replacement will demonstrate an initial period of decreased functionality, followed by improvement over several months' time. Such designs enable the nurse to counsel patients about what they can expect from a treatment in terms of both effects and timing (Melnyk & Fineout-Overholt, 2014). Time-series designs are also useful when a change is being implemented and the researcher is focused on the results of that change. For example, a unit might change its procedure manual to evidence-based practice guidelines and desire to measure the effects of the change. It is difficult, if not impossible, to construct a randomized trial focused on this type of change, but a comparison to a baseline helps the researcher infer which results were achieved.

Time-series studies often address questions such as "What is the effect over time?" or "When do effects occur?" Results of these studies are useful for practicing nurses in evaluating both what to expect from an intervention and when to expect it.

Time-Series Design Methods and Procedures

Time-series designs are carried out systematically in a way very similar to other quasi-experimental designs. Although subjects are not randomized to groups, other elements are controlled as much as possible so that the effects of extraneous variables are held to a minimum. In this way, rival explanations can be considered and reasonable conclusions drawn. The following steps are involved in a time-series design:

- *Identify the population of interest.* Because there will be only one group, describing the population of interest also describes the sample. Inclusion and exclusion criteria are important to minimize selection effects. A random sample may be drawn from an overall population, but more often an accessible sample of convenience is used.
- *Define the variables.* The independent variable is the intervention, as in other experimental and quasi-experimental designs, and the dependent variable is the outcome of interest. Both variables are operationally defined in a quantifiable way before the experiment begins.
- *Measure the baseline condition.* The outcome of interest and the subject characteristics are measured at the beginning of the study, before any intervention is applied. This may take the form of a single, point-in-time measure or multiple measures completed over a specified time period.
- *Apply the intervention.* Detailed protocols for implementation are used to apply the intervention. These protocols maintain the consistency of the intervention so that treatment effects can be isolated from experimenter effects.
- *Measure the outcome variables over time.* The variables are measured at specified intervals over an extended time period.
- *Perform quantitative analysis of differences in groups and time periods.* Statistics are applied to determine the magnitude of any effects that are identified from the baseline to each time period and between time periods. Any changes are evaluated for the probability that sampling error is responsible for the outcome. In addition, the data from time-series studies are analyzed for differences over time to determine which changes can be expected at each interval.

Strengths of Time-Series Designs

The use of a time-series design offers many advantages for the researcher:

- Fewer subjects are required to achieve adequate power. Time-series studies have substantial power because there are more observations per subject.
- The effects of the intervention over time can be quantified. This is particularly helpful for interventions that take some time to have an effect, such as lifestyle changes or conquering an addiction.
- Multiple data points can be collected both before and after the intervention. The extended time period for measurement strengthens the researcher's ability to attribute changes to the intervention.
- Time-series analysis can be applied to evaluate the effects of change on groups of individuals, such as organizational changes or cultural events.

CASE IN POINT Time-Series Design

Patients with prostate cancer often experience lower urinary tract symptoms after surgical treatment. A team of nurse researchers studied changes in lower urinary tract symptoms after open radical prostatectomy, laparoscopic radical prostatectomy, and brachytherapy for the treatment of prostate cancer (Li, Chen, Lin, & Chen, 2015). To do so, they used a time-series survey design with both descriptive and comparative variables. A total of 51 patients with prostate cancer were recruited, and data were collected at six time points: baseline, 1 week, 1 month, and 2, 3, and 8 months post treatment. A reliable, valid instrument was used to assess the patients' urinary tract symptoms.

The results showed no significant differences between the three treatment options in terms of the incidence of lower urinary tract symptoms. The timing of resolution was different between groups, however. The groups who underwent open radical prostatectomy and brachytherapy showed faster improvement, reporting reduced symptoms 1 month sooner than those undergoing laparoscopic radical prostatectomy. The time-series design used in this study is typical in that the associations of variables were measured over time. Specifically, the timing and occurrence of symptoms were measured relative to time in the postoperative period. These are helpful findings for counseling patients about what to expect after surgery and when to expect their symptoms to improve.

Limitations of Time-Series Designs

Although time-series designs offer many advantages, some of the disadvantages associated with their use include the following:

- The inability to include a meaningful control group limits the ability to determine cause and effect.
- Rival explanations may exist for observed outcomes.
- Attrition can be a particular problem because there is only a single sample. Loss of subjects over time may weaken the results of the study.

Reading Quantitative Research

The first step in the critique of the methods and procedures of a quantitative study is to determine the specific type of design used in the study. The design is generally specified in the abstract; if not, it should be explicitly identified in the beginning of the article or in the first few lines in the methods section. If a design is experimental, then the authors will almost certainly identify it as a randomized controlled trial, clinical trial, or experiment.

If the design is not explicit, the reader must infer the type of design by comparing its characteristics to those of a quantitative study. If the study uses numbers and measures differences between groups (or within a group over time), then it is a quantitative analysis. If these characteristics are present but the author does not specify the type of design, assume it is quasi-experimental (Girden & Kabacoff, 2010). Randomized trials are so difficult to carry out that authors are anxious to report their use of this design if they have managed to do so.

Enough detail should be provided so that the reader can judge the rationale for the design decisions made by the researcher. As with other designs, the specific type of study should be clearly linked to an appropriate research question. The research question should include all the elements required for a quantitative study: the population of interest, the intervention, a relevant comparison, and an outcome. It is helpful if the author reports a rationale for selection of the specifics of the study related to the demands of the question; there should be a clear link between the purpose of the study and the type of design used to achieve it.

If detail about the type of study is not reported clearly, then the reader may need to examine the article closely for evidence of the type of design that was employed. Clues to the specific design may be present in the research question, aims, purpose statement, or objectives. Words such as *affect, influence, change,* or *improve* may indicate that a quantitative design was used.

The reader can differentiate experimental designs from quasi-experimental ones by scrutinizing the group assignment procedure. If subjects are assigned to groups randomly and an intervention is applied, then it is a true experiment. If subjects are assigned any way other than randomly, it is quasi-experimental (regardless of how the author describes it). If only one group exists and measures are taken over time, then it is a time-series design. Groups may also be labeled as "convenience samples" or "accessible groups"; in either case, this descriptor indicates studies that involve intact groups rather than randomly assigned ones.

Quantitative studies often have the most detailed methods and procedures sections of any research reports. The reader should be able to ascertain the way samples were selected and assigned to groups, the protocol used to apply the intervention, the way outcomes were measured, and the way data were analyzed. It is not uncommon for the author to provide figures or photographs to demonstrate the intervention protocol or measurement procedures. Enough information should be provided that a reasonably informed researcher can replicate the study from that information. The authors should demonstrate a systematic and rigorous approach to controlling extraneous variables through controls of internal and external validity.

Finally, examine the conclusions section to ensure that the authors do not over-interpret or make inferences that go beyond what the results can support. Only experimental studies can result in a definitive statement about cause and effect. Although quasi-experimental, time-series, and intact-groups studies may be used to infer causality, readers should interpret these results with caution. Extraneous variables can be controlled only when subjects have been assigned to a control group in a way that ensures the baseline equivalency of treatment groups—and meeting that criterion requires randomization. Any other type of study yields information about the assumed effectiveness of interventions, but it cannot be considered to provide conclusive evidence of effects. These latter studies may suggest or imply causal relationships—and the authors may use quasi-experimental studies as pilot studies for later experiments—but causal relationships are supported only through studies utilizing experimental designs. Without the controls that are inherent in an experimental design, and without a randomly chosen comparison group, it is impossible to confirm all the conditions necessary for causality.

Even with all these caveats, quantitative designs produce some of the strongest evidence for nursing practice. Understanding the nature of the relationship between an intervention and its effects is a powerful way to ensure that nursing practices are, indeed, based on what is known rather than what is believed.

WHERE TO LOOK FOR INFORMATION ABOUT QUANTITATIVE DESIGNS

- A quantitative design is generally identified in a straightforward way in the abstract or the introduction. If it does not appear here, then it will be found in the initial statements in the "methods and procedures" section. The design should be easily identifiable and a major part of the research study write-up.
- If the write-up does not specify whether the study used an experimental design, then assume it is quasi-experimental. Experimental designs are so challenging that authors are quick to note when they have been able to carry one out.
- The specific methods and procedures should be clearly reported. The description may be concise, but it should have enough detail that an informed reader could replicate the study. If the intervention or measurement is complex, there may be a separate section for procedures, which may be labeled as such or called "protocols." This section may describe either the specific steps for applying the treatment or the steps for measuring its effects (or both).
- What is included in the methods section is not always standard. This section should have subheadings for the sampling strategy, research design, treatment protocols, measurement, and analytic plan.

Using Quantitative Research in Evidence-Based Nursing Practice

Quantitative designs—particularly when they are replicated and reported in aggregate—provide some of the strongest evidence for evidence-based nursing practice. The ability to determine causality and to measure the effects of interventions provides powerful information to support practice.

Quantitative evidence has a variety of uses in nursing practice. In particular, assessment, interventions, and evaluation of outcomes are supported by studies that are highly controlled and that link interventions to outcomes.

- *Assessment and diagnosis of patients:* Quantitative studies can help the nurse identify if particular assessment procedures are effective in detecting patient conditions. In particular, case-control studies help elucidate the relationships between risk factors and disease states, and these designs are helpful in determining if the nurse can expect that a given risk factor will result in a disease state or complication.
- *Interventions:* The test of interventions is where quantitative studies really shine. Whether the interventions are planned on an individual or group basis, quantitative studies allow the reader to draw definitive conclusions about cause and effect. These studies are considered some of the strongest scientific evidence for nursing practices. Quantitative studies can help the nurse discover interventions that prevent complications, quickly address problems, and help patients attain and maintain health.
- *Evaluation of outcomes:* Quantitative studies provide strong evidence to support outcome measurement and evaluation. Such studies enable the nurse to draw conclusions about the relationships between interventions and outcomes and, in the process, help develop operational definitions of these variables. These definitions can assist in standardizing the way patient outcomes are measured, collected, and reported.

In addition, quantitative studies let the nurse determine which outcomes can be expected from specific interventions. Time-series studies have the added benefit of contributing information about the timing of responses. Such studies are helpful in designing patient teaching and counseling because they enable the nurse to provide the patient with realistic expectations about treatments and procedures.

Generalizing the Results of Quantitative Studies

Quantitative studies are intended to provide the nurse with information about how well the sample represents the population. When samples are selected randomly, the chance that the sample will represent the population accurately increases, so experimental designs have especially strong external validity. The description of the sample characteristics and a clear definition of the population help the nurse determine if the study results could be expected to apply to his or her particular patients. Before using the results of quantitative studies in a specific population, the nurse is responsible for ensuring that the populations are similar enough that expecting similar results in the new population is reasonable.

The results of quantitative studies are stronger when they are confirmed in the aggregate. Reviews of multiple experiments enable the nurse to draw strong inferences about the usefulness of an intervention. Experimental designs conducted in multiple sites provide some of the strongest evidence for nursing practice. It is rare that a practice change is warranted after a single study. If the study has been replicated many times in various settings and with multiple populations, however, then the nurse can use the results more confidently.

CHECKLIST FOR EVALUATING A QUANTITATIVE STUDY

❑ The quantitative nature of the study is made clear early in the study and the specific design is identified.

❑ A rationale is provided for the choice of a design, and it is linked to the research question.

❑ A specific procedure is described for the application of the treatment or intervention.

❑ Instruments and measurement procedures are described objectively.

❑ The reliability of the instrumentation is described and supporting statistics are provided.

❑ The validity of the instrumentation is described and supporting statistics are provided.

❑ A detailed protocol for the use of each instrument in the measurement is described.

❑ Threats to internal validity are identified and controlled.

❑ Researcher bias and treatment effects are controlled by blinding.

❑ The authors provide sufficient information to determine whether their findings can be generalized to other groups or settings.

Creating Quantitative Research

Quantitative research is a widely used research method because it provides strong information about the effectiveness of interventions. It is difficult, however, to achieve the level of control that is required to definitively rule out rival explanations for an outcome. Indeed, this complexity of control means that pure experimental designs are uncommon. Nevertheless, quasi-experimental studies, studies of intact groups, and time-series designs can still provide compelling evidence for practice, particularly when they are replicated and reported in the aggregate. Achieving adequate control can be accomplished by using a systematic approach to consider the design decisions inherent in quantitative study:

- *Clarify the research question.* The question should have all the elements represented by the PICO (or PECO) approach: an identified population, an intervention (or exposure) of interest, a comparison, and an outcome.
- *Identify a specific design that will answer the question in the most efficient, effective way.* This choice depends on several factors: whether the independent variable can be manipulated, whether it can be delivered to individuals, whether it will be possible to randomly assign subjects to groups, and whether the outcome will be measured at a single point in time or over time. By clarifying these aspects of the question, the correct design will generally become evident.
- *Describe the population of interest, and determine inclusion and exclusion criteria for the sample.* Devise a sampling strategy that maximizes the representativeness of the population and will support the external validity of the findings.
- *Determine the way that subjects will be assigned to groups.* If random assignment to groups is possible, the researcher should take advantage of that approach, even if it requires extra effort. Random assignment strengthens a study in so many ways that it is worth the extra time and energy to implement it.
- *Clarify the variables of interest and write operational definitions for each one before selecting measurement instruments.* Identify which variable is the independent variable and which is the dependent variable. Brainstorm potential extraneous variables, and build in methods to control the foreseeable ones.
- *Devise a description of the intervention and write a protocol that is objective and detailed and that provides direction to the nurses who will apply it.* Use photographs or video recordings if they are appropriate. The protocol should identify when the treatment is applied, how it is applied, to which patients, and how often. Step-by-step directions for each element of the treatment should be provided in detail. Have nurses who are not involved in the research read the protocol to uncover confusing or misleading sections. Control of variability in treatments is one of the most important considerations in quantitative research design.
- *Determine a measurement procedure that will generate reliable, valid data.* If instruments or tools are to be used, ensure that they possess the appropriate psychometric properties for the specific study design that is proposed. Provide written directions for using the measurement instruments; provide word-for-word directions to read to subjects so they are consistently applied. Determine the inter-rater reliability of data collectors prior to beginning data collection.
- *Manage the data collection process carefully.* Data should be collected carefully to ensure their accuracy and completeness. Working with a statistician to create a data collection spreadsheet or an online database is helpful because it ensures that the researcher will not have to reenter or manipulate data prior to analysis. Apply a process for maintaining the integrity of the data set. Specific measures should be planned for restricting access and ensuring confidentiality, such as password-protected files and locked file cabinets. Incorporate periodic quality checks into the data management process.

- *Use the appropriate analytic tools for the question to be answered and the type of data being collected.* Consider the level of measurement of each variable, the number of groups to be compared, and the level of confidence needed in the outcome. Statistical analysis software is widely available; in fact, most common statistical tests can be done with Excel spreadsheets, so there is no need to manually calculate statistics. If statistical analysis becomes complicated, consult a statistician from a university or medical center.

- *Report the analysis accurately and completely; report each test that was run, even if it did not contribute to the overall outcome of the study.* This approach reduces the potential for selective retention of findings—which poses a threat to the study's validity. The results of statistical tests should be reported in a standard way that enhances their understanding across disciplines. The research report should include the results of each test using appropriate summary statistics in tables or figures; the meaning of each should be explained in the text of the research report as well.

- *Draw conclusions appropriate for the intent of the study and the results that were found.* Even with experimental designs, the author should resist the urge to over-interpret the data. Definitive conclusions about causality can be drawn only from pure randomized controlled trials. However, it is common to note the causal relationships that were indicated by the data or suggested by the findings, as long as the appropriate cautions are noted.

Developing a design for a study requires attention to each of these elements. Decisions must be made during each step that support the findings and provide a clear answer to the research question. These answers, in turn, provide some of the strongest scientific evidence for effective nursing practices.

GRAY MATTER

Quantitative evidence in nursing practice may be used for the following purposes:
- Identify whether particular assessment procedures are effective in detecting patient conditions.
- Discover interventions that prevent complications, quickly address problems, and help patients attain and maintain health.
- Draw conclusions about the relationship between interventions and outcomes.
- Determine which outcomes can be expected from specific interventions.

Strengthen Quantitative Studies

It is difficult to conduct a pure experimental design in an applied setting. Extraneous variables abound, and it is often unethical to withhold treatment from a control group. In addition, it is difficult to ensure that all members of the experimental group always get the treatment in exactly the same way. Time constraints and availability of individuals to collect data can hinder the validity of the experiment.

Although it may be challenging to conduct a true experiment in a working unit, the following strategies can strengthen the validity of applied quantitative studies:

- Use a comparison group of some kind. Although it may be difficult to randomly assign patients to groups, the use of a comparison group does strengthen the study's validity, even if it is just a convenience sample.
- If using a nonrandom comparison group, match the groups as closely as possible on potential extraneous variables (for example, age, severity of illness, and number of comorbid conditions).
- Clearly identify the independent and dependent variables, and write formal operational definitions of each. These definitions can help to determine criteria for inclusion in the study, treatment protocols, and measurement systems.
- Use simple, straightforward measurement methods whenever possible. Measure unobtrusively to minimize treatment effects.
- Take advantage of automated systems to capture data whenever possible, including the recording systems that are built into some patient care equipment, such as intravenous pumps, automated beds, and medication administration systems.
- If using a chart review to capture data, select a random sample of charts to limit the labor involved in data retrieval.
- Training is critical. Train those who will apply the treatment and those who will collect the data.
- Set up monitoring systems and random checks to ensure the treatment and measurement systems are working consistently.
- Hide the identity of the experimental and control groups from those who are collecting data whenever possible. Blinding of both subjects and data collectors minimizes several threats to validity, including treatment effects and researcher bias.
- Get help when designing the study. Universities and medical centers often have consulting statisticians available. Advanced practice nurses are also good sources of research support, as is an organization's evidence-based practice council or research team.
- Replicate the studies of others whenever possible. Finding a published study that reports an experiment can jump-start the nurse's own research plan by describing procedures and measures that a subsequent researcher might be able to use.

Summary of Key Concepts

- The purpose of quantitative research is to use measurement to determine the effectiveness of interventions.
- Quantitative research involves measuring objective characteristics or responses of subjects, and is reported using numbers.
- Quantitative studies are designed to provide high levels of control so confidence in the results is enhanced.
- Quantitative methods allow the researcher to measure the probability that some other factor caused the outcome—specifically, things such as extraneous variables, measurement error, or sampling error.
- Quantitative studies can help the nurse appraise the effectiveness of an intervention, determine the relationship between actions and patient responses, and measure changes over time.
- Quantitative research questions include variables that can be operationally defined and measured in a numerical way.

- The quantitative research question identifies the population of interest, the intervention under study, the comparison that makes up the control, and the outcome of interest.
- Quantitative studies have many characteristic elements, including an interest in variables, control over the experiment, the use of measurement to compare groups, and statistical data analysis.
- Quantitative studies utilize *a priori* designs, meaning that most design decisions are made before the research begins.
- Four common classifications of quantitative research in nursing are experimental designs, quasi-experimental designs, studies of intact groups, and time-series designs.
- Experimental designs are characterized by random assignment of subjects to groups, a manipulated independent variable, and an outcome of interest. Differences between groups at the end of the experiment are assumed to be due to the intervention.
- Quasi-experimental designs are very similar to experimental ones, except that subjects are assigned to groups in some way other than randomly.
- Studies of intact groups include ex post facto, causal-comparative, and case-control designs. These designs involve finding subjects with the variable of interest and matching them to a comparison group to discover relationships.
- Time-series designs enable the researcher to determine both the effectiveness of an intervention and the timing of its effects.
- Quantitative designs are considered some of the strongest scientific evidence for nursing practice.

CRITICAL **APPRAISAL EXERCISE**

Retrieve the following full-text article from the Cumulative Index to Nursing and Allied Health Literature or similar search database:

Lin, S., Huang, C., Shiu, S., & Yeh, S. (2015). Effects of yoga on stress, stress adaptation, and heart rate variability among mental health professionals: A randomized controlled trial. *Worldviews on Evidence-Based Nursing*, 12(4), 236–245.

Review the article, focusing on the sections that report the question, design, methods, and procedures. Consider the following appraisal questions in your critical review of this research article:

1. How do the authors describe the design of this study? Which characteristics of the study lead you to agree or disagree with their description? Describe the blinding method. Which kind of bias does this method control?
2. Discuss whether the design is the most appropriate for this research objective.
3. What is the independent variable? The dependent variable?
4. What were possible sources of measurement error in this study?
5. Was the treatment protocol described adequately for replication?
6. What are the strengths of the design, methods, and procedures of this study? Contrast them with its limitations.
7. How could this study be incorporated into evidence-based practice? To which groups could this study be generalized?

References

Conway, A., Rolley, J., Fulbrook, P., Page, K., & Thompson, D. (2013). Improving statistical analysis of matched case-control studies. *Research in Nursing & Health, 36*, 320–324.

Dawson, B., & Trapp, T. (2016). *Basic and clinical biostatistics* (5th ed.). New York, NY: McGraw-Hill.

Fain, D. (2013). *Reading, understanding, and applying nursing research* (4th ed.). Philadelphia, PA: F. A. Davis.

Gavalas, E., Kountouras, J., Boziki, M., Zavos, C., Polyzos, S., Vlachaki, E., . . . Deretzi, G. (2015). Relationship between *Helicobacter pylori* infection and multiple sclerosis. *Annals of Gastroenterology, 28*(3), 353–356.

Gianakis, A., McNett, M., Belle, J., Moran, C., & Grimm, D. (2015). Risk factors for ventilator-associated pneumonia. *Journal of Trauma Nursing, 22*(3), 127–131.

Girden, E., & Kabacoff, R. (2010). *Evaluating research articles from start to finish*. Thousand Oaks, CA: Sage.

Hall, H., & Roussel, L. (2012). *Evidence-based practice: An integrative approach to research administration and practice*. Burlington, MA: Jones & Bartlett Learning.

Li, H., Chen, K., Lin, Y., & Chen, T. (2015). Lower urinary tract symptoms of prostate cancer patients undergoing treatments over eight-month follow-up. *Journal of Clinical Nursing, 24*(15/16), 2239–2246.

McCusker, K., & Gunaydin, S. (2015). Research using qualitative, quantitative, or mixed methods and choice based on the research. *Perfusion, 30*(7), 537–542.

McKeon, J., & McKeon, P. (2015). PICO: A hot topic in evidence-based practice. *International Journal of Athletic Therapy & Training, 20*(1), 1–3.

Melnyk, B., & Fineout-Overholt, E. (2014). *Evidence-based practice in nursing and healthcare: A guide to best practice* (3rd ed.). Philadelphia, PA: Lippincott Williams & Wilkins.

Montejo, J., Duran, M., Martinez, M., Hilari, A., Roncalli, N., Vilaregut, A., . . . Ramos-Quiroga, J. (2015). Family functioning and parental bonding during childhood in adults diagnosed with ADHD. *Journal of Attention Disorders, 1557–1246*.

Ozden, D., & Gorgulu, R. (2015). Effects of open and closed suction systems on the haemodynamic parameters in cardiac surgery patients. *Nursing in Critical Care, 20*(3), 118–125.

Saadatmand, V., Rejeh, N., Heravi-Karimooi, M., Tadrisi, S., Vaismoradi, M., & Jordan, S. (2015). Effects of natural sounds on pain: A randomized controlled trial with patients receiving mechanical ventilation support. *Pain Management Nursing, 16*(4), 483–492.

Sanz, C., Matesanz, P., Nieri, M., & Pagliaro, U. (2012). Quality of reporting of randomized clinical trials in implant dentistry: A systematic review on critical aspects in design, outcome assessment, and clinical relevance. *Journal of Clinical Periodontology, 39*(Suppl. 12), 81–107.

Sathian, B., Sreedharan, J., & Mittal, A. (2012). *Case control studies in medical research: A practical approach*. London, UK: Lampert Academic Publishing.

Yin, T., Yang, L., Lee, T., Li, C., Hua, Y., & Liaw, J. (2015). Development of atraumatic heel-stick procedures by combined treatment with non-nutritive sucking, oral sucrose, and facilitated tucking: A randomised, controlled trial. *International Journal of Nursing Studies, 52*(8), 1288–1299.

Chapter 13

Analysis and Reporting of Quantitative Data

CHAPTER OBJECTIVES

The study of this chapter will help the learner to

- Compare inferential statistics to other types of quantitative analysis.
- Discuss the types of decisions that are made *a priori* and the rationale for making these choices prior to reviewing data.
- Describe the ways in which quantitative analyses are classified based on the goals of the analysis, the assumptions of the tests, and the number of variables in the study.
- Explain how sampling distributions relate to the calculation of inferential statistics and interpretation of the results.
- Summarize the usefulness of confidence intervals in interpreting quantitative data, and explain how they are used to judge clinical significance.
- Differentiate statistical significance from clinical significance.
- Differentiate the appropriate application of *t* tests, chi square tests, and analysis of variance.
- Evaluate the statistical section of a research report to determine its value as evidence for practice.

KEY TERMS

Bivariate analysis	Inferential analysis	Parametric tests
Confidence interval	Levels	Point estimate
Effect size	Magnitude of effect	Robust tests
Error of multiple comparisons	Multivariate analysis	Standard error
Factors	Nonparametric tests	Univariate analysis

It has been thoroughly demonstrated that regular physical activity is associated with better physical well-being and overall mental health. Since both of these outcomes are often identified as problematic to achieve in older adults, studying nursing interventions that can improve an older adult's health and well-being is important. Khazaee-pool et al. (2015) conducted a randomized controlled trial to determine if a program of regular exercise could improve happiness in older adults.

These nurse researchers recruited volunteers from a public park. Each person was then checked against inclusion and exclusion criteria, and a final sample of 120 adults was identified and randomly assigned to either the experimental group, who participated in an 8-week physical exercise program, or a control group, who received no specific physical activity recommendations.

Variables that were collected included demographic data and responses on the Oxford Happiness Inventory. The latter instrument takes a broad look at personal happiness, and its results have been determined to be a reliable and valid reflection of satisfaction with life, positive mood, mental health, self-esteem, and efficiency. The measure itself is an ordinal, Likert-type scale.

Some interesting data were revealed by the researchers' descriptive analysis. For example, a significant inverse relationship between age and level of happiness was identified before the experiment began, meaning older subjects were less happy. This lent credence to the need for interventions for this age group. Females were happier than males, but overall those persons with lower incomes reported being less happy. There was a significant inverse relationship between being dependent on others and lower happiness—a relationship that was found to reverse itself after the exercise program ended. This was a particularly important finding, in that older people who are active feel less dependent on others for their day-to-day care.

Almost all of the scale scores improved after members of the experimental group engaged in the 8-week program of physical activity. Self-esteem, life satisfaction, and global happiness showed the greatest improvements, but statistically significant differences were found in the results of all six scales that the researchers administered.

The results of this study were reported in a way that made their interpretation relatively easy. Two tables were used to display demographic characteristics of the subjects and the results of statistical tests. The authors reported test statistics as well as *p* values. They noted which findings were clinically significant and focused the discussion section on the nursing implications of the findings. Enough data were provided for the reader to get a general sense of the magnitude of differences and to determine which findings were large enough to be clinically important.

It has been clear for some time that participating in a regular program of physical activity has wide-ranging implications for health as we age. This study indicates that mental health and happiness can be improved through physical activity as well. These findings—the result of a single randomized trial—represent evidence that can support nursing practices in the care of older adults.

Khazaee-pool, M., Sadeghi, R., Majilessi, F., & Rahimi, F. (2015). Effects of physical exercise programme on happiness among older people. *Journal of Psychiatric & Mental Health Nursing, 22*(1), 47–57.

Introduction

If descriptive analysis answers the question "What is going on?", then inferential analysis answers the question "Are you sure?" The word *inferential* means that the reader can infer something about a population's response to an intervention based on the responses of a carefully selected sample. Inference requires the calculation of numerical values to enhance the researcher's and reader's confidence that the intervention resulted in the outcome and to rule out the possibility that something else did. In quantitative inferential analysis, that "something else" is error in all its forms—sampling error, measurement error, standard error, even random error—and inferential analysis allows the researcher to quantify its effect.

When reading quantitative analysis, it is important to focus on both the probability of error and the certainty of the estimates. When quantitative analysis is used as evidence for nursing practice, the nurse should also consider the size of the effect and determine whether it attains both statistical and clinical significance. When creating quantitative analysis, the focus is on choosing the correct test and making appropriate decisions about its application. All of these factors are critical for ensuring that the relationship between intervention and outcome is one that is defined with certainty so the results can be expected to be replicated in different settings among different people.

Some General Rules of Quantitative Analysis

Quantitative analysis is a highly systematic and organized process. Data for quantitative analysis are represented numerically, so the reliability of data collection, accuracy of data entry, and appropriateness of analytic processes are critical for drawing the correct conclusions. Because these types of analyses can be complex, a plan for analysis and reporting is determined when the research methods and procedures are designed. A wide variety of statistical tests are available, each of which has specific requirements for data preparation and analysis. There are, however, some general guidelines for conducting all types of quantitative analyses:

- *Select tests* a priori. The specific statistical tests that will be used for quantitative analysis are selected before the experiment begins. The selection of specific tests is based on the research question to be answered, the level of measurement, the number of groups, and the nature of the data. Selecting the tests before the data are generated reduces the chance that a researcher might use a test that is less conservative or more favorable by eliminating this source of researcher bias.
- *Run all the tests identified.* The researcher must run all tests that were identified *a priori*. Looking at the data and then deciding which tests to run can create bias. Although the specific version of a test may be dictated by the nature of the data (for example, using a test for non-normal data), the researcher should not pick and choose tests after reviewing the data.
- *Report all the tests that were run.* The researcher must report the results from each test that was run. Selectively reporting or retaining data to support a personal viewpoint is a form of researcher bias and is unethical.

Types of Quantitative Analysis

Quantitative analysis refers to the analysis of numbers. Quantifying the values of variables involves counting and measuring them; these counts and measures result in numbers that can be mathematically manipulated to reveal information. The researcher can think of quantitative analysis as an interpreter that takes raw data and turns it into something understandable.

Parametric tests:
Statistical tests that are appropriate for data that are normally distributed (that is, fall in a bell curve).

Nonparametric tests:
Statistical tests that make no assumptions about the distribution of the data.

Robust tests:
Statistical tests that are able to yield reliable results even if their underlying assumptions are violated.

Many types of quantitative analyses are possible. Those available to the researcher can be categorized in several ways: by the goals of the analysis, by the assumptions made about the data, and by the number of variables involved.

Goals of the Analysis

Quantitative analyses are useful for many research goals. In particular, research questions that focus on evaluating differences between groups (for example, between an experimental group and a control group) are amenable to quantitative analysis. This type of research leads to some of the strongest studies when it comes to presenting evidence for practice. Quantitative tests are appropriate to assess the nature and direction of relationships between subjects or variables, including the capacity to predict an outcome given a set of characteristics or events. Researchers also use quantitative methods to sort data; for example, a clinician may identify characteristics that enable him or her to differentiate people at risk for falls from those who are not at risk. Quantitative analyses aid in data reduction by grouping variables into overall classifications, which then helps researchers determine, as an example, which clusters of symptoms may predict complications.

Quantitative analyses are also classified as descriptive or inferential based on the aims of the study. Descriptive studies are concerned with accurately describing the characteristics of a sample or population. Inferential analyses are used to determine if results found in a sample can be applied to a population—a condition necessary for confidently generalizing research as a basis for evidence for nursing practice (Schmidt & Brown, 2012).

Assumptions of the Data

Quantitative analyses are generally grouped into two major categories based on assumptions about the data: parametric and nonparametric. The key differentiating factor for these categories is the assumptions made about the distribution, or shape, of the data. **Parametric tests** are based on the assumption that the data fall into a specified distribution—usually the normal (bell-shaped) distribution. This assumption holds only when interval- or ratio-level measures are collected or when samples are large enough to achieve normality. In reported healthcare research, parametric tests are the most common, even when doubt exists about whether the basic assumptions have been met. Other tests, however, are specific to data that are not normally distributed. If a normal distribution cannot be assumed, then such **nonparametric tests** are needed. This group of tests is "distribution free," meaning the tests do not rely on a specific distribution to generate accurate results. Nonparametric tests are becoming more common in research, particularly in health care, where many variables are not normally distributed.

Parametric tests are usually desirable because they are sensitive to relatively small differences, they are commonly available in most software packages, and they are readily recognizable by the reader. Nevertheless, they are sometimes applied erroneously to data sets for which the distribution of the data has not been shown to be normal; in such a case, they may result in misleading conclusions. Small deviations from normality may be acceptable with these tests because most parametric tests are **robust tests**, or capable of yielding reliable results even when their underlying assumptions have been violated. Nevertheless, some data are so non-normal as to require a test that makes no such assumptions.

Compared to parametric tests, nonparametric tests are not as commonly applied, are less recognizable, and are not always available in analytic packages. These tests are also relatively insensitive and require large samples to run effectively. When possible, researchers should strive to collect data in a form that can be expected to be normally distributed and to create sample sizes that allow them to use parametric tests. However, researchers should use the appropriate category of test for the data, meaning they should specifically evaluate the distribution of the results prior to making the final decision on which tests to use. Most parametric tests have a nonparametric counterpart, enabling researchers to apply the correct class of test to the data.

Number of Variables in the Analysis

Quantitative analyses can be classified in terms of the number of variables that are to be considered. In practice, such tests are usually classified by both the number and the type of variables involved.

Univariate analysis involves a single variable. Such analyses are the primary focus of descriptive and summary statistics. The term univariate analysis may also be applied when the study involves a single dependent variable or when only one group is included. For example, differentiating whether blood pressure is affected more by exercise in the morning or the evening is a univariate analysis; that is, even though two groups (morning and evening) are included in the study, the analysis focuses on a single dependent variable—blood pressure.

Bivariate analysis is the analysis of the relationship between two variables. The most common form of bivariate analysis is correlation. Bivariate analysis is also used to determine if a single variable can predict a specified outcome. For example, determining if blood pressure is associated with sodium intake is a bivariate analysis. In this case, two variables—blood pressure and sodium—are analyzed to determine any relationship between them.

Multivariate analysis is the simultaneous analysis of multiple variables. This endeavor may address the effects of multiple predictors on a single outcome, the differences between groups on several effects, or the relationships between multiple factors on multiple outcomes. For example, determining if blood pressure is different in the morning or evening, and is associated with sodium intake, weight, and stress level, is an example of a multivariate analysis.

These analyses become more sophisticated and complex as more variables are added to either side of the equation. On the one hand, a research study may require a simple univariate analysis to achieve a descriptive goal. On the other hand, an experiment may require the complexities of a full factorial multivariate analysis of variance—a calculation of the effect of multiple factors on multiple outcomes, taking into account both their main effects and the effects that occur when factors interact. Quantitative analyses can accommodate the complexity of human responses to interventions and illness by reflecting the multivariate nature of health and illness.

An Overview of Quantitative Analysis

Inferential analysis is undertaken to determine if a specific result can be expected to occur in a larger population, given that it was observed in a sample. In statistics, a sample (part of the population) is used to represent a target population (all of the population); the

Univariate analysis: Analysis of a single variable in descriptive statistics or a single dependent variable in inferential analysis.

Bivariate analysis: Analysis of two variables at a time, as in correlation studies.

Multivariate analysis: The simultaneous analysis of multiple variables.

Inferential analysis: Statistical tests to determine if results found in a sample are representative of a larger population.

question then becomes whether the same results found in the sample would be found in the larger target population. Quantitative research as evidence for practice is useful only when it can be generalized to larger groups of patients than those who were directly studied in the experiment. Inferential analysis allows the nurse to recommend that an intervention be used and to do so with an identified level of confidence that it is evidence based.

Inferential analysis is fundamentally an analysis of differences that occur between samples and populations, between groups, or over time because something changed. In experimental research, the change is an intervention. In case-control studies, the "change" is a risk factor; in causal-comparative studies, it is a characteristic or an event. Inference is used to determine if an outcome was affected by the change.

It is not enough, however, to see a difference between two samples and assume that the difference is the same as would be expected in a larger population. Samples, by their very nature, are different than the populations from which they were drawn. Samples are made up of individuals and, particularly in small samples, we cannot be sure that the sample exactly matches the population's characteristics. These differences—the ones that are due to the sampling process—are quantified as **standard error**. One might view standard error as the differences between samples and populations that are expected simply due to the nature of sampling.

Statistical Significance

Historically, researchers were interested in finding an objective way to decide if differences between treatment groups and control groups were important. Comparing the differences to standard error made sense; it told the researcher if the change was real. For many decades, researchers have relied on the statistic that is yielded by this comparison—the probability of standard error—to determine if changes are different from random errors (Scott & Mazhindu, 2014). This comparison of observed differences to standard error forms the basis for most inferential tests.

The certainty with which a researcher can say "these effects are not due to standard error" is subject to rules of probability. The calculations produce a p value, or the probability the results were due to standard error. If the p value is very small, then the probability that the results were due to error is very small, and the researcher can be very confident that the effects of the intervention are real. The largest a p value can be, and still be considered significant, is 0.05, or 5%. If the p value is very large (greater than 0.05 or 5%), then the probability that the results were due to error is very large, and the researcher cannot conclude that the intervention had an effect greater than would be expected from random variations. When the p value is very small, indicating that the probability the results were due to chance is also very small, then the test is said to have *statistical significance*. It is the comparison of differences to standard error and the calculation of the probability of error that give inferential analysis its strength. Nevertheless, statistical significance is just one of the important measures that determine whether research is truly applicable to practice. Many readers rely solely on the p value to determine whether results are useful as evidence for practice; this value is often misinterpreted as scientific evidence of an effect, when it is actually a measure of error. Significance testing does not eliminate the need for careful thought and judgment about the relevance of the findings for clinical practice.

Inferential analysis yields more than a *p* value, and it is these other statistics—the test statistic, confidence intervals, and difference scores—that enable the researcher to quantify whether the difference is important (clinical significance). Statistical significance tells us the findings are *real*; clinical significance tells us if the results are *important for practice*. This type of analysis forms the basis of some of the strongest scientific evidence for effective nursing practices.

Clinical Significance

In evidence-based practice, the concern for statistical significance has been augmented with a broader focus on clinical significance. Clinical significance is generally expected to reflect the extent to which an intervention can make a real difference in patients' lives. Clinicians are more frequently interested in these kinds of findings than in whether the result was due to chance. However, while well-established means are available to assess statistical significance, no single measure can identify a result's clinical significance. Nevertheless, several statistics can inform the clinical evaluation of the importance of a finding, including confidence intervals, minimum important difference (MID), and effect size.

Estimates of population values can be expressed as **point estimates** or interval estimates. A point estimate represents a single number. In other words, a researcher measures a value in a sample, calculates a statistic, and then concludes that the population value must be exactly that number. In reality, samples rarely produce statistics that exactly mimic the population value (called a parameter). In this respect, a point estimate is less accurate than an estimate that includes a range of numbers. The likelihood that a single point will match the population value is quite small; the likelihood that the actual value could be captured in a range of numbers is considerably better. This range of numbers represents a **confidence interval** and is used to estimate population parameters.

A confidence interval enables the researcher to estimate a specific value, but it also provides an idea of the range within which the value might occur by chance. It is defined as the range of values that the researcher believes, with a specified level of confidence, contains the actual population value. Although it sounds counterintuitive, confidence intervals are more accurate in representing population parameters than are point estimates because of the increased likelihood that an interval will contain the actual value.

Confidence intervals are helpful in quantitative analysis in several ways. The calculation of a confidence interval takes into account the effects of standard error, so the probability that the interval actually contains the population value can be determined. Confidence intervals allow the measurement of sampling error on an outcome and express it in numeric terms. They provide more information than *p* values do; they enable the evaluation of magnitude of effect so the nurse can determine whether results are large enough to be of clinical importance. Confidence intervals are constructed using several pieces of information about the data, combined with a decision made by the researcher regarding how much confidence is necessary. Although such intervals may be constructed around any statistic, the mean is typically used for this purpose. Confidence intervals for mean estimates and for estimates of the mean differences between groups are popular ways to measure experimental differences, and they represent a critical aspect of application of research as evidence for practice. Their construction requires that the researcher calculate

Point estimate:
A statistic derived from a sample that is used to represent a population parameter.

Confidence interval:
A range of values that includes, with a specified level of confidence, the actual population parameter.

the mean value and then determine the range around the mean that is due to standard error. This range is affected by the level of confidence in the results that the researcher must have (usually 95% or 99%), the amount of variability among subjects, and the size of the sample.

FIGURE 13.1 indicates how a confidence interval of the mean is constructed. At the most fundamental level, confidence intervals show the range of possible differences in effect caused by the intervention. They help the nurse determine whether the observed differences suggest true benefits or just minor changes. The confidence interval is particularly helpful in determining how close the treatment came to *no difference*. For example, a confidence interval for a weight-loss strategy might be from 0.25 to 2.0, meaning that the strategy could result in a loss of as much as 2 pounds or as little as 0.25 pound. Such an interval is helpful in judging evidence about which treatment might be statistically sound but has little clinically meaningful effect.

An additional advantage of the confidence interval is that it is reported on the same relative scale as the outcome itself. In other words, a *p* value of 0.02 tells us nothing about how effective a treatment was; its scale matches that of probability, ranging from 0 to 1.0. The confidence interval, in contrast, is reported on the original scale of the outcome measure, so it is more meaningful (Pandis, 2013). For example, knowing that "the weight lost as a result of the treatment was between 3.5 and 6 pounds" gives the nurse valuable information for counseling patients and judging the success of an intervention. Table 13.1 explains the interpretation of confidence intervals.

A measure of clinical significance that is being more commonly reported in study write-ups is the MID. This clinically derived number represents the smallest difference in scores between the experimental and control groups that would be of

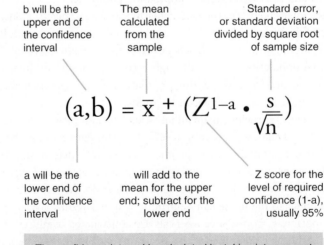

b will be the upper end of the confidence interval

The mean calculated from the sample

Standard error, or standard deviation divided by square root of sample size

$$(a,b) = \bar{x} \pm \left(Z^{1-a} \cdot \frac{s}{\sqrt{n}}\right)$$

a will be the lower end of the confidence interval

will add to the mean for the upper end; subtract for the lower end

Z score for the level of required confidence (1-a), usually 95%

The confidence interval is calculated by taking into account the amount of error in the sample and the level of confidence required. This creates a range above and below the sample mean that we are confident contains the population mean.

FIGURE 13.1 What Makes Up a Confidence Interval?

Table 13.1 Confidence Intervals Interpreted: An Example

Statistic	Confidence Interval	What It Means
Mean number of distressful symptoms reported by patients with terminal cancer	3.5 to 4.1 symptoms	Patients with terminal cancer have, on average, between 3.5 and 4.1 distressful symptoms, inclusive.
Proportion of patients with terminal cancer who report distressful symptoms	79.2% to 88.7%	Between 79.2% and 88.7% of patients with terminal cancer report distressful symptoms, inclusive.
Mean difference between number of symptoms experienced by men and women as distressful	−0.24 to 1.4 symptoms	The average difference between the number of symptoms reported as distressful by men and women could be nothing (zero, which appears in this interval). There are no statistical differences between these groups.
Mean difference between number of symptoms experienced by members of a treatment group and members of a control group	−1.2 to −0.3 symptoms	A nursing intervention had the effect of reducing the number of symptoms perceived as distressful. The decrease could be as little as 0.3 of a symptom or as much as 1.2 symptoms. There is a significant effect, but it is very small.
Mean difference between number of symptoms experienced by those with early-stage disease and those with late-stage disease	2.1 to 4.3 symptoms	People late in the terminal stages of cancer experience more distressful symptoms than those in early stages of the same disease. They could experience as few as 2.1 symptoms or as many as 4.3 symptoms, which demonstrates a significant effect of considerable magnitude. This is a clinically meaningful finding.

interest as evidence for practice. For example, a weight change of 4 ounces may be of no importance in a study of adult males, but it would most certainly be clinically notable in a sample of preterm infants. There are three commonly accepted ways to find the MID:

1. Compare the change in the outcome to some other measure of chance (anchor based).
2. Compare the change to a sampling distribution to determine its probability.
3. Consult an expert panel (Fethney, 2010).

Effect size:
The size of the differences between experimental and control groups compared to variability; an indication of the clinical importance of a finding.

The MID is determined prior to statistical analysis. The confidence interval is reviewed; if it contains the MID value, then the results are clinically significant. If the confidence interval does not include the MID, however, then the results are not considered clinically significant, whether they are statistically significant or not.

To see how the MID is used in practice, suppose a researcher testing the effects of massage therapy on hypertension consults the literature and an expert panel and determines that a change of 5 mm Hg in blood pressure would be considered clinically significant. If the confidence interval for the change were 1 to 3 mm Hg, the interval does not include 5 mm Hg, so the result is not clinically significant. If the confidence interval were 2 to 10 mm Hg, however, then the researcher could conclude that the findings were clinically significant.

Clinical importance can also be represented by **effect size**, meaning the size of the differences between experimental and control groups. Effect size can provide the nurse with a yardstick by indicating how much of an effect can be expected and, therefore, it provides more information for evidence-based practice than statistical significance alone.

Effect size is calculated in many different ways, but all have in common a formula that takes into account the size of differences and the effects of variability. Interpreting effect size is relatively easy: Larger numbers represent a stronger effect, and smaller numbers represent a weak one. Effect size can also be discerned from a confidence interval. If the confidence interval for a mean difference includes zero or nears zero on one end, for example, then the difference could be nothing. In such a case, clinical significance becomes a critical consideration.

Both statistical significance and clinical significance are needed to ensure that a change in practice is warranted based on the study results. A change in practice should not be recommended if the researcher cannot demonstrate that the results are real—in other words, that the results are statistically significant. Change also is not warranted if the results are not important enough to warrant the effort involved in changing a practice. Effect size is needed to draw this conclusion. No single statistic can be used to establish the usefulness of a study; all of the results taken together provide the nurse with evidence that can be applied confidently.

Designs That Lend Themselves to Quantitative Analysis

Some research questions naturally lend themselves to quantitative analysis. Experimental, quasi-experimental, causal-comparative, and case-control designs are all particularly well suited to inferential analysis, for example. A research question must lend itself to collection of numerical data to be appropriate for quantitative testing, and a relationship, difference, or effect must be the focus of the study. Qualitative studies are not appropriate candidates for statistical testing because—unlike quantitative research—they do not involve analysis of numbers.

Predictive and correlation studies also yield statistics, but they do not necessarily focus on differences in groups. A correlation coefficient yields a p value that represents the probability that the relationship observed is not due to standard error. That relationship, however, may be a weak one, so statistical significance is less important for a correlation study than interpretation of the size and direction of the coefficient. Predictive studies involving regression also yield quantitative output. The regression itself is compared to the mean to determine the value of the prediction. Thus a *p* value in a regression simply indicates that the values are related in a linear way and that the regression line is a better predictor than the mean.

The primary consideration in any quantitative analysis is appropriate interpretation. That is, the researcher's interpretation of the results should not exceed what the data will support. Appropriately reporting statistical tests and associated effect sizes, along with confidence intervals, is a complete and accurate way to draw conclusions about evidence for nursing practice. All three of these results should be incorporated into the quantitative research report.

Selecting the Appropriate Quantitative Test

Conducting an appropriate quantitative analysis depends on the ability of the researcher to select the appropriate statistical test. This is often the most daunting part of the analysis process because many tests are available to the nurse researcher. Each has specific requirements and yields particular information, which may then be appropriate in specific circumstances. The researcher must make decisions about the appropriateness of a statistical test based on the following factors:

- The requirements of the research question
- The number of groups to be tested
- The level of measurement of the independent and dependent variables
- The statistical and mathematical assumptions of the test

Each of these elements is considered in determining which group of tests to select and, from that group, which particular version will best answer the question without producing misleading results. Questions about differences between two groups, for example, will be answered with different tests than would be used with three or four groups. Likewise, interval data, which are assumed to be normally distributed, are tested differently than nominal data, which must be represented as proportions or rates. All statistical tests have assumptions; the data must meet the assumptions for the results to be interpreted correctly.

The tests most commonly used in intervention research are tests of means and proportions. When dependent variables are measured as interval numbers (for example, heart rate, length of stay, and cost), then the mean value can be calculated and compared. When dependent variables represent nominal or ordinal data, then frequencies, rates, or proportions are tested. In each case, tests may be conducted to determine if differences exist between two, three, or more groups.

Tests of Differences Between Two Group Means

Frequently, the research question of interest is whether an intervention, risk factor, or condition made a difference in a specific outcome between two groups. The typical experiment, in which the outcomes for a treatment group are compared to those for a control or comparison group, falls into this category. If the outcome can be expressed as a mean, then a *z* or *t* test is appropriate to use for these differences. These statistical tests indicate whether the differences in mean values between two groups are statistically significant and clinically important. **FIGURE 13.2** depicts the decision process that results in a *z* or *t* test for a quantitative analysis.

The two tests essentially accomplish the same end: They generate a statistic that reflects the differences between the groups compared to standard error—a *p* value that quantifies the probability that standard error is responsible for the outcome and a confidence interval for mean differences that enables the quantification of effect size. The *z* test

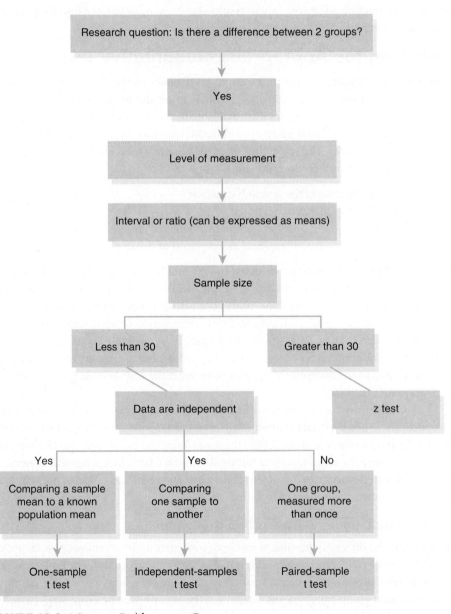

FIGURE 13.2 A Decision Tool for a *z* or *t* Test

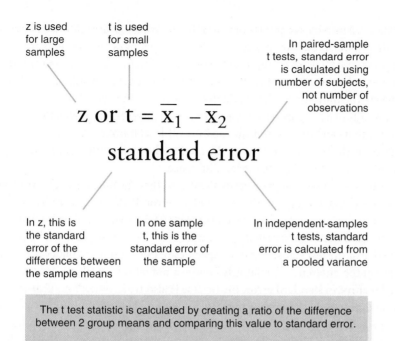

z is used for large samples

t is used for small samples

In paired-sample t tests, standard error is calculated using number of subjects, not number of observations

$$z \text{ or } t = \frac{\overline{x}_1 - \overline{x}_2}{\text{standard error}}$$

In z, this is the standard error of the differences between the sample means

In one sample t, this is the standard error of the sample

In independent-samples t tests, standard error is calculated from a pooled variance

The t test statistic is calculated by creating a ratio of the difference between 2 group means and comparing this value to standard error.

FIGURE 13.3 What Makes Up a *t* Test?

is appropriate for large samples or when testing an entire population. The *t* test is best used with smaller samples, generally including fewer than 30 subjects (Hoffman, 2015). **FIGURE 13.3** shows how the *t* test is calculated and the calculations that are represented by each part of the formula.

Because most experiments involve samples, the remainder of this discussion will focus on the *t* test. There are essentially three versions of this test that can be applied to determine differences in mean values:

- The one-sample *t* test quantifies the difference between a mean value in a sample and a mean value in the larger population. For example, a one-sample *t* test could test the difference between a hospital's mean length of stay and the national average.
- The independent-samples *t* test quantifies the difference between the mean in one group and the mean in another group. An example would be a test to determine if mean lengths of stay were different for rural and urban hospitals. This *t* test variant could also be used as a test of effectiveness by comparing the mean in an experimental group to the value for a control group. For example, an independent-samples *t* test would be appropriate to determine if units that relied on standard orders sets had a shorter length of stay than units that did not.
- The paired-samples *t* test quantifies the difference between a mean value measured in the same group over time. For example, a paired-sample *t* test could be used to answer questions about average length of stay before and after a change in Medicare reimbursement.

Table 13.2 provides examples of research questions that are addressed by each type of *t* test. In general, *t* tests are appropriate when two groups or time periods are compared against some value that is well represented by a mean. Data must be normally distributed to lend themselves to a *t* test; therefore, interval or ratio data (or ordinal data from large samples) are the only appropriate variables evaluated with such a test.

The results of a *t* test are used to determine if an intervention is effective in achieving an outcome that can be measured with an interval-level number. Appropriately reported results include the test statistic (*t* or *z*), the *p* value, the mean difference between groups, and a confidence interval for the mean difference.

If the results of a *t* test are statistically significant, then the differences observed between the groups are real and are not due to standard error. If the results are not statistically significant—in other words, if the *p* value exceeds 0.05—then the remaining numbers in the output need not be interpreted. In contrast, if the results are statistically significant, then the size of the test statistic and the specifics of the confidence interval give clues as to the size of the difference. A relatively large test statistic means that a greater effect was achieved relative to standard error; the reverse is also true. When a confidence interval has one end near zero, that means the difference could be near nothing, so a smaller effect is expected. Conversely, if the ends of the confidence interval are some distance from zero, then the effect is likely quite large. More detailed statistical texts—specifically, those by Hulley, Cummings, Browner, Grady, and Newman (2013) and Galin and Ognibene (2012)—provide formulas for calculating effect size.

Table 13.2 Research Questions Answered by the *t* Test

Question	Characteristics	*t* Test
Is there a difference between mean costs per patient-day in an urban-based rehabilitation hospital and the national average for rehabilitation hospitals?	Comparing a sample mean to a known population value	One-sample *t* test
Is there a difference in mean costs per patient-day in urban-based rehabilitation hospitals and rural rehabilitation hospitals?	Comparing the mean value in one group to the mean value in another group; the groups have no influence on each other	Independent-samples *t* test
Is there a difference in mean costs per patient-day for patients in rehabilitation hospitals who are managed with a pharmacist/nurse/physician team and patients who are managed with a traditional model?	Comparing the mean value in one group to the mean value in another group; the groups have no influence on each other	Independent-samples *t* test
Is there a difference in mean costs per patient-day before and after Magnet designation of a rehabilitation hospital?	Comparing the mean value in a group measured over time; a value in the first sample can be "paired up" with a value in the second sample	Paired-samples *t* test

The *t* test is widely used in health care, is relatively simple to calculate, and is easily interpreted. It is included in most introductory statistics classes, so it is meaningful to a wide range of readers. The *t* test is also robust, meaning it may still be effective even if data are not normally distributed, and it works well even with small samples. This relatively simple test cannot accommodate multiple independent or dependent variables, however, so it is used primarily for univariate analysis.

Researchers are often interested in outcomes that are summarized as average scores, although by no means does this description encompass the entire range of tests that nurse researchers may wish to use. Often, variables in health care are expressed as rates, frequencies, proportions, or probabilities, and these values do not lend themselves to analysis with a *t* test. If a dependent variable must be expressed as a nominal or ordinal number (for example, gender, satisfaction, or presence of a risk factor), then a *t* test is not appropriate. In these cases, the nonparametric chi square test is a good choice.

Tests of Differences in Rates and Proportions

As just noted, healthcare variables are often expressed as rates or proportions. Events that either do or do not occur (e.g., a medication error), characteristics that are either present or absent (e.g., risk factor or no risk factor), and variables that describe characteristics in a categorical way (e.g., ethnicity or gender) cannot be expressed as intervals. These variables are not expressed as means, so they are inappropriate for tests using the *z* or *t* distribution. **FIGURE 13.4** depicts the decision process leading to selection of a

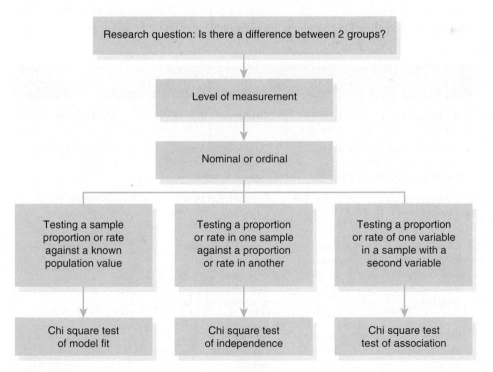

FIGURE 13.4 A Decision Tool for the Chi Square Test

chi square test for quantitative analysis. In this case, tests that are based on a chi square distribution are appropriate.

Three kinds of chi square tests are commonly used in hypothesis testing:

- The chi square test of model fit is used to determine if a sample proportion is independent of a population; it is analogous to the one-sample t test and is used for the same purposes. For example, a chi square test of model fit could be used to determine if a hospital's infection rate were the same as the national rate.
- The chi square test of independence is used to determine if two samples are independent of each other. It is analogous to the independent-samples t test and is used for the same reasons. An example of an appropriate application of the chi square test of independence would be to determine if the infection rate in one nursing home is the same as the infection rate in another nursing home.
- The chi square test of association is used to determine if there is an association between the presence or absence of a characteristic and the occurrence of an event. It is analogous to the paired-samples t test. A chi square test of association could be used to determine if there is an association between the infection rate on a unit and attendance at a unit-based educational event.

Table 13.3 provides examples of research questions that are addressed by each type of test. The chi square test essentially determines an occurrence rate that is expected, based on prior probabilities, or (alternatively) by assuming equal distribution across all groups. These expected rates are then compared to the rates observed in the experiment. A probability is calculated for the differences between observed and expected values, which yields a p value. This p value is interpreted identically to the way it is used in z tests,

Table 13.3 Research Questions Answered by the Chi Square

Question	Characteristics	Chi Square
Is the proportion of patients who fall the same on a rehabilitation unit as it is for the rest of the hospital?	Comparing a sample proportion to a known population value	Chi square test of model fit
Is the proportion of patients who fall the same on the day shift as it is on the night shift?	Comparing a sample proportion to another sample's proportion	Chi square test of independence
Is the proportion of patients who fall the same on a shift that received Internet-based training and a shift that received coaching-based training?	Comparing a sample proportion in an experimental group (coaching-based training) to a comparison group (Internet-based training)	Chi square test of independence
Is there an association between falls and the use of diuretics?	Comparing two characteristics of a single sample	Chi square test of association

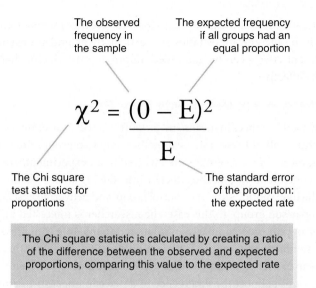

The observed frequency in the sample

The expected frequency if all groups had an equal proportion

$$\chi^2 = \frac{(0 - E)^2}{E}$$

The Chi square test statistics for proportions

The standard error of the proportion: the expected rate

The Chi square statistic is calculated by creating a ratio of the difference between the observed and expected proportions, comparing this value to the expected rate

FIGURE 13.5 What Makes Up a Chi Square?

t tests, and other hypothesis tests. If the *p* value is less than the preset alpha value, then the fit, association, or independence is considered statistically significant and the differences are real. **FIGURE 13.5** demonstrates the calculation and meaning of a chi square statistic.

The chi square test is based on the assumption that the data are not normally distributed and that variables are measured in a categorical manner. Therefore, only nominal or ordinal data (or interval data that have been turned into categories) are appropriate for this test.

Several different versions of the actual chi square statistic exist. The version used and a rationale for its selection should be provided. The test statistic (the chi square) should be reported, along with the *p* value for the test. Confidence intervals are not generally reported for chi square tests, but proportions in each group should be specified.

Chi square is a simple test to run. It is available in nearly all statistical analysis software, and it is a readily recognizable and interpretable. On the downside, chi square is a relatively insensitive test due to its nonparametric nature. Large samples are needed to ensure avoidance of Type II error, and the results provide very little information. Aside from the proportion of a variable and a *p* value, little else is generated from these tests. Even so, the chi square test is widely used for assessment of research involving everything from risk prediction to model testing; therefore, it is a versatile test for the healthcare researcher.

A specific test for categorical data that is highly useful for evidence-based practice is the odds ratio. This statistic is often reported in clinical intervention studies—for example, drug studies, studies of the effectiveness of procedures, and treatment studies. Such studies generally are designed to measure the effects of some treatment and report the probability, or "odds," that an intervention will change an outcome (Wassertheil-Smoller & Smoller, 2015). Larger odds ratios mean larger effects. An odds ratio of 1.0 means that the group

Error of multiple comparisons:
The increased error associated with conducting multiple comparisons in the same analysis; the 5% allowable error for each test is multiplied by the number of comparisons, resulting in an inflated error rate.

Factors:
Independent variables in an ANOVA that are measured as categories.

that gets the treatment and the group that does not get the treatment are equally likely to achieve a given outcome. Odds ratios are particularly helpful as evidence for practice because treatment effects can be quantified, improving the chance that the change in practice will be effective.

Tests of Differences in Means with Many Groups

Although tests for differences in means and proportions will answer many evidence-based research questions, all of these tests assume that only two groups are being compared. In some cases, more than two groups are involved in an experiment. For example, a researcher may control for the placebo effect by introducing an intervention to one group, withholding the intervention from the control group, and delivering a "sham" intervention to a third comparison group. In this case, the researcher is interested in comparing the intervention group to each comparison group and then comparing the two controls to each other. Differences between the intervention groups and the nontherapeutic groups will support the existence of a treatment effect; differences between the control and comparison groups support the emergence of a placebo effect. If treatment effects are identified without placebo effects, the results of the study represent particularly strong evidence for practice.

The analysis of more than two groups creates a problem, however. Each statistical test is based on the idea that there is less than a 5% chance that the results are due to standard error. The key word here is *each*. When three groups are involved, three comparisons are needed: (1) group 1 compared to group 2, (2) group 2 compared to group 3, and (3) group 1 compared to group 3. Each of these tests is associated with a 5% error rate. Thus, when we make three comparisons instead of a single comparison (as we would do with two groups), the error rate triples from 5% to 15%. This **error of multiple comparisons** affects statistical analysis in which multiple tests are carried out within the same analysis. Analysis of variance, better known by its acronym ANOVA, avoids this problem when an interval outcome is compared in more than two groups (Wassertheil-Smoller & Smoller, 2015).

ANOVA is one of the most frequently used statistical tests in evidence-based research studies. It is a staple for testing the effectiveness of interventions because of its versatility and its capacity to produce a tremendous amount of information. It is effective in studies utilizing experimental and quasi-experimental designs, particularly those such as the Solomon four-group design, which (as the name suggests) tests four groups simultaneously. ANOVA is helpful when the research involves more than two groups. Studies that compensate for placebo effects or that test for extraneous variables are also suitable for ANOVA. In addition, ANOVA and its variants may be used to determine if factors have interaction effects. **Factors** in ANOVA are the broad categories by which subjects are categorized into levels (for example, gender is a factor in which there are two levels—male and female). Research questions that search for the interactions between characteristics, events, and responses are well addressed with the full-factorial versions of ANOVA. A full-factorial ANOVA can be used to test all the main effects and interactions involved in an experiment with multiple groups. **FIGURE 13.6** depicts a decision tool for the application of ANOVA.

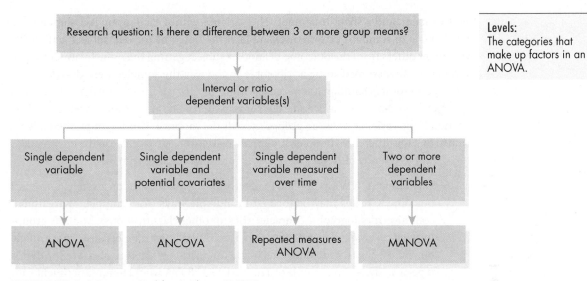

FIGURE 13.6 A Decision Tool for Applying ANOVA

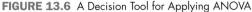

Levels:
The categories that make up factors in an ANOVA.

For example, a researcher may be interested in determining if guided imagery can reduce preoperative anxiety. In a study of this issue, the researcher might randomly assign preoperative patients to one of three groups: a group that receives formal training in guided imagery, a group that receives nonspecific guidance in relaxation, and a group that receives no formal intervention. The differences among these three groups would be classified as a main effect. Finding a difference between the guided imagery group and the two comparison groups would provide evidence that the imagery worked. In contrast, finding a difference between the control group and the group receiving nonspecific relaxation guidance would provide evidence of a placebo effect. If the researcher were concerned that gender might influence the acceptability of guided imagery, the researcher could test for an interaction effect between gender and group membership. Testing both main effects and interaction effects makes up a full-factorial ANOVA and enables the researcher to appraise both the effects of the intervention and its interaction with other variables.

ANOVA is used for data that meet some fundamental assumptions. Although this technique is focused on the ANOVA, it is actually a test of means. Therefore, the dependent variable must be numerical and its data must be approximately normally distributed. ANOVA possesses a considerable amount of robustness and can still generate good conclusions even if this assumption is somewhat violated. It also depends on a random sample to ensure the generalizability of results. Unless a special version of the test is used, ANOVA data must be independent, meaning the score at each level has no effect on other scores. In other words, the data must not be repeated measures.

ANOVA is used to determine if the differences between multiple groups are greater than standard error. The test accomplishes this goal by comparing the variance between treatment groups to the variance within each group. The variance between treatment groups is assumed to be attributable to the different applications of the intervention, called levels. As an example, levels of an intervention might be an experimental treatment, no treatment, and a sham treatment. The variance within each group is assumed to be attributable to standard error. For example, if the outcome for one subject getting the treatment differs from the outcome of another subject getting the same treatment, these differences are assumed to be attributable to the way the samples were drawn. If this description sounds familiar, it is because within-groups variation is considered and used in ANOVA in the same way standard error is used in a *t* test—as a surrogate for random chance. If the variance between groups exceeds the variance within groups, then it is assumed that the differences between groups are real and are attributable to the intervention.

Four basic kinds of ANOVA are useful for evaluating experiments:

- Univariate ANOVA is applied to determine if groups differ on a single numerical outcome. Groups may be formed in multiple ways (for example, by treatment condition, demographic characteristics, or other classifications). Multiple groupings with a single dependent variable are called univariate because only a single outcome is measured. Main effects and interaction effects are measured with this type of analysis. An example of a univariate ANOVA would be an experiment with treatment, sham, and control conditions measured with respect to gender on an outcome such as time to treatment for chest pain.
- Repeated-measures ANOVA is used to determine if time is a factor in treatment conditions. Because these data are not independent, a different version of ANOVA must be applied. For example, a study of the differences in functionality between a treatment group and a control group at four different time periods of recovery would be analyzed with repeated-measures ANOVA.
- Analysis of covariance (ANCOVA) is used to determine if a covariate—commonly an extraneous variable—has an impact on the experiment. For example, a researcher might want to determine if socioeconomic status—rather than the treatment condition—was a reason for the poor outcome in a treatment group.
- MANOVA, the multivariate version of ANOVA, is the most complex version of the test. MANOVA can accommodate multiple groups and multiple dependent variables, and it is particularly useful when the researcher believes that multiple dependent variables are related to one another. For example, a researcher could use MANOVA to determine if a combination of music therapy and relaxation techniques affected anxiety and panic attacks during painful procedures.

Table 13.4 provides examples of research questions answered by ANOVA. This test and its variants are powerful tools for quantitative analysis. ANOVA is a robust test with broad applicability, and it is familiar to the reader of research. It enables the researcher to determine the effects of multiple variables on multiple outcomes, and to do so in a way that minimizes error associated with multiple comparisons. However, it can be a complex test to carry out. As more variables and interactions are considered, the size of the required sample increases. Beyond a fundamental univariate ANOVA, specialized software and training are required to run and interpret the analysis. Nevertheless, ANOVA remains one of the most widely used tests in healthcare research and yields high-quality evidence for practice.

The results of an ANOVA test are reported similarly to the results of other tests of group differences. The *p* value indicates whether the overall model is statistically

Table 13.4 Research Questions Answered by Analysis of Variance (ANOVA)

Question	Characteristics	ANOVA
Is mean length of stay in a rehabilitation facility different for children who have constant parental presence, periodic but daily parental presence, or periodic but not daily parental presence?	Comparing a mean value among three groups	Analysis of variance (ANOVA)
Is mean length of stay in a rehabilitation facility different for children who have constant parental presence, periodic but daily parental presence, or periodic but not daily parental presence? Is this relationship mediated by socioeconomic group?	Comparing a mean value among three groups while controlling the effects of a potential extraneous variable	Analysis of covariance (ANCOVA)
Are mean length of stay and mean functional status on discharge different for children who have constant parental presence, periodic but daily parental presence, or periodic but not daily parental presence?	Comparing mean values on two outcome variables among three groups	Multivariate analysis of variance (MANOVA)
Does functional status after discharge from a pediatric rehabilitation facility change the most in the first month, between 1 and 3 months, between 3 and 6 months, or after 6 months?	Comparing a mean value over time periods	Repeated measures analysis of variance

significant—in other words, whether the differences between groups are greater than one would expect from standard error alone. If the p value for the ANOVA is less than 5%, however, it simply indicates that some group mean is different. If this is the case, then post hoc tests, or tests that look for specific group means, are appropriate. Post hoc tests allow for all groups to be freely compared to all other groups, and for all interactions to be tested, while overall error is controlled. If no statistical significance is determined for the overall ANOVA, however, then any group differences are due to standard error and no additional testing is required.

Tests for Non-normal Data

Although most data questions can be addressed with statistical tests intended for normally distributed data, some data do not conform to this standard. A moderate violation of the assumptions of a statistical test may still yield accurate results; indeed, many tests that depend on normal distributions are "robust" in this way. Other data are so skewed as to be inappropriate for tests intended for normally distributed data. If there are no "tails" in the distribution, for example, then finding statistical significance is a more challenging proposition.

For these data—data that are ranked, ordinal data, or data that are skewed—nonparametric tests are available. These tests are "distribution free," meaning they make no underlying assumptions about the way the variables are distributed. As such, they can be useful in cases of non-normality. However, these tests are also less sensitive, leading to more Type II error. Avoiding error requires large samples. Further, these tests produce little information (for example, they do not yield confidence intervals), so their application is limited.

Tests for non-normal data depend on the ability to rank data, so they are well suited for ordinal data. Examples of these tests include the Mann-Whitney U, the Wilcoxon Signed Rank test, and the Kruskal-Wallis test. The choice of specific tests depends on whether the data are independent or paired-sample data.

Reading the Analysis Section of the Research Report

The statistical analysis of a research study provides the tools to determine if interventions do, indeed, make a difference. Without statistical analysis, a researcher cannot quantify if results are attributable to the experiment or to some random effect. Yet the statistical section of a research article is the one area that is often a mystery—a collection of daunting tables, figures, and numbers that seem to confuse more than they clarify. In turn, clinicians often focus on the methods and then flip the pages to the discussion and conclusion section, taking it on faith that the statistics are reported appropriately.

This approach is insufficient to critically evaluate the value of a research study as evidence for practice. Studies do get into print with faulty statistical conclusions; errors (both Type I and II) are made; authors go beyond what the statistics will support in interpreting output (Girden & Kabacoff, 2010). The nurse must be able to review the statistical section of a research report both to judge the quality of the article and to decide if the findings should be applied to practice.

There is little reason to be intimidated by the statistical section of a research article. Numbers in research are just tools that are used to convert raw data into information. Statistics are used in research to measure the effects of sampling, to quantify the amount of error in measurement, and to put a value on the effects of chance. These numbers in a research study can help determine if the findings are clinically relevant. Whether a finding is of practical use depends on the magnitude of the effect, and confidence intervals help to evaluate effect size. Such numbers provide a yardstick against which to assess whether estimates are precise and useful. Fundamentally, the numbers in a research study help determine if the results are credible and ultimately if they should be applied to practice.

That is not to say that the nurse must understand every variant of every statistical test. Understanding the ways numbers are used, combined with a focus on some of the most important numbers, can shed light on whether the results can be trusted. A quality evaluation of a research study should address the appropriateness of tests and those numbers that provide critical information. The following are the most common types of numbers reported in the quantitative results section:

- Descriptive statistics about the sample and variables
- Analysis of sample subgroups for group equivalency
- Statistics to evaluate the role of error in measures and results
- Statistics to evaluate the magnitude of effect (if there is one)
- Statistics to determine the level of confidence in the findings

Descriptive Statistics About the Sample and Variables

Quantifying characteristics of the sample is important for many reasons. Numbers provide information about the size of the sample and the way the adequacy of the sample size was determined. Descriptive and summary statistics familiarize the reader with the characteristics of the subjects, their baseline conditions, and their responses to treatments. The initial part of the results section should provide sufficient descriptive statistics about the sample and each variable so that the reader develops a good sense of the characteristics of this sample in this study. This information provides a basis for understanding how these subjects responded to treatment and supports generalization of the study results to other groups.

WHERE TO LOOK FOR QUANTITATIVE RESULTS

- The text of the section labeled "Methods and Procedures" should include a description of each test that was planned and run. If plans were modified, this fact should be clearly identified, along with the reasoning for changing the *a priori* plan.
- The report of quantitative analysis will be clearly identified as a separate section of the report, typically called "Results" or "Findings."
- The text of the "Results" section should include a description of the most important results, along with numbers that are critical for understanding the nature of the findings. For each test, these values should include at least the test statistic and the *p* value. Many authors also report degrees of freedom (a number reflecting the effects of sample size) and confidence intervals for the results.
- Look for confidence intervals to help determine how "close" the results were and to estimate the

magnitude of effect. The inclusion of confidence intervals is becoming more common—and, in fact, is required by some journals—and indicates the completion of a thorough report on the part of the authors.
- The "Results" section will often include detailed tables, graphs, and figures to support the text, which generally includes only the most important results. These elements often make the results more understandable, so take the time to review them individually.
- The *p* values may be reported as the actual, calculated probability of error, or they may be identified as "*p* < 0.05" or "*p* < 0.01," which is acceptable. The latter forms are more common when a single table reports multiple test results, or when a large number of insignificant results are mixed with significant ones. Authors may also simply note nonsignificant results as "NS" or "n.s."

Analysis of Sample Subgroups for Group Equivalency

Numbers related to the sample can tell us whether the experimental and control groups are similar enough that extraneous variables are controlled. Deciding whether results are due to a treatment requires eliminating the other potential explanations for a result.

Differences in key characteristics of subjects (for example, age, severity of illness, activity level, or ethnicity) may compromise internal validity.

Many researchers provide statistics to document the similarity of the treatment groups on key characteristics that might affect the outcome. The effects of these extraneous variables can be minimized if they are distributed equally between the experimental and control groups; thus, documenting this equivalence statistically enhances confidence in the study's results. When groups have been evaluated for comparability, the researcher should provide the results of inferential tests to determine how well the groups match on key characteristics. In this case, the statistical tests should *not* be statistically significant, meaning that any differences between groups are due to chance. When tests of group comparability are provided in a research study, look for a *p* value that is *greater* than 0.05, meaning the groups are statistically identical.

SKILL BUILDER   Reading Statistical Tables and Graphs in Research Reports

Details of quantitative analyses are often displayed in tables and graphs to present them more efficiently and so the text can focus on the most important findings. Although this organization is an effective way to present a large volume of results, the various elements can be difficult to sort through and evaluate. Tables may be filled with confusing numbers, and results often have to be read and reread to determine their importance. The wide array of graphical presentations that are available means that the reader may have to figure out exactly what the graph itself represents before determining the implications of the results. A key challenge for the reader is the lack of a universal method for reporting data in tabular or graphical form, either in style manuals or in authors' guidelines. Because no such standards exist, authors generally provide the numbers in a way that makes sense to them—which does not always translate into an interpretable approach from the reader's perspective.

A systematic approach to evaluating tables and figures can help the nurse reader determine if the results are represented accurately in the discussion and conclusions; this is essential to the critical evaluation of a research report. Do not expect that every study write-up will report every statistic in the same way. It takes some persistence on the reader's part to track down the numbers that are important for his or her evaluation of the study as effective evidence for practice.

Although tables present numbers efficiently, the reader should begin his or her evaluation by looking at the words in the text. When reading the results that are reported in the text, refer to the tables at the same time to determine the meaning of the findings. For example, if the authors note that a finding was "statistically significant at 0.01," then expect to find more detailed data in the table that match the text report. Use the text to guide reading of the data in the table, and refer back to the table to expand understanding of the information provided in the text.

Do not rely solely on the numbers in the table to draw conclusions. The titles of tables and footnotes that accompany them often illuminate the most critical information from the table. Footnotes often contain information about statistical significance, particularly if they are reported in aggregate form. Check each column and row heading to determine the information that is being reported and match it with the text description.

Information in tables and graphs should always be consistent with the textual report; discrepancies between the numbers found in a table and those reported in the text are cause for grave concern about the accuracy of the researcher's conclusions. It can be helpful to write in the article margin what each test means so that an aggregate of all the findings can be reviewed prior to reading the author's conclusions.

Statistics to Evaluate the Role of Error in Measures and Results

If a researcher could enroll every member of a population in his or her study, then sampling error would be nonexistent. That is rarely possible, however, so it is inevitable that some differences in the characteristics of a population and the characteristics of the sample will emerge, no matter how carefully the sample is drawn. These differences, which are quantified as standard error, are directly affected by variability and indirectly affected by sample size. In other words, as samples get larger, standard error gets smaller.

How big is an unacceptable standard error? There is no easy answer to that question; standard error is a relative number, specific to the measures that are used and their scale. However, when standard error is very large relative to the mean value, you can draw the conclusion that a lot of sampling error is present in the experiment. Standard error is, in general, the comparison value used to determine statistical significance, so it may be difficult to find statistically significant results when standard error is large. The researcher can reduce standard error by using a sound sampling strategy and drawing a sample that is as large as is practical.

Even when sampling error is small and the sample size is large, misleading results may be caused by error associated with the measurement itself. Measurement error can be directly evaluated by scrutinizing the reliability of the measures; subtracting the reliability coefficient alpha from 1 results in an approximation of the amount of error contributed by the measure. For example, a measure with a coefficient alpha of 0.72 is contributing 28% measurement error to the experiment.

Random events can also create error. All of these factors taken together provide a rough estimate of the chance of concluding that an intervention caused an effect when it did not. The probability of a Type I error is reflected in the p value that is reported with test statistics. When the p value is very small, then the role of error is also very small. Conversely, a large p value indicates a large probability that error is responsible for the result. The p value is not the sole number of interest in a statistical report, but it should be one of the first that is appraised when reading research.

The p value actually tells the reader very little about the effectiveness of an experiment, but it does reflect whether any effects that were demonstrated were due to chance. If the probability that error is responsible for the outcome is very large, then any other calculations are irrelevant and should be dismissed. In contrast, if the probability of error is very small, then the chances that the results are real is very high and the reader should move on to look for signs of effect size and clinical importance.

Statistics to Evaluate the Magnitude of Effect

Studies that include inferential tests report several numbers. One of these, the test statistic, enables the reader to judge the **magnitude of effect**, or the size of the differences between groups. Armed with this information, the nurse can conclude whether the difference is large enough to be of practical use. The magnitude of effect helps the nurse make the critical decision of whether to use the results with specific patients. Magnitude of effect can be calculated, but often it is just "eyeballed" by appraising the relative size of the test statistic. Keep in mind that the test statistic is generally a ratio of the effect of treatments

Magnitude of effect: The size of the differences between experimental and control groups; it supports clinical significance of the findings.

to error. As such, this number can provide a rough idea of the importance of any differences identified in the study.

How do you know when a test statistic is large? Again, this is a relative judgment. In general, the larger the test statistic, the greater the effect. Test statistics that are decimal values or low single digits may signal that the intervention has very little practical effect, even if the *p* value shows statistical significance. Test statistics that are in the tens or hundreds usually indicate a good deal of effect. When test statistics show a great deal of effect, then the final consideration is how much confidence the nurse has that this statistic can estimate the effect on another population with accuracy. It may be difficult to judge magnitude of effect from the test statistic, however. In particular, chi square yields a test statistic that is difficult to interpret directly. It is becoming more common to report confidence intervals for mean differences, however, and these data provide a great deal of information about the size of an effect as well as its direction.

Numbers That Reflect Confidence in Estimates

When a test statistic is reported, the researcher should report confidence intervals for the results. Confidence intervals indicate the precision with which the researcher has been able to estimate various characteristics or differences between groups. Confidence intervals become larger as they get more precise; they become smaller as they get more accurate.

Looking at a confidence interval in tandem with the test statistics can give the reader an idea whether the results were close or whether they are precise enough for generalization. For example, if the confidence interval for a mean difference is "0.01 to 6.5," it means the average difference could be as little as one-hundredth of a unit or as big as six and a half units. In other words, the difference could be next to nothing. In contrast, if a confidence interval for a mean difference is identified as "12.6 to 12.8," there were quite a few units of average difference between groups and the estimation of the difference is very precise.

Kalinowki and Fidler (2010) recommend the reader of research keep three principles in mind when interpreting quantitative results as evidence for practice:

1. *A p value does not measure effect size.* The *p* value refers to the probability of error, and nothing more. It means the results are statistically *real*, but it provides little information about the meaning of the results. Effect sizes offer more information about the magnitude of response.
2. *Effect size is not a measure of importance.* Instead, this factor reflects importance only if a bigger response is better. Conversely, even very small effects may be of importance if the condition is lethal or if the population is large.
3. *Statistical significance does not mean replicability.* This value does not give any direct information about the chance that the results will be repeated. Its interpretation is solely focused on the probability that the results could have happened by random chance.

Although quantitative results can appear daunting, a systematic appraisal of the most important numbers can provide the nurse with enough information to determine if the findings should be applied in practice. When evaluating research as evidence for practice, both statistical significance and clinical importance must factor into the nurse's final judgment. Indeed, the usefulness of clinical research depends on clinical importance even more than statistical significance. Once it has been determined that effects are statistically significant, then the focus of evaluation should turn to the size of effects, confidence in the results, and descriptions that enable appropriate generalization of findings.

Using Quantitative Results as Evidence for Practice

Statistical significance is a requirement for using evidence in practice: If results are due to error, then their application is irrelevant. At the same time, statistical significance tells the nurse little about whether the results will have a real impact in patient care. To make this assessment, the nurse must focus on measures of magnitude of effect and clinical significance.

Even with that caveat, inferential results are some of the strongest evidence for practice. Considered the "top of the heap" in most evidence hierarchies, experimental designs provide evidence about the effectiveness of interventions that can be used with a great deal of confidence.

When considering the application of inferential results, nurses should evaluate whether the effects make sense in light of the kinds of patients and outcomes encountered in their specific practice. In other words, can the results be generalized to the setting in which the reader is practicing? All the numbers in the study, taken together, help to answer that question. A systematic appraisal of quantitative information about the sample, the role of error, and the size of effects is required to draw a conclusion about the appropriateness of using quantitative research as evidence.

CHECKLIST FOR EVALUATING QUANTITATIVE RESULTS

❏ The statistical tests are appropriate for the research question and the goals of the analysis.

❏ The statistical tests are appropriate for the level of measurement of the variables.

❏ Assumptions of the data were tested and meet the requirements of the tests used.

❏ If groups were compared, inferential analyses were used.

❏ If more than two groups were compared, the researcher compensated for the error of

multiple comparisons by running a test such as ANOVA.

❏ Tables and graphs are clear and labeled correctly.

❏ Results reported in tables and graphs are consistent with the summary report in the text.

❏ The researcher reports findings objectively and accurately.

Creating a Quantitative Analysis

Creating a quantitative analysis requires selecting the right test, using software correctly, interpreting the output, and reporting the results appropriately and completely. Decision trees in this chapter have provided guidance in choosing the correct test. In general, selection of a test is based on the research question, the level of measurement, the specific statistics used to represent the variables, and the number of groups to be compared.

Research Question

Specific research questions dictate use of specific methods of analysis. If words such as *relationship* or *association* appear in the research question, then correlation or chi square statistics should be used. If terms such as *differences* or *cause and effect* are inferred by the research question, then inferential tests of group differences are required, such as *t* tests, ANOVA, or Mann-Whitney U. If words such as *explanation* or *prediction* appear in the research question, then regression tests should be used. The research question will also drive the choice of variables and the level at which they are measured.

Level of Measurement

Not all numbers are created the same, and not all numbers in a research study can be treated the same way mathematically. Whether data are nominal, ordinal, interval, or ratio will drive the specific tests that can be applied. For example, nominal data can be expressed only as frequencies, proportions, or rates, so the tests used in the analysis must accommodate these numbers. Interval and ratio data can be analyzed using a wide range of tests, but they are not appropriate for tests of frequency. An early step for the researcher is to identify the unit of analysis and the level of measurement of each variable so the correct statistical tests can be selected.

Statistics Used to Represent the Variables

The selection of a specific test depends on the statistics used to represent the variables. For example, when testing interval-level data, means are often used to represent a typical response. Tests of means include several varieties of the *t* test and ANOVA. Frequencies, proportions, and rates are tested with chi square tests. In addition, the choice of test should consider the relationship that is expected between variables. Associations and relationships, for example, are tested with different statistics than are the effects of treatments. Sample size will also support or limit the selection of a specific test.

Number of Groups to Be Compared

When only two groups are compared, the role of error is not an issue. When more than two groups are compared, however, the error of multiple comparisons should be controlled. This can be done by restricting the alpha level considered statistically significant. More commonly, the tests applied are intended to be used as omnibus tests that avoid the multiple comparisons error. It is important, then, that one of these two approaches be applied when more than two group comparisons will be carried out.

Availability of Statistical Software

From a practical standpoint, the final selection of a statistical test is based on access to software that supports the particular analysis chosen. Statistical analysis is much less burdensome when adequate statistical software is used to conduct it. Many packages are available for inferential analysis (indeed, even Excel will perform most common statistical tests), so researchers have little motivation to perform manual calculations.

The selection of a specific software package depends on many factors, including the user's skill and knowledge, financial resources, and statistical acumen. Some software, such as AnalyzeIt and StatsDirect, is simple to run and inexpensive; these packages support analysis of the most common types of questions. More sophisticated software, such as SPSS (Statistical Package for the Social Sciences) and SAS (Statistical Analysis Software), requires substantial training and investment to maximize its usefulness. Keep in mind that even though the software SPSS was originally intended for analysis of social science studies, it is now widely used and accepted in other areas of research, including research conducted for biomedical purposes.

Regardless of the complexity of the analysis programs, statistical software is simply a tool. Unless the appropriate decisions and interpretations are made, software will be of little assistance in evaluating data.

Summary of Key Concepts

- Inferential analysis is the analytic tool most commonly used in quantitative studies; it enables a researcher to draw conclusions about a population given the results from a sample.
- Quantitative tests should be selected *a priori*; all identified tests should be run and reported.
- Parametric tests are appropriate for normally distributed data; otherwise, nonparametric tests should be used.
- Statistical analyses can be univariate, bivariate, or multivariate, depending on the nature and number of variables involved.
- Statistical significance indicates that a result is not due to standard error; therefore, the effect can be assumed to be real.
- Standard error is the amount of variability in the sample that is due to the sampling procedures; it is directly affected by variability and indirectly affected by sample size.
- Statistical significance should be evaluated in tandem with clinical significance, which determines the usefulness of the results as evidence for practice.
- Clinical significance can be judged by estimation, confidence intervals, minimally important difference, and effect size.
- A confidence interval is a way of reporting results so the precision and accuracy of the estimates can be evaluated as well as the size of the effect.
- Effect size is a better basis for determining clinical importance than for assessing statistical significance. It indicates the relative size of differences that can be expected under similar circumstances.
- The appropriate statistical test will take into account the requirements of the research question, the number of groups to be tested, the level of measurement of variables, and the assumptions of the statistical test.
- The *z* or *t* test is appropriate for analyzing differences between means; as a consequence, these tests are useful when differences in interval-level variables are contrasted in two groups.
- The chi square test is appropriate for analyzing differences between proportions; as a consequence, it is useful when differences in a nominal- or ordinal-level variable are contrasted between two groups.

- The ANOVA test is appropriate for analyzing differences among three or more group means and is applied to avoid the error of multiple comparisons.
- Some data are so non-normal that they require tests that do not rely on a specific distribution. These tests are described as nonparametric, require large samples, and are not as sensitive as other tests.
- When reading the quantitative analysis section of a research report, the nurse should focus on the appropriateness of the statistical selection and key numbers that reflect the role of error and the amount of certainty that exists in the estimates.

CRITICAL **APPRAISAL EXERCISE**

Retrieve the following full-text article from the Cumulative Index to Nursing and Allied Health Literature or similar search database:

Saadatmand, V., Rejeh, N., Heravi-Karimooi, M., Tadrisis, S., Vaismoradi, M., & Jordan, S. (2015). Effects of natural sounds on pain: A randomized controlled trial with patients receiving mechanical ventilation support. *Pain Management Nursing, 16*(4), 483–492.

Review the article, focusing on the sections that report the results of the quantitative analyses. Think about the following appraisal questions in your critical review of this research article:

1. Identify the inferential tests that were used in the analyses of data in this study. How are they appropriate for the research questions?
2. List the variables that were measured by the researchers. For each, identify the level of measurement represented by the variable.
3. The authors note that the visual analog scale may be considered a continuous (i.e., interval) measurement scale. Look up a visual analog scale and decide whether you agree or disagree with the authors; provide your rationale.
4. Review the demographic characteristics of the samples. Do you agree that the groups were statistically similar? Why or why not? Was each demographic variable reported with the appropriate summary statistic?
5. Which inferential test was performed to determine whether the intervention made a difference between groups? Was this the appropriate test to use? Why or why not?
6. Discuss whether the authors use tables and graphs appropriately to represent the data. How could the results reported in the tables be clearer?
7. Do the authors draw appropriate conclusions? Are the data over-interpreted, under-interpreted, or appropriately reported in the discussion and conclusion sections?

References

Fethney, J. (2010). Statistical and clinical significance, and how to use confidence intervals to help interpret both. *Australian College of Critical Care Nurses, 23*, 93–97.

Galin, J., & Ognibene, F. (2012). *Principles and practice of clinical research*. Waltham, MA: Academic Press.

Girden, E., & Kabacoff, R. (2010). *Evaluating research articles from start to finish*. Thousand Oaks, CA: Sage.

Hoffman, J. (2015). *Biostatistics for medical and biomedical practitioners*. Cambridge, MA: Academic Press.

Hulley, S., Cummings, S., Browner, W., Grady, D., & Newman, T. (2013). *Designing clinical research*. Philadelphia, PA: Lippincott Williams & Wilkins.

Kalinowki, P., & Fidler, F. (2010). Interpreting significance: The differences between statistical significance, effect size, and practical importance. *Newborn & Infant Nursing Reviews, 10*(1), 50–54.

Pandis, N. (2013). Confidence intervals rather than *p* values. *American Journal of Orthodontics & Dentofacial Orthopedics, 143*(2), 293–294.

Schmidt, N., & Brown, J. (2012). *Evidence-based practice for nurses: Appraisal and application research*. Burlington, MA: Jones & Bartlett Learning.

Scott, I., & Mazhindu, D. (2014). *Statistics for healthcare professionals: An introduction*. Thousand Oaks, CA: Sage.

Wassertheil-Smoller, S., & Smoller, J. (2015). *Biostatistics and epidemiology: A primer for health and biomedical professionals* (4th ed.). New York, NY: Springer.

Part VI

Research That Describes the Meaning of an Experience

Guillaume Razumovo/Shutterstock

Chapter 14

Qualitative Research Questions and Procedures

CHAPTER OBJECTIVES

The study of this chapter will help the learner to

- Discuss the purpose of qualitative research as evidence for nursing practice.
- Define characteristics of the qualitative research question.
- Relate sampling strategies and data collection procedures to qualitative design.
- Determine the ways in which credibility, confirmability, dependability, and transferability are demonstrated in qualitative design.
- Review the classifications of common qualitative traditions, including appropriate questions, methods, strengths, and limitations of each.

KEY TERMS

Audit trail	Habituation	Reflexivity
Bracketing	Integrative review	Saturation
Case research methods	Investigator triangulation	Snowball sampling
Constant comparison	Member checking	Stratified purposive sampling
Constructivist research	Method triangulation	Theory triangulation
Data source triangulation	Participant observation	Traditions
Ethnography	Phenomenology	Transferability
Extreme case sampling	Prolonged engagement	Triangulation
Field notes	Purposeful sampling	
Grounded theory	Qualitative meta-synthesis	

An Introduction to Qualitative Research

Research that focuses on the effectiveness of interventions is critical evidence for nursing practice, but it is not the only evidence that is important. The definition of evidence-based practice places equal emphasis on scientific studies, clinical experience, and the preferences of patients. It is these last two sources of information—clinical experience and patient preferences—that are commonly addressed by qualitative studies. Qualitative research is grounded in the belief that reality can never be completely known because it is constructed by each individual (Creswell, 2013). Attempts to *measure* reality are limited to methods that aim to define variables and find manifestations of them. Much of the human experience is not easily defined, however, and outward expressions may be difficult, if not impossible, to detect. For instance, although blood pressure and circulating blood volume are relatively easy to define and measure, experiences such as grief and quality of life are much more difficult to assess.

There are fundamental reasons why qualitative research is important in nursing practice. Nursing is a humanistic, holistic approach to promoting health and minimizing the effects of disease. Indeed, the profession of nursing is based on these fundamental elements of care. Understanding the human experience of health and disease is central to appreciating how to help patients manage them.

The impetus behind qualitative research is to discover the meaning of the phenomenon under study; in quantitative research, determining cause and effect is the main goal. Qualitative research, by comparison, integrates the use of language, concepts, and words rather than numbers to produce evidence. This type of research can be either descriptive or interpretive (Denzin & Lincoln, 2011). Descriptive qualitative research is used in a preliminary way to establish basic knowledge about a group's or individual's response to health and illness. Interpretive qualitative research is a more complex form of analysis that involves extracting meaning from data in a way that requires inductive thought on the part of the researcher. It emphasizes understanding the meaning that individuals ascribe to their actions and to the reactions of others (Thorne, Stephens, & Truant, 2016). This type of research also emphasizes process and context in understanding the meaning of an experience (Nicholls, 2009). The point of qualitative research is to elicit a description of a social experience that is so detailed and insightful that someone who has not experienced the phenomenon can understand and appreciate its nuances. The researcher accomplishes the research goals by establishing a relationship with informants and by considering the contextual issues that may shape inquiry into the research question.

In many ways, qualitative research is the polar opposite of quantitative research. Designs are not preplanned; the details of a particular study are "emergent," meaning the specifics of the study adapt to the emerging characteristics of the data. Qualitative research seeks to understand the meaning of an event, rather than measure effects, so issues of internal validity, control, and avoidance of bias are not central concerns. Instead, trustworthiness is the key issue when appraising the validity of a qualitative study (Thomas & Magilvy, 2011; Whitting & Sines, 2012). Sampling strategies, analysis procedures, and reporting of results are all considerably different for qualitative studies than for quantitative research.

Despite these differences, qualitative and quantitative researchers also share many characteristics in common. Both employ a rigorous approach to elicit the best possible answer to a research question, and both engage in disciplined inquiry aimed at finding the truth.

SCENES FROM THE FIELD

Young adults are not immune to grief. In fact, research suggests that as many as 30% of college students experience the death of a family member or friend during their college years. These losses can be particularly difficult to deal with: College students are away from home, often have poorly developed support systems, and face expectations that they will continue to attend class, even when they have suffered overwhelming bereavement.

Social media have changed the way that the current generation of college students communicates and keeps track of friends. Pennington (2013) used qualitative methods to determine how college students used the Facebook accounts of their deceased friends to deal with their grief.

The theory behind this study is compelling. Experts in grief communication have found that the attachment felt toward a deceased person can be understood as continuing a bond. Those who feel loss do not desire to sever all ties with the one they loved. Rather, successfully navigating grief requires the bereaved person to find ways to renegotiate and reframe the relationship now that the friend has passed on. Pennington (2013) proposed that using social media may be one way to effectively support this transition.

The author interviewed a total of 43 college students about their use of Facebook to interact with their deceased friends. Rather than investigating Facebook memorial pages—which are created by survivors to memorialize the deceased—she asked these students to discuss how they accessed a dead friend's page—that is, the page that the friend created before his or her death. The study participants were asked to log into their Facebook account and go to the profile page of the friend who had died to help them explain their experience. Reviewing the profile page and the content were important aspects of the experience of remembering their friend through media.

"Maintaining the friendship" was an important use of Facebook in dealing with grief. None of these participants had cut their ties with the deceased; indeed, they visited their dead friends' pages frequently. When asked why they had done so, the responses were consistent: *You do not defriend the dead.* In fact, these respondents described the experience as extending the memorial and honoring their dead friend's memory. They also found it comforting to connect with the people who also loved their friend, and as a means to comfort each other.

Even among those participants who struggled with the page and rarely visited it, none considered "defriending" them; they reported that they could not take the step of removing the deceased individual from their friends list. Nevertheless, most of these students did not actively engage with the site; for various reasons they did not feel it appropriate to continue to post on their friend's wall. Those who did so used this interaction as a way of coping with their own grief; they saw it as a way of maintaining a connection with the deceased. The students found photographs to be the most helpful aspect of the page. They found it least helpful when a parent maintained the page and responded to posts.

This study provided a contemporary view on the ways college-age people use social media to help cope with grief. This evidence could serve as the basis for designing coping strategies and therapeutic communication to help them deal with an unexpected death in a positive way (Pennington, 2013).

The Purpose of Qualitative Research

Qualitative research seeks to gather data that illuminate the meaning of an event or phenomenon. The main purpose in doing so is to develop an understanding of meaning from the point of view of the informants. Data are gathered directly from informants or through the investigator's observations. Qualitative research has also been called **constructivist research** because it is grounded in the assumption that individuals construct reality in the

Constructivist research: Research that attempts to discover the meaning and interpretations of events, phenomena, or experiences by studying cases intensively in their natural settings and by subjecting data to analytic interpretation.

form of meaning and interpretation (Denzin & Lincoln, 2011). Such research attempts to discover the meaning and interpretations of events, phenomena, or experiences by studying cases intensively in their natural settings and by subjecting the resulting data to analytic interpretation. Qualitative designs answer questions about the human experience by exploring motives, attitudes, reactions, and perceptions.

Qualitative designs are particularly useful in evidence-based practice for determining patient needs, preferences, and motives. Although quantitative studies are useful in determining the *effectiveness* of an intervention, qualitative studies are helpful in describing the *acceptability* of an intervention. Interventions that require lifestyle adjustments, attitude changes, or behavioral alterations are particularly well suited to qualitative studies. Nursing practices that support adaptations on the part of the patient are well addressed by qualitative studies, as are counseling and therapeutic communication. Qualitative research is an appropriate means of addressing a wide variety of research questions that focus on the needs, responses, and experiences of patients.

The Uniqueness of Qualitative Research

Qualitative inquiry is unique in terms of the researcher's beliefs about the nature of reality and in the methods and procedures used to describe the informant's worldview. Although quantitative researchers focus on a single, objective reality, the lens of a qualitative researcher is based on a social construction of reality in which multiple realities are acceptable. In the world of the qualitative researcher, all variables are dependent on each other, and the context of the study is naturalistic. Control and validity are less salient than credibility and trustworthiness.

Integration of Qualitative Research into Evidence-Based Practice

In the past, evidence-based practice focused on the medical model, with an overall emphasis on experimental designs that yielded an evaluation of the effectiveness of an intervention. Discovery of this evidence came through systematic reviews of quantitative studies or meta-analysis of aggregate effect size. Nursing is a profession focused on the human experience, however, and relying solely on experimental designs produces evidence that can lack understanding of the human dimension. As a result, evidence of nursing practice has expanded to include qualitative studies that illuminate the nature of the patient's experience.

In current practice, researchers now realize that, to gain a full understanding of the needs of patients, they must integrate quantitative and qualitative research. Whereas quantitative evidence is widely incorporated into practice, however, qualitative evidence is less commonly used. Even so, both types of inquiry can prove helpful in determining best practices. The nurse must examine scientific evidence to determine the best nursing interventions, but he or she must also be able to see a social or human problem through the eyes of the patient (Lavoie-Tremblay et al., 2012). Qualitative research provides a depth of understanding and adds another dimension to quantitative evidence: one based on the human experience.

Evidence of nursing practice is often discovered through methods that integrate both quantitative and qualitative studies in what is referred to as qualitative meta-synthesis and integrative review. A **qualitative meta-synthesis** is analogous to a systematic review; it is based on a preestablished set of selection criteria and a systematic appraisal of study quality. An **integrative review** encompasses both quantitative and qualitative studies, resulting in a practice guideline that incorporates elements of both types of research. This integrative perspective focuses on the effectiveness of an intervention as well as on the effects of the treatment on the patient's life; both are required to assess efficacy (Pearson, 2011).

Attaining health depends on developing and maintaining health-promoting behaviors, lifestyle adaptations, knowledge, and an attitude that supports these efforts. Qualitative research is used to discover how the nurse can support the patient's health-promoting actions. Such studies are helpful in addressing complex problems, such as perceptions of care or quality of life. In essence, qualitative research helps to explain the experiential and behavioral components of illness and health care.

The Qualitative Research Question

The fundamental characteristics of the research question will determine whether it is best answered with a qualitative approach. Questions that reflect exploration of feelings, perceptions, attitudes, motives, quality of life, and other subjective experiences are well addressed with qualitative inquiry. Table 14.1 provides examples of research questions that are well suited to qualitative study and the specific designs that are appropriate to answer them.

Qualitative meta-synthesis: The development of overarching themes about the meaning of human events based on a synthesis of multiple qualitative studies.

Integrative review: A methodology that synthesizes quantitative, qualitative, and comparative effectiveness research to provide a comprehensive understanding of the human condition.

Table 14.1 Examples of Qualitative Research Questions

Research Question	Design Used to Answer It
How do patients with chronic pulmonary hypertension respond to a lung transplant?	Case research methods
How do nurses on a neonatal unit respond to a medication error causing a death?	Case research methods
How are nurses portrayed in the media?	Content analysis
What are the perceived barriers for ethnically diverse students in nursing programs?	Content analysis
What is the nature of moral distress in nurses related to witnessing futile care in the critical care unit?	Phenomenology
What are the long-term implications for intimacy of couples in which the husband has been treated for prostate cancer?	Phenomenology
Which cultural issues emerge during a merger between a for-profit hospital and a not-for-profit hospital?	Ethnography
What is the culture of the waiting room for the open-heart surgery unit?	Ethnography
Which relationships and interactions affect intimate-partner violence?	Grounded theory
Which relationships and reactions lead to teen pregnancy?	Grounded theory

Traditions:
Particular designs or approaches in qualitative research used to answer specific types of study questions.

In qualitative designs, researchers specifically state questions—not objectives, aims, or hypotheses. There is often a central, broad question and several subquestions. The central question is written in such a way that it accommodates the emerging design that is characteristic of qualitative inquiry. Consequently, it is typically written in broad terms and is open-ended. Such questions commonly begin with words such as *what* and *how* to convey the researcher's open mind and lack of preconceived notions. The verbs in the research question are exploratory and do not reflect directionality; they do not indicate any expectation of demonstrating cause and effect. Thus qualitative research questions often include verbs such as *discover* and *explore.*

This broad, general approach to the topic conveys the expectation that specifics of the study will emerge during the course of the research. It is also likely that the question itself may evolve and change as the study progresses. The continual review and reformulation of the research question are characteristic of qualitative inquiry. The question should, however, focus on a single phenomenon or concept; a lack of specificity should not be construed as a lack of focus. The researcher should be clear about the fundamental purpose of the study. Qualitative studies frequently identify more specific subquestions that address particular areas of interest. These subquestions narrow the focus and become the explicit topics that are explored through interviews, focus groups, observations, and other sources (Creswell & Clark, 2011).

Although the qualitative research question may evolve as the study progresses, the researcher must start with a general approach that can remain consistent throughout the study. The specifics of the research question guide the selection of a particular design that is best used to address it. Research designs are sometimes called traditions when they refer to qualitative approaches; each tradition is intended to answer a particular kind of question.

The way a question is worded determines the specific tradition the researcher will select to fully answer it. For example, phenomenology focuses on determining the essence of a lived experience. The following are two examples of questions that might be answered with phenomenology: "What is it like to be wheelchair bound?" and "What is it like to be a freshman student in an urban university?" Nurse researchers use ethnography to examine the interrelationships among people, environment, culture, and health: "What is the culture of the department of nursing and how does it affect the university as a whole?" and "How do the health beliefs and practices of Asian Americans integrate with Western medicine?" Another type of question that lends itself to qualitative research is steeped in examining processes, interactions, and interrelationships through grounded theory: "What are the social processes that nursing students must attend to if they are to be successful in the nursing program?" An identifiable link should be apparent between the research question and the specific question used to answer it, even though the details of the design may take some time to emerge.

Characteristics of Qualitative Research Methods

Qualitative research is a systematic approach to understanding the experiences of others. This type of research is characterized by sampling procedures, data collection processes, and analytic processes that seek to achieve this understanding. Although internal validity and external validity are not paramount for qualitative researchers, concern for

Table 14.2 Comparison of Quantitative and Qualitative Characteristics

Element	Quantitative Version	Qualitative Version
Research question	Specific; includes identification of population, variables, and outcome	General and broad; may be stated as a purpose instead of a question
Design	Preplanned and specific	Emergent in response to data collection and ongoing analysis
Sample selection	Random selection to achieve maximum representation of the identified population	Purposeful selection to achieve maximum information about the topic of interest
Inclusion/exclusion criteria	Strictly adhered to; based on demographic or other characteristics	Loosely applied; based on shared experience or group membership
Sample size	Based on power calculation	Based on achievement of saturation
Data collection	Achieved through measurement of a quantifiable characteristic	Achieved through observation, interaction, or document review
Instrumentation	Measurement instruments are calibrated or otherwise determined to be reliable and valid	The researcher is the measurement instrument
Analysis of data	Preplanned; does not begin until all data have been collected	Emergent; data are analyzed as they are collected and compared to previous results

Purposeful sampling: A technique used in qualitative research in which the subjects are selected because they possess certain characteristics that will enhance the credibility of the study and because they can reliably inform the research question.

trustworthiness is critical (Whitting & Sines, 2012). Strong qualitative research studies pay attention to actions that can support confidence in their results.

Table 14.2 contrasts the characteristics of quantitative and qualitative research processes.

Sampling Strategies

In qualitative research, subjects are referred to as "informants," "respondents," or "participants." As in other types of research, the qualitative sampling strategy deals with how participants are selected and how many are enough to meet the goals of the research. The way these two elements of the strategy are addressed is unique to qualitative research.

The first element of the qualitative sampling strategy is the selection procedure. Qualitative samples are most commonly selected using a purposeful sampling method. In purposeful sampling, the researcher identifies criteria for the type of informant most likely to illuminate the research question, actively seeks out these individuals, and personally invites their participation. These criteria often involve a shared experience, membership in a specific demographic group, or simply a willingness to share information with the researcher. The researcher is usually the person who approaches the accessible informants, informs them about the study, and obtains their consent to participate. Informed consent is as important in qualitative research as in quantitative research; concerns for confidentiality,

Stratified purposive sampling:
Sampling of individuals who meet certain inclusion criteria, and who are then stratified according to other criteria (e.g., age, gender, and ethnicity).

Snowball sampling:
A nonprobability sampling method that relies on referrals from the initial subjects to recruit additional subjects. This method is best used for studies involving subjects who possess sensitive characteristics or who are difficult to find.

Extreme case sampling:
Sampling of unusual or special participants who exhibit the phenomenon of interest in its extremes.

Saturation:
The point at which no new information is being generated and the sample size is determined to be adequate.

anonymity, and protection of privacy likewise remain important. These issues may be of particular concern because of the often sensitive nature of the subject matter.

The researcher is involved in each step of the sampling process. Selection bias is not a concern if clear criteria are used and the researcher is aware of his or her own biases. Qualitative researchers acknowledge the potential for bias and assume that it is inherent in any study of an interpretive nature. This active process of identifying biases and making them explicit constitutes a control for validity called bracketing (Creswell & Clark, 2011).

Most qualitative samples are purposeful, but several other types of sampling strategies may be employed. **Stratified purposive sampling** involves sampling participants who meet certain inclusion criteria and then stratifying them according to age, gender, ethnicity, and other criteria. For example, the researcher may be interested in how older women react to an unplanned pregnancy, so he or she might stratify the sample by age. **Snowball sampling** is useful when the researcher cannot locate a list of individuals who share a particular characteristic. With this sampling technique, as participants are identified, they in turn are asked to identify others who meet the inclusion criteria; in this way, the sample "snowballs." Snowball sampling is a common approach when working with sensitive populations such as drug addicts or pregnant teens. **Extreme case sampling** focuses on unusual or special cases; these individuals exhibit the phenomenon of interest in its extremes. This approach may be useful for studying the characteristics of individuals who exhibit superior abilities or those who are considered worst cases. An example of the former might be a study of the characteristics of nurses who have zero errors; the latter might be apparent in a study of nurses who made serious errors resulting in patient death.

In addition to the selection procedure, a second consideration is sample size. Qualitative studies are not intended to be generalized to broader populations, and they are not tests of cause and effect. Moreover, issues such as power and Type I and II errors are not applicable to this kind of research. Instead, the researcher must make the final determination: When is the sample big enough? **Saturation** is the key consideration for the sample size in a qualitative study (Creswell & Clark, 2011; O'Reilly & Parker, 2013; Roy, Zvonkovic, Goldberg, Sharp, & LaRossa, 2015). Saturation is reached when themes become repetitive, suggesting no new input is needed. The sample size is not predetermined, although the researcher may consider a general sample size as a goal at the beginning of data collection. Once the study has been initiated, recruitment of informants and data collection continue until the researcher finds that no new information has been elicited. This so-called point of saturation is the standard for determining the adequacy of the sample size. Saturation may be achieved with as few as five or six informants, or it may take a considerably larger number of participants in studies of complex or sensitive topics. Determination of saturation is up to the researcher, but it should be reported that it was reached.

Data Collection Methods and Procedures

Data may be collected through a variety of methods. Qualitative data are usually collected through a combination of methods, including observation, interaction, and document review. Interaction data may be collected via essay questions, interviews, focus groups, and conversation. These data are often recorded on audiotape and transcribed for analysis purposes. Some researchers employ photographic methods to capture observations, document interactions, and even stimulate discussion (Lachal et al., 2012). Video may also be used with individuals or focus groups to capture both verbal and nonverbal responses to questions.

With most qualitative research traditions, analysis occurs simultaneously with data collection—another significant departure from quantitative research. This method of analysis, called **constant comparison**, is widely used in the qualitative traditions. Data are reviewed and analyzed as they are gathered, and new data are compared to what has been interpreted to support or disprove earlier conclusions. This process results in an emergent analytic process that evolves and changes focus as more data are gathered. The analytic process involves coding units of meaning into themes.

Observations of body language, the surroundings, and other factors are also an important part of the data collection. Often referred to as **field notes**, they enrich the data interpretation process with detailed descriptions of the context, environment, and nonverbal communications. These observations are generally inserted into the transcripts as soon as possible to ensure they are recollected correctly and completely. In addition, the researcher may maintain a personal journal to capture his or her individual responses and reactions to the research process.

The qualitative researcher must be highly attentive to how the data are collected. For example, when the study addresses sensitive issues, the researcher needs to create an environment of safety and trust for the participants. Conducting interviews in natural settings (for example, observing and speaking with nurses in the unit conference room or meeting with an informant in the informant's home) is appropriate for qualitative studies and can elicit the most natural responses. The researcher must strive to engender mutual respect and maintain confidentiality throughout the data collection process.

Constant comparison: A method of analysis in qualitative research that involves a review of data as they are gathered and comparison to data that have been interpreted to support or reject earlier conclusions.

Field notes: Detailed descriptions of the context, environment, and nonverbal communications observed during data collection and inserted by the researcher into the transcripts to enrich the data interpretation process.

Enhancing the Trustworthiness of Qualitative Studies

Qualitative research is not subject to concerns about internal or external validity because these studies do not focus on cause and effect, and they are not intended to be generalized to larger populations. Nevertheless, rigor and truth remain key concerns—no researcher wants his or her findings to be misleading or in error. The rigor of qualitative research, however, is judged differently from quantitative research. The seminal work of Guba and Lincoln (1989) advanced the notion that qualitative research is based on trustworthiness rather than reliability and validity.

Trustworthiness includes the following specific characteristics:

- *Credibility:* The results of the study represent the realities of the participants as much as possible.
- *Confirmability:* The researcher attempts to enhance objectivity by reducing bias in methods and procedures.
- *Dependability:* Repetition of the study with similar subjects in similar circumstances results in consistent findings.
- *Transferability:* Results can be transferred to situations with similar subjects and settings.

Methods to support these characteristics should be built into the study methods and procedures.

Table 14.3 Methods Used to Achieve Trustworthiness in Qualitative Inquiry

Consideration	Qualitative Version	Methods to Achieve This Characteristic
Internal validity	Credibility: Can the results be believed?	Prolonged engagement Researcher reflexivity Bracketing of researcher bias Member checking Triangulation
External validity	Transferability: Can the results be transferred to other people and situations?	Purposeful sampling Inclusion/exclusion criteria Thick description of the setting In-depth description of informants
Reliability	Dependability: Would the results be similar if the study was repeated with similar subjects in similar circumstances?	Audit trail Researcher journal Detailed descriptions of research methods Triangulation Peer examination of procedures and results Measures of inter-rater reliability
Objectivity	Confirmability: Was objectivity enhanced by reducing bias?	Bracketing of researcher bias Researcher reflexivity Triangulation

One of the most common threats to credibility of a study is bias. For example, drawing premature conclusions, basing themes on isolated responses, and incorrect interpretations can all influence the strength of a qualitative study. The nurse researcher can limit the effects of bias through bracketing, prolonged engagement, triangulation, member checking, and audit trails. Some of these processes are built into the design of a qualitative study; others are initiated during analysis of results. Table 14.3 identifies the methods used to achieve trustworthiness in qualitative inquiry. Separating the specific strategies that are used in each phase of a qualitative study can prove difficult, however, because emergent design and data analysis often overlap in this type of research. These controls are discussed in this chapter as they relate to design.

GRAY MATTER

Threats to the credibility of qualitative research may include the following errors:
- Drawing premature conclusions
- Basing themes on isolated responses
- Incorrectly interpreting data

Bracketing—one method of limiting the effects of researcher bias—is a means of demonstrating an awareness of the potential assumptions and preconceived notions of the researcher. Bracketing includes three phases:

1. The researcher examines and reflects on his or her own perspective regarding the topic.
2. The researcher identifies his or her own assumptions, based on theory or experience.
3. The researcher explicitly identifies the process for setting aside, suspending, or holding at bay personal biases (Creswell & Clark, 2011).

Qualitative researchers must be sensitive to the ways in which both the researcher and the research process have shaped the data (Lanford & Young, 2013). This sensitivity, which is referred to as **reflexivity**, is based on introspection and acknowledgment of biases, values, and interests. Reflexive introspection is a key component of bracketing and requires maturity and honesty on the part of the researcher.

Prolonged engagement with the participants involved in the study enhances the credibility of the researcher's conclusions. Extended contact with informants and the setting serves as a means of controlling the biases that might otherwise result in premature conclusions. Included in this process is the investment of sufficient time in the data collection process so that the researcher gains an in-depth understanding of the culture, language, or views of the group under study. Sustained involvement also helps build the trusting relationships and rapport that are necessary to elicit accurate and thorough responses.

Triangulation is another useful strategy for the enhancement of credibility. In triangulation, at least three sources of information are used to support each major conclusion. The qualitative researcher uses a variety of methods or informants to capture a more complete and insightful portrait of the phenomena that are being studied. Four types of triangulation have been described by Denzin and Lincoln (2011):

- **Data source triangulation** involves the use of multiple data sources in a study (e.g., interviewing diverse key informants to give credence to the findings).
- **Investigator triangulation** employs more than one person to collect, analyze, or interpret a set of data.
- **Theory triangulation** involves gaining and using multiple perspectives from other researchers or published literature.
- **Method triangulation** entails the use of multiple data collection methods (e.g., interviews, observation, and document review).

Performing external checks on the data and their interpretation is a common method of ensuring validity via member checking. In **member checking**, researchers ask participants to review and comment on the accuracy of transcripts, interpretations, or conclusions. Member checking requires that contact be made with each informant twice: once to collect data and a second time to review those data's accuracy and completeness.

An audit trail also supports the dependability of a study and its analysis. An **audit trail** is a thorough, conscientious reflection on and documentation of the decisions that were made, the procedures that were designed, and the questions that were addressed during

---

Bracketing:
A method of limiting the effects of researcher bias and setting them aside by demonstrating awareness of potential suppositions of the researcher.

Reflexivity:
A sensitivity to the ways in which the researcher and the research process have shaped the data; based on introspection and acknowledgment of bias.

Prolonged engagement:
Investment of sufficient time in the data collection process so that the researcher gains an in-depth understanding of the culture, language, or views of the group under study.

Triangulation:
A means of enhancing credibility by cross-checking information and conclusions, using multiple data sources, using multiple research methods or researchers to study the phenomenon, or using multiple theories and perspectives to help interpret the data.

Data source triangulation:
A type of triangulation in which multiple data sources are used in a study.

Investigator triangulation:
A type of triangulation in which more than one person is used to collect, analyze, or interpret a set of data.

Theory triangulation:
A type of triangulation in which multiple perspectives are obtained from other researchers or published literature.

Method triangulation:
A type of triangulation in which multiple data collection methods are used, such as interviews, observations, and document review.

Member checking:
A method of ensuring validity by having participants review and comment on the accuracy of transcripts, interpretations, or conclusions.

Audit trail:
Detailed documentation of sources of information, data, and design decisions related to a qualitative research study.

analysis. A thorough record of the emerging design decisions helps other researchers confirm the findings.

Although qualitative research has a subjective focus, it does not lack rigor. Methods of ensuring trustworthiness enable the researcher to support the validity and usefulness of his or her conclusions. These strategies should be evident throughout the research process and documented in the research report.

Some contemporary qualitative researchers suggest that more traditional means of evaluating studies should be applied to qualitative as well as quantitative or survey methods. Morse (2015) argues that reliance on the term "trustworthiness" reduces the applicability of qualitative research to practice, as practitioners are likely to lean toward applying quantitative results that are tested with greater rigor. She recommends grouping the key qualitative trustworthiness characteristics into groups that mirror the aspects of quantitative evaluation. Thus, in Morse's approach, a qualitative research study would be considered *valid* if it had prolonged engagement, persistent observation, and thick description. A study would be considered *reliable* if triangulation and inter-rater reliability were present. *Generalizability* would be evident through bracketing, negative case analysis, member checking, and external audits.

The conversation continues as to which elements in a qualitative research study reflect its strength as evidence for practice. Regardless of the terminology used to describe the study's quality, qualitative researchers are in a search for truth, and that search can take on many forms.

Classifications of Qualitative Traditions

Multiple strategies are available to the qualitative researcher. The selection of a particular tradition depends on the purpose of the research and the nature of the research question. Some traditions are more common in nursing and health care in general. These designs, which include those in the following list, are regularly used because they answer questions about human reactions and interactions:

- *Case research methods:* Intense study of a single subject or small group of subjects
- *Content analysis:* Interpretation of the meaning in verbal responses or in documents
- *Phenomenology:* Investigation of the meaning of a phenomenon among a group who have experienced it
- *Ethnography:* Study of the features and interactions of a given culture
- *Grounded theory:* Research aimed at developing a theory of process, action, and interaction

Although these are the most commonly encountered qualitative methodologies, often no specific tradition is identified. Rather, a researcher's report may simply refer to a study as "qualitative research" without identifying the specific approach employed. Shin, Kim, and Chung (2010) reviewed more than 500 articles in two qualitative nursing research journals to determine the most common methods identified. In nearly 30% of the articles, no specific method was identified. Thus qualitative design principles may be applied with no specific methodology identified. Even so, specific methodologies should be matched appropriately to research questions when possible, and guidelines have been developed to address these situations.

GRAY MATTER

The following traditions are commonly used in qualitative studies by nurses:
* Case research methods
* Content analysis
* Phenomenology
* Ethnography
* Grounded theory

Case research methods:
The meticulous descriptive exploration of a single unit of study such as a person, family group, community, or other entity.

Case Research Methods

Research often seeks to understand entire populations, but nursing practice is concerned with the health of *individuals*. Case research methods involve the in-depth study of a single participant or a single group over an extended period of time with the goal of describing the impact of health and illness on an individual. Multiple data collection methods may be used, including observation, interviewing, and instrumentation (Creswell & Clark, 2011). Mixed methods, which combine qualitative and quantitative data collection, are also widely used. Case research is an appropriate method for studying the responses of individuals and small groups related to interventions, health behaviors, and perceptions of illness. It may be the only way to study individuals with rare conditions (Secomb & Smith, 2011).

Case research methods are often the basis for teaching strategies. For example, "grand rounds" had its roots in the medical model, but it has evolved into a valuable teaching tool in all health professions. Using in-depth analyses of individuals and groups helps illuminate the human dimension of the healthcare experience and enables a rich, multidimensional picture of the subjects to emerge.

Questions That Are Addressed with Case Research

Research questions that focus on the effects of treatments or conditions for individuals are appropriately answered with case studies. The case research method is valuable in these situations because it can generate evidence about the impact of health and illness for an individual who represents a unique or interesting subject. Often these cases are ones that present challenges for nursing care. Exploratory questions and questions that are intended to produce potential interventions for later testing are also well addressed with case research methods. Because case research allows for a thorough analysis of a rare or uncommon situation, it often leads to the discovery of relationships that were not obvious or observed prior to the experiment (Cardwell & Elliott, 2013; Crowe et al., 2011).

Methods and Procedures for Case Research

Case research is an intensive investigation designed to analyze and understand factors that are important to the cause of health problems, care of patients, and outcome of interventions (Creswell & Clark, 2011). In this type of research, an individual is identified who meets the criteria or (more often) presents himself or herself as a patient with a challenging or unusual condition. Data are collected over an extended period of time using multiple data collection methods. The case analysis begins with a description of the patient's history and demographic, social, and environmental factors that are relevant to the subject's health care. Data collected via observation and interactions are usually qualitative, but quantitative data may also be collected to augment the subjective responses.

Strengths of Case Research

Case research methods have some clear strengths in generating evidence for nursing practice:

- Case research is a practical method for studying individuals or small groups.
- Case research has direct applicability to patient care.
- Case research demonstrates the impact of health and illness on individuals.

Limitations of Case Research

Case research methods also have some inherent limitations:

- In-depth analysis requires extended contact and involvement in the research; attrition of the subjects limits the usefulness of the entire study.
- Studies apply only to individuals and are not generalizable to other groups or people.
- These studies have an inherent lack of control over extraneous variables, so researchers can draw any conclusions about the effects of treatments.

Case research is a useful methodology for determining how individuals in unique circumstances respond to their health and disease conditions. It is also an effective way to communicate with colleagues and teach others about challenging cases.

CASE IN POINT   A Case Research Method Example

An injury during a military deployment disrupts more than the soldier's life—it is a major trauma to the soldier's family and its overall life functioning. These changes may last a lifetime. Gorman et al. (2016) used a comparative case study model to provide an in-depth examination of three injured National Guard soldiers, and to demonstrate how their unique experiences navigating multiple systems to obtain treatment resulted in different outcomes for them and their families.

This study was unique in that the sample was drawn from a larger longitudinal study of soldiers deployed to Afghanistan. This sampling technique enabled the case researchers to integrate pre-deployment survey data into the study to provide a baseline for comparison of later coping. The researchers used both inclusion and exclusion criteria to draw the sample; they wanted to assure that active mental illness or sui-

cidal ideation was not disproportionately present in the sample. A larger sample was interviewed, and the case research was limited to those soldiers who reported a significant injury as a contributing factor to their difficult recovery of a familiar life. The researchers also used pre-deployment surveys, and readministered them 90 days and one year post return. Other measures used included a mental health analysis, a reflection on marital health, treatment history, and a measure of resilience.

The study findings demonstrated that a delay in diagnosis, long waiting times for treatment, and a lack of integrated care led to a critical mass of stress. This stress affected the soldier's physical and mental health, as well as the financial stability of the family and its overall well-being. These problems appear to be system-level issues that are not easily resolved. The researchers were able to demonstrate that resilience on the part of the soldier and his or her family could alter the trajectory from one that represented poor adjustment to a more positive resolution.

Gorman et al.'s (2016) study was typical of case research in that a limited number of "cases" were studied in depth—specifically, soldiers and their families. Multiple sources of both interview and survey data were used to achieve triangulation, supporting the study's credibility. Verbatim quotes were used to demonstrate the themes, which were described in sufficient detail that the reader could understand the experiences of these soldiers and their families. This study had a particularly well-done sampling strategy, with strong use of both inclusion and exclusion criteria to enable comparisons across the three cases.

Content Analysis

Content analysis is technically not a specific qualitative research design; it is more accurately described as a data analysis method. Nevertheless, this term is commonly attached to designs that rely on data collected via interviews or document analysis and that use interpretive coding to arrive at themes and patterns. Such designs are sometimes referred to as descriptive qualitative designs—but even that term is misleading, because these studies may be interpretive as well. In reality, content analysis is often used when no other classification "fits."

The purpose of content analysis is to discover and interpret the meaning imbued in the words of respondents or in historical or written documents. Content analysis as an analytic method may be used in any of the other traditions, but when a qualitative study does not neatly fit into one of the more formal classifications, it is often referred to simply as a content analysis study.

Questions That Are Addressed with Content Analysis

The primary application of content analysis is to answer a research question that explores feelings, perceptions, thoughts, attitudes, or motives related to a concept of interest to the researcher. Content analysis can be used for either descriptive or interpretive studies.

Methods and Procedures for Content Analysis

Content analysis requires the researcher to gather in-depth data in word form. Purposeful sampling is used to identify and recruit appropriate informants who can best help the researcher answer the specific research question. General interview questions are designed and document retrieval guidelines are developed. Although interviews and focus groups are widely used to gather data for content analysis, document review may be the focus of the study. Many researchers use all three strategies as a method of triangulating the data. Interviews and focus groups are more commonly employed in phenomenological studies or research focused on subjective aspects of a concept. Document review is more widely used in studies that involve historical reviews, biographies, or secondary data analysis.

To prepare for content analysis, data are collected and transcribed in their entirety, and thematic coding is applied to draw meaning from the content. Procedures for data management and maintenance of confidentiality are critical in the design of content analysis studies.

CASE IN POINT   A Content Analysis Example

Intimate-partner violence (IPV) puts patients at risk of physical injury as well as threatens mental health. These risks are heightened when the woman involved is pregnant. Alhusen and Wilson (2015) used interviews and simple content analysis to determine the perceptions of pregnant women about the experience of IPV as it affects maternal and fetal health.

The sample selection for this study was unique, in that it was pulled from a much larger study of the effects of mental health on maternal-child bonding. During the analysis completed for the larger study, a theme of IPV emerged as a threat to both mother and child. Alhusen and Wilson (2015) used inclusion criteria to identify eight women who reported experiencing IPV during their pregnancies. These women were then interviewed in depth using exploratory interviewing.

Three major themes emerged from the content analysis. The strongest theme was the drive to love and protect their unborn children while managing the effects of violence. The women had learned means to keep conflict from escalating to full-blown violence, and often developed new behaviors and coping mechanisms in an effort to protect their babies. A second theme was a concern that the unborn child would be aware of the violence, with the pregnant women expressing a concern that the child could sense the stress of the mother. They described their fetuses as balled up, quiet, tensed, tightened, or curled up. One of the informants had ended her romantic relationship and was concerned about longer-lasting effects on the baby. A third theme was concern for the fetus's well-being—specifically, the possibility that the baby would not grow well. In addition, the informants were concerned that stress had affected their ability to eat well and prepare for a healthy birth. The authors had multiple recommendations for how nurses could support pregnant women whom they suspect are experiencing IPV.

This study was typical of a content analysis in that interviews were the sole source of data, and themes were determined from analysis of units of meaning—in this case, phrases from the informants' own words. Because content analysis is a tool, rather than a design, this strategy is encountered in many qualitative studies that use a general approach to explore a topic of interest about which little has been published. Alhusen and Wilson's (2015) study was unique in that it arose from a secondary analysis of cases from a larger study that would not have revealed the specific concerns of this subgroup.

Strengths of Content Analysis

Content analysis is widely applied to answer qualitative research questions. It has some definite advantages as an approach to qualitative inquiry:

- Content analysis is relatively uncomplicated to carry out.
- Extended time periods of observation are generally not needed; saturation may be achieved with relatively few interviews or focus groups.
- Content analysis results in identification of general themes that allow the researcher to report and answer the question in a straightforward, concise way.

Limitations of Content Analysis

Content analysis is not appropriate for all studies because it has the following limitations:

- Content analysis relies on the informant's recall, ability to report, and willingness to talk.
- Selection effects may come into play because those individuals who agree to participate in interviews may not be representative of all of those who are affected.
- The researcher's bias may affect the interpretation and coding of themes in the data.

Content analysis is a popular technique in nursing and healthcare research, and it is considered one of the less complex qualitative methods. It is useful in identifying themes, patterns, and common experiences among individuals related to their health and disease.

Phenomenology

Phenomenology is concerned with the lived experiences of humans in relation to a shared phenomenon. Researchers use this tradition to describe how unique individuals respond to the circumstances of their health and illness. Phenomenology may be either descriptive or interpretive. It is based on a philosophical premise that it is possible to capture and articulate the "essence" of an experience that can be explored and understood (Flood, 2010). Phenomenology is defined as a research methodology that is rigorous, critical, and systematic in its investigation of a human experience in context (Fain, 2013). It is useful for understanding the way in which patients react and respond to both everyday experiences and unique events. It is also useful for obtaining evidence of nursing practices that support and enhance the ways patients respond to the challenges in their health care.

> **Phenomenology:** Investigation of the meaning of an experience among a group whose members have lived through it.

Questions That Are Addressed with Phenomenology

Phenomenological research always focuses on a variation of the following question: "What is this experience like?" The goal of this research is to develop rich, detailed, insightful descriptions of the way individuals react to the experiences in their lives. It is particularly helpful when an experience of interest has been poorly defined or explored. Phenomenology can also identify interventions that might support or enhance the experiences of patients who are facing healthcare decisions or conditions.

Methods and Procedures for Phenomenology

A phenomenological study begins with the articulation of an experience of interest. This becomes the focus of the research question, sample selection, and data collection. In this sense, phenomenological research questions are specific to a single experience. Although the exact nature of the study and data collection may evolve and change, the focus on the experience of interest does not.

CASE IN POINT A Phenomenology Example

Technology is unavoidable in the critical care unit. But it plays a paradoxical role in this setting: It is simultaneously lifesaving and anxiety generating for patient and nurse alike. While most of the care in a critical care unit focuses on the patient's medical condition, the psychological disturbance to and recovery of the individual's mental health should also be considered. Nurses play a key role in addressing this psychological disturbance, but some evidence shows that the use of technology in health care may lead nurses to dehumanize their patients and may serve as a distraction. Sayt,

Seers, and Tutton (2015) undertook a phenomenology study to investigate patients' experiences of technology in an adult intensive care unit (ICU). In their study, the researchers interviewed 19 informants who had experienced stays in a critical care unit.

These subjects perceived the technology used and the care delivered as inseparable during the critical care episodes. While the technology was to be "endured," respondents described an attitude of "getting on with it" by "being good" and "being invisible." These patients were able to get through the experience by focusing on technology's benefit as a "necessary evil." These patients found the experience full of paradoxes—alienating yet reassuring, uncomfortable yet comforting, impersonal yet personal. To minimize the invasive and isolating nature of technology in the critical care unit, the authors recommend that nurses maintain a close and supportive presence, and provide personalized comfort to their patients in the ICU.

This phenomenological study was typical in that subjects were selected because they had a shared experience (stay in a critical care unit) and were willing to discuss the experience. It is a good example of the use of phenomenology to build evidence for nursing practices. The authors arrived at their recommendations for staff nurse interventions based on the perceptions of the informants who had experienced this phenomenon.

Once a research question has been articulated, the researcher must identify informants who have experienced the phenomenon. Subjects are purposefully selected based on this central characteristic, although other criteria may also be specified, such as demographic, social, or relationship roles. Samples are often small in phenomenological studies, although data collection should continue until saturation is achieved (Connelly, 2010).

In phenomenology, the researcher acts as the primary data collection instrument. It is important, then, for the researcher to conduct a reflective self-assessment for the purposes of bracketing prior to initiation of data collection. Phenomenological studies require that an individual be able to reflect on and report reactions to a specific phenomenon in his or her life. Data collection generally takes place through interviews or focus groups. When gathering the data, there is less concern for recording the facts of an experience than for uncovering the meaning of these facts to the people experiencing them. A general interview guide may be developed for data collection, but the interviewing process is guided by the respondent, as the interviewer follows the thoughts and ideas of those who have experienced the phenomenon. Data are transcribed and analyzed using coding and content analysis.

Phenomenology generates large amounts of data, so the research procedure should include a method for filing, coding, and retrieving data. Analysis proceeds through constant comparison, so continuous reflection on the meaning of the data, use of analytic memos, and comparison of emerging data with existing data are essential in determining the essence of the experience for informants.

Strengths of Phenomenology

Phenomenology has several advantages as an approach to generating evidence for nursing practice:

- The phenomenological tradition can be used to study a wide range of phenomena, including both common and uncommon experiences.
- The interviewing process that is characteristic of phenomenology enables exploration of a wide range of responses.
- Phenomenology lends itself well to focus groups and, as such, may yield results that are more transferable than other types of qualitative study.
- The procedures for phenomenological research are relatively straightforward, and questions are usually more focused than for other types of qualitative study (Flood, 2010).

Limitations of Phenomenology

Phenomenology is a valuable source of evidence for nursing practice, but it also has some limitations:

- Phenomenology generates large amounts of data that must be carefully managed. Because the reports of experiences may be sensitive, protection of confidentiality is paramount.
- Bias is a potential problem in drawing conclusions and exploring experiences. Bracketing of researcher bias may be difficult to accomplish if the researcher is inexperienced or has strong feelings about the subject of interest.
- The interview process in phenomenology requires a high level of skill in eliciting clear and accurate responses from informants.
- Respondents must be able to reflect on their experience and report their responses, and recall and sharing of sometimes painful events may be stressful for participants.

In general, phenomenology requires a skilled researcher who is capable of identifying and setting aside his or her bias about an experience. The analysis of the essence of an experience requires reflection and careful interviewing techniques. The outcome can represent a valuable addition to the evidence base regarding the way individuals respond to events and the meaning of their lived experiences.

Ethnography

Ethnography focuses on the culture of a group of people. The assumption underlying this tradition is that every group of individuals evolves a culture that guides the way members structure their experiences and view the world (Creswell & Clark, 2011; Cruz & Higginbottom, 2013). This qualitative approach to inquiry gives the researcher an opportunity to conduct studies that attend to the needs and relationships of members of a culture. In ethnography, **participant observation** is the norm. That is, the researcher is more than an observer, but actually becomes an active participant in the culture under study to more thoroughly understand its experiences and worldview. As such, the ethnographic researcher's aim is to learn from, rather than study, the members of a culture (Cruz & Higginbottom, 2013). This does not mean the researcher attempts to have an effect on the members of the culture; instead, using an approach rooted in anthropology, the ethnographic researcher attempts to understand a culture without changing it.

Questions That Are Addressed with Ethnography

Ethnographic research questions are unique in that they focus exclusively on understanding the culture of a group of individuals (De Chesnay, 2015a). Many ethnographic questions are addressed in large-scale studies (e.g., What is the culture of a Samoan village?). Nursing research usually involves smaller, more narrowly focused cultural studies (e.g., What is the culture of a critical care waiting room?).

Methods and Procedures for Ethnographic Study

Ethnographers engage in extensive fieldwork to learn about the culture under study; ethnography is a time-consuming and labor-intensive type of research. One of the goals of such studies is to reveal information that is so embedded in a culture that it may not

Ethnography:
A study of the features and interactions of a given culture.

Participant observation:
Involvement of the researcher as an active participant in the culture under study to more thoroughly understand the culture without changing it.

be discussed. In fact, members may not even be aware of the cultural implications of their lived experiences. This level of understanding of a group requires an extended period of participant observation, multiple methods for collecting data, and rigorous data analysis procedures.

Gaining entry into the cultural setting may pose the greatest challenge in an ethnographic study. No strict rules have been established regarding how to enter a field setting to make observations; the procedures for gathering data are based on the characteristics of the field setting, its members, and where the researcher intends to situate himself or herself on the continuum from complete participant to participant-observer (Cruz & Higginbottom, 2013).

Much as in phenomenology, the concept of researcher as instrument is inherent in ethnography. The study of a culture requires rapport, trust, and, ultimately, intimacy with the members of the culture. The researcher plays a significant role in forging relationships that will result in reflection on the part of members of the culture and a willingness to share thoughts, feelings, and perceptions.

Ethnographers begin with general questions about the nature of reality for a given culture. Three types of information are usually collected for analysis:

- *Cultural behavior:* Collected via extended observation, this information is used to describe what members of a culture do, how they interact, and which outcomes are achieved.
- *Cultural artifacts:* These items are the objects and materials that the members of the culture make, use, and consider valuable. Information about cultural artifacts is also collected by observing, but historical artifacts may be described by informants.
- *Cultural speech:* As the term implies, information on cultural speech is gathered verbally through interaction with members of the culture (Cruz & Higginbottom, 2013).

As this description suggests, the ethnographer relies on multiple sources of information and a variety of data collection methods. Although some of these approaches may be preplanned, most are discovered during extended observational periods. Data are collected in the form of detailed field notes, and they may include words as well as drawings. Some ethnographers use audio or video recordings of activity as well. Observers should strive to collect field notes that are detailed and concrete rather than vague and overgeneralized. This type of data collection supports credibility and reduces bias in reporting. Ethnographers analyze the data they have collected by constructing rich and detailed descriptions and interpretations of the culture. These interpretations may include descriptions of normative behaviors, reactions and interactions among members, and observable social patterns.

Strengths of Ethnography

Ethnographic studies provide rich information about a culture and insight into its reactions and interactions. The following are some of the strengths of this design:

- These studies can provide insight into the way unique groups react to health and illness and give the nurse information with which to design effective interventions that will support health.

- Ethnography is a naturalistic inquiry that enables the nurse to draw conclusions about how health and illness are addressed in "real life."
- Many different kinds of cultures can be defined for the purposes of ethnography. This approach lends itself to groups as small as "children in a third-grade health class" as well as to groups on a grander scale, such as "members of an ethnic subgroup."

Limitations of Ethnography

Ethnography can help nurses understand how cultural groups respond to health and illness, but these studies have some limitations as well:

- Ethnographic studies are labor intensive and time consuming. Achieving the rapport and intimacy necessary for honest sharing of the lived experience may require years of involvement on the part of the researcher. Some researchers spend their entire professional lives studying a particular culture.
- The researcher must take extreme care not to over-interpret his or her observations but rather report them objectively; otherwise, biased, incorrect conclusions may result.
- Members of the culture may react to the observer's presence, inhibiting accurate conclusions about natural behavior. Extended contact enables **habituation**, or a reverting to natural behaviors, as members of the culture come to disregard the observer's presence and no longer see the researcher as an intruder.
- Observers may become so immersed in the culture that they change the cultural behaviors of the members. This outcome is a particular concern in the study of developing groups or groups who have not had contact with outsiders.

Habituation:
A process that occurs when an observer has extended contact with the subjects of a study. The subjects revert to natural behaviors and come to disregard the observer's presence.

CASE IN POINT   An Ethnography Example

A large proportion of children with chronic illnesses or serious disabilities are cared for at home by their families. These children's conditions are not one-time stressors on families; rather, chronic illness and disability are experiences within an illness trajectory that changes as the child matures. Given this long-term nature of such conditions, it is important to understand the evolving roles and challenges faced by parents of these children so as to better support them. Woodgate, Edwards, Ripat, Borton, and Rempel (2015) used an ethnographic approach to understand the roles that parents assume in parenting their children with complex care needs.

In total, 68 parents from 40 families were recruited to participate in Woodgate et al.'s (2015) study. Data collection strategies included two ethnographic methods—interviewing and photo-voice methods. All of the families responded to an initial interview; 29 of them participated in a second follow-up interview, and 20 were interviewed a total of three times. The researchers also used photo-voice methods by asking parents to take pictures of objects, people, places, and events that represented their everyday life. In a follow-up interview, the parents were asked to explain what was happening in each photograph and how it related to their lives. The meanings attached to these artifacts were also analyzed.

The overarching theme that the researchers discovered in their study was "intense parenting." This description referred to the extra efforts parents had to commit to in raising their children with complex care needs. Parenting was described as labor intensive and emergent—that is, parents had to be available for care provision at any time. The intense parenting left minimal time for addressing any other needs in the parents' lives or the lives of their other children. Some of the parents also indicated the complexity and intensity of their child's care needs were taking a toll on their own personal health.

Overall, these parents took on more roles and worked more intensely at those roles. The authors had substantial recommendations for the kind of support these families would value and the resources they require.

This study used an ethnographic approach, in that the researchers collected a variety of data using interviews and artifacts. The use of narratives to describe photos was a unique approach to real-time data collection that minimized the amount of time during which the researcher had to conduct actual observations. The period of time over which the data were collected was lengthy. This approach allowed the researchers to become "participants" in the family's life with an actual presence, and resulted in those observed becoming habituated to the data collection process quite quickly. Such habituation is a hallmark of ethnographic research. The rich description and volumes of data that resulted lent credibility to the findings and encouraged application of the findings to other settings.

Grounded Theory

Grounded theory is the discovery of theory from data systematically obtained through qualitative means. It does not begin with theory, but rather leads to development of a theory to explain the phenomenon. The intent of grounded theory is to discover a pattern of reactions, interactions, and relationships among people and their concerns (Moore, 2010). This complex type of qualitative research requires a high level of skill and the capacity to suspend bias related to the topic of interest.

Questions That Are Addressed with Grounded Theory

Grounded theory is rarely undertaken to answer a central research question. Instead, the research problem is discovered, as is the process that resolves the problem (Fain, 2013). Because the purpose of such research is to develop theory, the grounded theory study begins with a general area of interest and proceeds to explore how individuals frame the problem, which variations arise as a result, and how people deal with it. Grounded theory provides evidence about the ways people react and interact with one another and with their own health and illness (Hernandez, 2010). The basic elements of grounded theory include answering the following questions: "What is the chief concern of people regarding this area of interest?" and "What accounts for the way people deal with this concern or problem?"

Methods and Procedures for Grounded Theory

Grounded theory: Research aimed at discovering and developing a theory based on systematically collected data about a phenomenon. The intent is to discover a pattern of reactions, interactions, and relationships among people and their concerns.

Grounded theory studies are the least preplanned of any of the qualitative methods. The researcher begins with a general research problem, selects individuals who are most likely to illuminate the initial understanding of the question, and collects data using a variety of methods. Interviewing, observation, and document review may all be used in establishing grounded theory.

The researcher interprets and codes data constantly and at each stage decides which types of data to collect so as to continue developing the theory. After initial identification of a purposeful sample, data collection, and analysis, the emerging theory drives subsequent decisions about the subsequent data collection and analytic processes. Additional sampling may be undertaken based on this preliminary analysis of results. The later samples may have relaxed inclusion criteria, thereby enabling the researcher to gather data that possess more variability and expose relationships. Use of such a theoretical sample is characteristic of this tradition.

The sample size, data collection, and analytic processes in grounded theory are not planned and finite, but rather emerge throughout the study. Rather than making the study easier to conduct, this lack of guidelines for implementation calls for a highly skilled and competent researcher to accomplish the study's purpose.

Strengths of Grounded Theory

Grounded theory is a method for developing the very basis of nursing practice via the proposition of theories for subsequent testing. The following list highlights some of its strengths:

- Grounded theory provides the basis for testing theories about reactions and interactions.
- Grounded theory enables the exploration of human actions and interactions related to subjects for which very little knowledge is available.
- Grounded theory allows researchers to determine what *is* rather than suggesting what should be.
- These studies help build models that can be used to assess human reactions to nursing interventions.

Limitations of Grounded Theory

Grounded theory is essential for the development of nursing theory, but it has significant limitations, particularly for a novice researcher:

- Grounded theory is difficult to conduct well and requires a high level of competence on the part of the researcher.
- Theoretical development is a complex process and has many points at which the investigator's bias may interfere with accurate theory development.
- Grounded theory studies are lengthy, are time intensive, and require a great deal of effort and skill on the part of the researcher (De Chesnay, 2015b).

Reading Qualitative Research Studies

Qualitative research as evidence for nursing practice is appraised for its trustworthiness, just as quantitative research is evaluated for reliability, validity, and generalizability. However, considerable controversy exists regarding the standards used to evaluate qualitative research. Most qualitative researchers focus on the elements of trustworthiness described earlier in this chapter. Other researchers, though, argue that the same standards that are applied to quantitative research should be used to appraise qualitative studies. Contemporary thinking is that evaluation of qualitative research should rely on some combination of the two approaches, and begin to use common verbiage. When qualitative research is sought as support for evidence-based practice, the evaluation typically relies on criteria that are specific to qualitative inquiry rather than quantitative study. To determine if the results of a qualitative study apply in a specific patient care situation, the standards for design, implementation, and analysis of qualitative inquiry must be used as a basis for appraisal.

Because qualitative research does not deal with testing hypotheses about cause and effect, issues of internal validity, measurement reliability, hypothesis testing,

Transferability:
The ability to apply qualitative research findings in other settings or situations.

and statistical analysis are not of concern. No attempt is made to evaluate effect size, so power is also not of concern. Likewise, generalizability is not a goal; qualitative research is either descriptive or interpretive, and it is not intended to generate conclusions that can be generalized to entire populations. As a result, random sampling is unnecessary and generation of confidence intervals, probability of error, and *p* values is not of concern.

Instead, the methodological rigor of the sampling strategy is assessed by evaluating how well the researcher used purposeful sampling to select those participants who could best inform the question. Appropriate selection criteria should be reported, and methods of recruiting and informing subjects of their rights should be described. Although power is not the primary issue in evaluating sample size, saturation of data may indicate that an adequate sample was accessed. The researcher should report both the way saturation was evaluated and the number of participants required to reach it.

Although internal validity is not a concern with qualitative research, the credibility and trustworthiness of the conclusions are. The researcher should report the ways in which credibility and reliability were maintained. Discussion of the bracketing method and the use of triangulation, extended contact, and member checking enhance reliability of the conclusions. An audit trail suggests that decisions and design processes were systematically recorded and supports the confirmability of the study.

Several tools have been developed to appraise the validity of qualitative research studies. The primary focus of these tools has been to translate qualitative research into evidence for nursing practice, specifically for the development of practice guidelines. Hannes, Lockwood, and Pearson (2010) compared three online appraisal instruments used for this purpose: the Joanna Briggs Institute (JBI) tool, the Critical Appraisal Skills Programme (CASP), and the Evaluation Tool for Qualitative Studies (ETQS). All three instruments were comprehensive and rigorous in their respective standards. The JBI tool requires completing a series of statements about the research; the CASP and ETQS rely on questions to guide an appraisal. **Table 14.4** indicates the type of validity tested by each instrument and identifies the criteria that make up the evaluation.

Although the reader of qualitative research should not broadly generalize the results to his or her population, qualitative research *is* transferable. **Transferability** refers to the ability of the nurse to transfer the findings to patients who are in similar situations and who have similar characteristics (Houghton, Casey, Shaw, & Murphy, 2013). Describing the sample carefully enables the nurse to have more confidence in transfer of the findings to other practice settings or patients. The extensive description that is characteristic of qualitative research reporting gives the reader sufficient information to be able to judge the applicability of the findings to other settings and people.

Using Qualitative Research Studies as Evidence

The integration of qualitative research findings into nursing practice is a strategy receiving increasing attention (Lavoie-Tremblay et al., 2012; Leeman & Sandelowski, 2012; Pedro-Gomez et al., 2011). Qualitative research can help the nurse better understand the nature of the effectiveness of interventions. In other words, what about the intervention

Table 14.4 Types of Validity Addressed in the Critical Appraisal Instruments

Types of Validity	Description	Criteria	Appraisal Instruments
Descriptive validity	The degree to which descriptive information such as events, subjects, setting, time, and places is accurately reported	Impact of investigator Context	Evaluated in JBI, CASP, and ETQS
Interpretive validity	The degree to which participants' viewpoints, thoughts, intentions, and experiences are accurately understood and reported by the qualitative researcher	Believability	Evaluated in JBI and ETQS
Theoretical validity	The degree to which a theory or theoretical explanation informing or developed from a research study fits the data and, therefore, is credible and defensible	Theoretical framework	Evaluated in JBI and ETQS
Generalizability	The degree to which findings can be extended to persons, times, or settings other than those directly studied	Value and implications of research	Evaluated in CASP and ETQS
Evaluative validity	The degree to which an evaluative framework or critique is applied to the object of study	Evaluation/ outcome	Evaluated in JBI and ETQS

Note: JBI = Joanna Briggs Institute; CASP = Critical Appraisal Skills Programme; ETQS = Evaluation Tool for Qualitative Studies.
Reproduced from Hannes, K., Lockwood, C., & Pearson, A. (2010). A comparative analysis of three online appraisal instruments' ability to assess validity in qualitative research. *Qualitative Health Research, 20*(12), 1740. Reprinted with permission of Sage Publications, Inc.

was helpful to the patient? What was clear? What was unclear? How did the patient respond to the treatment? Conversely, qualitative research can be invaluable in determining why an intervention did not work. What about the treatment was unacceptable to the patient? What affected his or her life in an adverse way? What caused complexity or confusion or was not sustainable? A treatment may be shown to be effective in a controlled setting, such as a randomized controlled trial, but not sustainable in a natural setting. Interventions may produce side effects that are not tolerated or that are undesirable. Quality of life may be affected in a way that is not acceptable to the patient or that is difficult to manage on an everyday basis. Qualitative research is helpful in discovering the ways that nursing interventions affect the everyday life experience of an individual, in both positive and negative ways. As such, these studies provide the evidence that is needed to help patients sustain their treatments and get the most benefit from them (Perry et al., 2011).

Qualitative research adds a dimension to interventional studies that cannot be attained through the measurement of variables alone. Much of the human experience—particularly in regard to health and illness—is affected by motivation and perception as much as by therapies. These aspects are some of the qualities most suited to qualitative inquiry.

Audrey (2011) and Young, Gomersall, and Bowen (2012) identified some of the ways in which qualitative research can be linked to interventional analysis. They note that qualitative study can help nurse researchers do the following:

- Identify the needs of a target population
- Design interventions that are most likely to be acceptable to patients
- Address the process and implementation issues associated with an intervention
- Improve the understanding of the impact of an intervention in a natural setting
- Understand the reasons for attrition, cessation of treatment, or lack of adherence to a treatment protocol

These are all ways that the nurse can integrate qualitative research into the evaluation of interventions and the design of evidence-based practices. It is particularly important to recognize the humanistic, holistic nature of nursing practice, and qualitative research is invaluable in adding this facet to the evidence that serves as the basis for nursing knowledge.

How does one determine whether to use a qualitative research study as sound evidence for practice? Kirkpatrick, Wilson, and Wimpenny (2012) recommend the use of four rules when determining whether to include qualitative research studies in evidence-based practice:

- *The study satisfies the general assumptions for the development of a practice guideline.* The study supports the topic under study and meets the inclusion criteria, and it is retrieved from a peer-reviewed journal.
- *The study meets the qualitative screening criteria.* The study involves observation of social or human problems in a natural setting, and observations are interpreted by the researcher. The study is conducted in conformance with ethical principles for research.
- *The study meets the criteria for trustworthy qualitative evidence.* The study is designed and carried out in a way that supports its credibility, transferability, dependability, and confirmability.
- *The strength of recommendations is based on the quality of the evidence.* Qualitative studies are graded according to their strength, and subsequent recommendations are consistent with the level of the evidence.

Qualitative studies are valuable additions to the evidence that supports nursing practice. These studies are subjected to the same appraisal process as quantitative studies, albeit one that is based on characteristics that are specific to qualitative research (Lavoie-Tremblay et al., 2012; Pedro-Gomez et al., 2011).

WHERE TO LOOK FOR INFORMATION ABOUT QUALITATIVE METHODS

- Some qualitative research reports do not explicitly report the type of research design employed in the study. In such a case, it may be up to the reader to infer the specific type of design that was used. The study may simply be described as "qualitative" or "content analysis." The types of research questions that were asked, the informants selected, and the methods used to collect and analyze data may provide hints as to the precise type of study design.
- The conversational style of qualitative writing, which is often reported in first person, and the liberal use of quotations from informants make the report an interesting one to evaluate. This is not a weakness, but rather a characteristic of qualitative reports. The insights provided by qualitative research are engaging and can provide the reader with personal insights as well, increasing the value of the reading experience.
- Conversely, the lack of consistent criteria for evaluating these studies and the controversy surrounding the use of standards for evaluating their reliability and validity frequently make such reports more difficult to evaluate. The use of criteria specific to qualitative research can reduce the level of frustration and enhance the reader's confidence in the findings.
- The sequence of information in a qualitative report may be quite different from that of a quantitative report. This is not a drawback, but rather an inherent characteristic of such studies. The literature review may appear at the beginning or during interpretation. The methods and procedures are often clearly described but may not be labeled as such. The reader must thoroughly review the entire study before determining that a particular aspect has been omitted.
- Whether labeled as such or not, a qualitative study should outline the sampling procedure, any inclusion criteria, the data collection technique, and an overview of analysis. These elements may not be standard, but they should be recognizable.
- Information about efforts to establish credibility, trustworthiness, dependability, and confirmability may appear nearly anywhere in the article, but in general:
  - Bracketing is described near the beginning of a research study.
  - Purposive sampling, inclusion criteria, and saturation will likely be described in the sampling strategy.
  - Triangulation, member checking, and peer debriefing are usually described with the data analysis procedure.
  - Documentation of an audit trail may appear anywhere in the report, although it is frequently mentioned near the end of the procedures section.

CHECKLIST FOR CRITICALLY READING A QUALITATIVE RESEARCH STUDY

- ❏ The central phenomenon, event, experience, or conceptual basis of the study is clearly stated in the research question.
- ❏ The research tradition that is chosen is linked to the research question and the nature of the information that is sought.
- ❏ The study participants are chosen using a purposeful method based on established criteria.
- ❏ Evidence of saturation is provided to justify sample size.
- ❏ The researcher provides evidence of bracketing of personal preconceptions and biases to mitigate their effects.
- ❏ The study includes a description of methods to enhance trustworthiness. For example:
  - Prolonged engagement
  - Triangulation
  - Member checking
- ❏ The author mentions the documentation of an audit trail to support dependability.
- ❏ Sufficient description is provided of the context and informants to determine the transferability of the findings to other settings or people.

Creating Qualitative Evidence

The creation of qualitative research requires patience, persistence, and a passion for the subject under study. Although qualitative studies are emergent designs, they are no less rigorous because of this factor. The lack of preconceived design elements does not mean the study is unfocused. It does mean that extended contact is required, so the nurse researcher must devote substantial time and effort to carrying out the study effectively. Analysis can be a complex process, and the software that supports statistical analysis has no utility in qualitative coding. Software is available for qualitative analysis, but it does not analyze the data for the researcher; these processes still require substantial time and skill to complete.

With that said, qualitative research enables the nurse researcher to identify rich, interesting, and insightful information about the experiences of patients. Health and illness are humanistic considerations, and qualitative inquiry is well suited to help the nurse understand them.

GRAY MATTER

The following key steps help create a strong qualitative study:
1. Identify a broad research question.
2. Select a research tradition.
3. Determine criteria for selection of participants who can best inform the question.
4. Locate a source of participants and invite their participation through informed consent.
5. Design general data collection procedures.
6. Transcribe data in their entirety and add field notes.
7. Analyze data as they are collected.
8. Develop a codebook of themes and code units of meaning.
9. Check the conclusions with participants.
10. Report the themes with supporting examples from informants.

The approach to a qualitative study is not preconceived, but it is systematic. The following steps can help the nurse researcher create a qualitative study that meets standards for trustworthiness and makes a strong addition to the evidence for nursing practice:

1. *Identify a broad research question.* The central question is broad and general, but it should focus on a single phenomenon or concept. Subquestions can add detail to the central question but may evolve and change as the study emerges; these often provide guidance for the development of specific interview guides, procedures, or sampling considerations.

2. *Select a broad research tradition.* A specific classification of qualitative research is selected next, based on the match between the research question and the characteristics of the tradition. This classification generally does not change and evolve with the study.

3. *Determine criteria for selection of participants who can best inform the question.* These criteria may be characteristics (for example, gender or age), experiences (for example, recent diagnosis of breast cancer), or membership in a particular group (for example, drug addicts). Criteria may also be developed that support the methodology and conduct of the study. For example, in a study of teen attitudes toward drug rehabilitation, the willingness of the teen participant to talk with an adult about his or her experience is paramount.

4. *Locate a source of informants and invite their participation through informed consent.* The researcher must find an accessible group of informants who meet the criteria created in step 3. An invitation is then issued, and participants are thoroughly informed about the nature of the study, associated risks, and benefits.

5. *Design general data collection procedures.* If the data collection process consists of interviews, then a general interview guide should be designed. No more than a handful of questions should be predetermined. The interviewer should, in essence, "go where the informant goes." Being bombarded with too many questions may lead the informant to espouse the researcher's preconceived conclusions. In contrast, open-ended questions that enable exploratory interviewing are recommended for beginning interviews. Focus group and observation guides should similarly be broad and enable exploration on the part of the researcher. Table 14.5 provides an example of an interview guide for a qualitative study.

Table 14.5 Example of a Qualitative Interview Guide

Purpose of the Study

Determine the aspects of nursing work that are considered "caring."

Interview Guide

Which kinds of things do you do for patients that you consider "caring"—that is, not tasks or procedures?

What are the characteristics of patients that you have found mean they will require more caring?

What are the characteristics of patients that you have found mean they will not require as much caring?

Which kinds of responses do you get from patients when you have exhibited caring behaviors?

Which kinds of responses do you find in yourself when you have exhibited caring behaviors?

6. *Transcribe data in their entirety and add field notes.* Data of any type—interviews, focus group recordings, or observational records—should be transcribed in their entirety. This step requires a high level of organization and data management because a large volume of data will be generated during qualitative studies. The researcher should add field notes to the transcribed data as soon as possible after the experience to capture contextual issues and nonverbal responses while they are still fresh in his or her mind.

7. *Analyze data as they are collected.* Analytic memos, or short notes indicating the potential for emerging themes or exemplar quotations, should be added to the data as they are collected and reviewed. As new data are collected, they should be compared to the existing data to determine the themes that are supported (or not).

8. *Develop a codebook of themes and code units of meaning.* The development of a codebook supports reliable coding of units of meaning—whether they are words, phrases, or observations—into overall themes that make up the key components of the conclusions.

9. *Check the conclusions with participants.* Member checking ensures that the researcher's interpretations are valid and that his or her assumptions and preconceived ideas have not affected the analysis of the data.

10. *Report the themes with supporting exemplars from informants.* Reporting themes and using the words of informants to support these conclusions is the accepted way to report qualitative studies. The use of direct quotations enables the reader to judge the credibility of the interpretations of the researcher.

Qualitative studies are invaluable tools for adding to the body of evidence that supports nursing practice. A systematic approach and attention to methodological rigor are not unique to quantitative research, but serve the qualitative researcher equally well. Qualitative research provides a rich dimension to the design of nursing interventions and gives voice to patients' needs, preferences, and concerns.

Summary of Key Concepts

- The impetus behind qualitative research is to identify the meaning of a phenomenon, event, or experience for an individual.
- Evidence of clinical experiences and patient preferences is often discovered through qualitative research.
- Qualitative research is grounded in the belief that reality can never be completely known because it is constructed by each individual, so meaning must be discovered by using methods that do not rely on measurement.
- Qualitative research is important in nursing because nursing is a humanistic, holistic profession in which knowledge of human reactions to illness and health is important.

- Qualitative research may be descriptive or interpretive; it does not result in conclusions about cause and effect, but rather understanding of meaning.
- The point of qualitative research is to elicit a description of a social experience that is so detailed and insightful that someone who has not had the same experience can understand and appreciate its nuances.
- Qualitative research involves an emergent design in which details of the research unfold as the study progresses. It is based on rigorous principles focused on credibility, trustworthiness, and confirmability.
- Qualitative data are gathered directly from informants via interview or focus groups, through researcher observation, or through review of documents and artifacts.
- Interventions that require lifestyle adjustment, attitude changes, or behavioral alterations are particularly suitable for qualitative study.
- Questions that reflect exploration of feelings, perceptions, attitudes, motivation, quality of life, and other subjective experiences are well addressed with qualitative inquiry. The central question is written in such a way that it accommodates the emerging design that is characteristic of qualitative inquiry.
- Qualitative research designs are sometimes referred to as "traditions." Each tradition is intended to answer a particular kind of question.
- Qualitative samples are most commonly selected using a purposeful sampling method.
- Saturation, or the point at which no new information is being generated, is the standard for sample size in a qualitative study.
- In qualitative research, data are analyzed using a constant-comparison method in which data are reviewed and analyzed continuously as new data are compared to existing data to confirm or disprove emerging themes.
- Qualitative researchers are concerned with credibility and trustworthiness, which are supported by the following methods:
  - Bracketing of the researcher's biases to "set them aside"
  - Triangulation of conclusions based on at least three separate data sources
  - Prolonged engagement with participants
  - Member checking to ensure that conclusions accurately represent the thoughts of informants
  - An audit trail to enable confirmability of the study
- Qualitative research is not intended to be generalized, but rather transferred to similar situations and individuals.
- The traditions that are commonly used as evidence for nursing practice include case studies, content analysis, phenomenology, ethnography, and grounded theory. In many cases, however, no specific tradition is explicitly identified in a qualitative study report.

CRITICAL APPRAISAL EXERCISE

Retrieve the following full-text article from the Cumulative Index to Nursing and Allied Health Literature or similar search database:

Berg, G., Harshbarger, J., Ahlers-Schmidt, C., & Lippoldt, D. (2016). Exposing compassion fatigue and burnout syndrome in a trauma team: A qualitative study. *Journal of Trauma Nursing, 23*(1), 3–12.

Review the article, focusing on the sections that report the question, tradition, methods, and procedures. Consider the following appraisal questions in your critical review of this research article:

1. What is the purpose of this research?
2. Which methodology (case research, content analysis, phenomenology, or ethnography) did these authors use to answer the question? Discuss how this question could have been studied using other qualitative methodologies.
3. Describe the data collection methodology. Which other data collection methods could have been used in this study? Were there sufficient data types to achieve triangulation?
4. How was the sample selected? Which inclusion and exclusion criteria were evident? Was the sampling purposive and focused on specific informants who could best answer the question?
5. How did these researchers ensure the credibility and trustworthiness of the data? Were these methods sufficient to support confidence in using these results as evidence for practice?
6. Which analytic process was used? How could the description of the analysis method be more fully developed?

References

Alhusen, J., & Wilson, D. (2015). Pregnant mothers' perceptions of how intimate partner violence affects their unborn children. *Journal of Obstetric, Gynecologic, & Neonatal Nursing, 33,* 210–217.

Audrey, S. (2011). Qualitative research in evidence-based medicine: Improving decision-making and participation in randomized controlled trials of cancer treatments. *Palliative Medicine, 25*(8), 758–765.

Cardwell, F. S., & Elliott, S. J. (2013). Making links: Do we connect climate change with health? A qualitative case study from Canada. *BMC Public Health, 13*(208), 1–12.

Connelly, L. (2010). What is phenomenology? *MedSurg Nursing, 19*(2), 127–128.

Creswell, J. W. (2013). *Qualitative inquiry and research design: Choosing among five approaches.* Thousand Oaks, CA: Sage.

Creswell, J. W., & Clark, V. L. (2011). *Designing and conducting mixed methods research.* Thousand Oaks, CA: Sage.

Crowe, S., Cresswell, K., Robertson, A., Huby, G., Avery, A., & Sheikh, A. (2011). The case study approach. *BMC Medical Research Methodology, 11*(100), 1–9.

Cruz, E. V., & Higginbottom, G. (2013). The use of focused ethnography in nursing research. *Nurse Researcher, 20*(4), 36–43.

De Chesnay, M. (2015a). *Nursing research using ethnography: Qualitative designs and methods in nursing*. New York, NY: Springer.

De Chesnay, M. (2015b). *Nursing research using grounded theory: Qualitative designs and methods in nursing*. New York, NY: Springer.

Denzin, N. K., & Lincoln, Y. S. (2011). *Qualitative research*. Thousand Oaks, CA: Sage.

Fain, J. (2013). *Reading, understanding, and applying nursing research* (4th ed.). Philadelphia, PA: F. A. Davis.

Flood, A. (2010). Understanding phenomenology. *Nurse Researcher, 17*(2), 7–15.

Gorman, L., Huebner, A., Hirschfeld, M., Sankar, S., Blow, A., Guty, D., ... Ketner, J. (2016). A comparative case study of risk, resiliency, and coping among injured National Guard. *Military Medicine, 181*(5), 70–78.

Guba, E., & Lincoln, Y. (1989). *Fourth generation evaluation*. Newbury Park, CA: Sage.

Hannes, K., Lockwood, C., & Pearson, A. (2010). A comparative analysis of three online appraisal instruments' ability to assess validity in qualitative research. *Qualitative Health Research, 20*(12), 1736–1743.

Hernandez, C. (2010). Getting grounded: Using Glaserian grounded theory to conduct nursing research. *Canadian Journal of Nursing Research, 42*(1), 150–163.

Houghton, C., Casey, D., Shaw, D., & Murphy, K. (2013). Rigour in qualitative case-study research. *Nurse Researcher, 20*(4), 12–17.

Kirkpatrick, P., Wilson, E., & Wimpenny, P. (2012). Research to support evidence-based practice in COPD community nursing. *British Journal of Community Nursing, 17*(10), 487–492.

Lachal, J., Speranza, M., Taieb, O., Falissard, B., Lefevre, H., Qualigramh, M. R. M., & Revah- Levy, A. (2012). Qualitative research using photo-elicitation to explore the role of food in family relationships among obese adolescents. *Appetite, 58*(3), 1099–1105.

Lanford, R., & Young, A. (2013). *Making a difference with nursing research*. Boston, MA: Pearson.

Lavoie-Tremblay, M., Richer, M. C., Marchionni, C., Cyr, G., Biron, A. D., Aubry, M., ... Verzina, M. (2012). Implementation of evidence-based practices in the context of a redevelopment project in a Canadian healthcare organization. *Journal of Nursing Scholarship, 44*(4), 418–427.

Leeman, J., & Sandelowski, M. (2012). Practice-based evidence and qualitative inquiry. *Journal of Nursing Scholarship, 44*(2), 171–179.

Moore, J. (2010). Classic grounded theory: A framework for contemporary application. *Nurse Researcher, 17*(4), 41–48.

Morse, J. M. (2015). Critical analysis of strategies for determining rigor in qualitative inquiry. *Qualitative Health Research, 25*(9), 1212–1222.

Nicholls, D. (2009). Qualitative research: Part three—methods. *International Journal of Therapy and Rehabilitation, 16*(12), 638–647.

O'Reilly, M., & Parker, N. (2013). Unsatisfactory saturation: A critical exploration of the notion of saturated sample sizes in qualitative research. *Qualitative Research, 13*(2), 190–197.

Pearson, A. (2011). Evidence-based healthcare and qualitative research. *Journal of Research in Nursing, 15*(6), 489–493.

Pedro-Gomez, J. D., Morales-Asencio, J. M., Bennasar-Veny, M., Artigues-Vives, G., Perello-Campaner, C., & Gomex-Picard, P. (2011). Determining factors in evidence-based clinical practice among hospital and primary care nursing staff. *Journal of Advanced Nursing, 68*(2), 452–459.

Pennington, N. (2013). You don't de-friend the dead: An analysis of grief communication by college students through Facebook profiles. *Death Studies, 37*, 617–635.

Perry, L., Bellchambers, H., Howie, A., Moxey, A., Parkinson, L., Capra, S., & Byles, J. (2011). Examination of the utility of the promoting action on research implementation in health services framework for implementation of evidence based practice in residential aged care settings. *Journal of Advanced Nursing, 67*(10), 2139–2150.

Roy, K., Zvonkovic, A., Goldberg, A., Sharp, E., & LaRossa, R. (2015). Sampling richness and qualitative integrity: Challenges or research with families. *Journal of Marriage & Family, 77*(1), 243–260.

Sayt, L., Seers, K., & Tutton, E. (2015). Patients' experiences of technology and care in adult intensive care. *Journal of Advanced Nursing, 71*(9), 2051–2061.

Secomb, J. M., & Smith, C. (2011). A mixed method pilot study: The researchers' experiences. *Contemporary Nurse, 39*(1), 31–35.

Shin, K., Kim, M., & Chung, S. (2010). Methods and strategies utilized in published qualitative research. *Qualitative Health Research, 19*(6), 850–858.

Thomas, E., & Magilvy, J. K. (2011). Qualitative rigor or research validity in qualitative research. *Pediatric Nursing, 16,* 151–155.

Thorne, S., Stephens, J., & Truant, T. (2016). Building qualitative study design using nursing's disciplinary epistemology. *Journal of Advanced Nursing, 72*(2), 451–460.

Whitting, M., & Sines, D. (2012). Mind maps: Establishing "trustworthiness" in qualitative research. *Nurse Researcher, 20*(1), 21–27.

Woodgate, R., Edwards, M., Ripat, J., Borton, B., & Rempel, G. (2015). Intense parenting: a qualitative study detailing the experiences of parenting children with complex care needs. *BMC Pediatricts, 15,* 1–15.

Young, A., Gomersall, T., & Bowen, A. (2012). Trial participants' experiences of early enhanced speech and language therapy after stroke compared with employed visitor support: A qualitative study nested within a randomized controlled trial. *Clinical Rehabilitation, 27*(2), 174–182.

Chapter 15

Analyzing and Reporting Qualitative Results

CHAPTER OBJECTIVES

The study of this chapter will help the learner to

- Describe the challenges facing the qualitative research analyst.
- Discuss the importance of developing an organized approach to managing qualitative data.
- Summarize the steps that make up the overall approach to qualitative analysis.
- Explain the purpose and process of constant comparison as an analytic technique.
- Express the process for coding data and development of a codebook.
- Review methods for establishing the trustworthiness of qualitative conclusions.
- Describe how qualitative data are reported and presented for publication.
- Discuss the implications of the analytic method on use of qualitative research as evidence.

KEY TERMS

Codebook
Codes
Cohen's kappa
Constant comparison
Decision trail
Dictionary

Editing analysis
Immersion/crystallization
  analysis
Inquiry audit
Margin notes
Parsimonious
Peer debriefing

Recontextualizing
Schematic
Template analysis
Themes
Theoretical sampling
Unit of analysis

Introduction to Qualitative Analysis

The qualitative analyst is much like the leader of a jazz band. Although he or she may start out with a general idea of what is to be accomplished, the band leader follows each musician as he or she improvises on a basic theme. The music is not exactly composed, but rather emerges. Much the same can be said about qualitative analysis: The final product of the analysis emerges as the researcher follows the informants as they illuminate the question more and more.

Jazz compositions are often longer than traditional compositions. Chasing interpretations of themes takes time and effort, so a lot of music is generated. Likewise, qualitative studies result in volumes of information. The thick description and prolonged engagement that produce credible, trustworthy results also generate a tremendous number of words. The sheer volume of data that is characteristic of qualitative inquiry creates challenges in both data management and drawing sensible conclusions. This factor explains why qualitative data analysis is sometimes referred to as data reduction. In essence, the researcher's goal is to reduce the data to meaningful units that can be described, interpreted, and reported in an understandable way. The analysis of numerical (quantitative) data is relatively straightforward: The correct statistical test is selected and applied, and results are interpreted. Qualitative analysis, in contrast, requires a different skill set—even a different state of mind—and the methods that are used are not standard, even within a single tradition.

The intent of data analysis, regardless of the approach applied, is to organize, provide structure to, and draw out meaning from the data collected. In performing such analysis, the qualitative researcher faces three types of challenges.

First, qualitative analysis offers no single standard for the analytic process. On its surface, this absence might seem to simplify analysis, but in the execution of such research, the lack of clearly defined steps often results in false starts and backtracking, and it requires an enormous amount of time. Even within traditions, recommendations may vary widely as to the appropriate steps to take. Some authors argue that simply having steps means that preconceptions exist, whereas the avoidance of a systematic process enables more creative and insightful conclusions to be drawn. Regardless, the qualitative researcher faces a perplexing array of possibilities for approaching the analytic process.

The work of the qualitative researcher is further complicated by a second characteristic of qualitative inquiry: the enormous quantity of data that must be thoughtfully reviewed, reflected on, and summarized. The researcher must make sense of pages and pages of narratives, observations, and transcripts to carry out the analysis process. Managing these reams of data, tracking the source and type of each piece, triangulating findings, and locating supportive quotations are all complex due to the sheer quantity of material that must be reviewed.

The last challenge centers on the need to reduce or put the data into a manageable format for dissemination of the findings. For the richness of the data to be maintained, the researcher must be thorough and use the words of informants, yet reporting and publication restrictions necessitate development of a concise report. Balancing rich description with focus presents a challenge for every qualitative researcher.

Qualitative analysis is difficult and complex when done well, mainly because of these challenges. It requires patience, persistence, and a good deal of self-discipline. While sometimes onerous, this effort may bring rich rewards: Soundly drawn qualitative conclusions enhance the evidence for a holistic view of nursing practice. Ensuring the findings are trustworthy is the job of the qualitative analyst.

SCENES FROM THE FIELD

Nursing is a human services profession, and one that interacts with people at their most vulnerable. This often translates into bad behavior on the part of patients, particularly in the form of verbal abusiveness. Many studies have reported the existence of verbal abuse in nursing care units, but a gap exists in understanding the specific nature and type of abuse many nurses endure.

Jackson and colleagues (2013) undertook an observational qualitative study in which they observed and classified verbal abuse targeted at nurses during the course of delivering care. The study was conducted within inpatient and emergency department settings in a large urban hospital. The researchers observed patient–nurse interactions in the thoroughfares and waiting areas of the hospital at all hours of the day and on all shifts. More than 1100 hours of observation resulted in data on 220 patients who displayed aggressive behaviors. The researchers recorded their observational notes on a predetermined template that included a checklist of 17 behavioral cues indicating aggression. This checklist included space for recording additional observational data, including the observed outcome of the interchange. Additional data included the time and duration of the event; the location, situational context, and participants; and the actions and reactions of the nurse and the patient. Nonverbal behavior, gestures, and language were recorded when related to the incident. Text from the observational tool was transcribed and analyzed for words and phrases denoting verbal violence and abuse. Threats, raised voices, swearing, humiliation, and degrading language were all categorized as verbal abuse.

Most of the verbal abuse occurred in the emergency department. This abuse took a variety of forms and occurred in the everyday interactions among nurses, patients, and persons accompanying patients. After analysis, three major content areas emerged:

- *Gendered verbal abuse that was largely sexual in nature.* Language was used in a way that was demeaning to female nurses and their character as women. This abuse originated primarily from patients, rather than from their families or others present. It included taunts and insults that were conveyed via stereotypical gendered assumptions about nurses and women. Often, these insults were made in public spaces in front of others. The attacks implied that nurses were sexual deviants in some way and denigrated their intelligence. In many cases, the abuse was used by patients to gain dominance or control over a situation.
- *Hostility, threats, and menacing language.* Both verbal and nonverbal hostility were displayed in interactions. Nonverbal hostility included damaging property, glaring at staff, and other signs of disrespect. Threats of complaints to administration or legal action were involved in several incidents. Using cell phones to record interactions was common. Both patients and families equally issued threats of violence against the nurses, as well as targeting other caregivers such as physicians and ambulance staff.
- *Insults, ridicule, and unreasonable demands.* Verbal abuse without a gendered undertone was also observed. This abuse involved insults, demeaning comments, ridicule, and sarcasm, often displayed in the presence of others. Ridicule that called into question the competence of the nurse was a common form of this abuse. Nurses were regularly subjected to swearing.

Most inpatient units have "zero tolerance" policies, yet those policies appear to be insufficient to address verbal abuse aimed at nurses. Nurse managers need to help their staff learn to deal with verbal abuse and should ensure intervention strategies to minimize nurses' exposure to aggression are in place. An interesting suggestion made by the study authors was to train all hospital staff in "bystander intervention strategies" that could empower multiple staff members to come to the nurses' aid. The findings from this qualitative study have implications for the development of overall intervention programs and policy frameworks that address aggression and verbal abuse in the hospital (Jackson et al., 2013).

Constant comparison:
A method of analysis in qualitative research that involves a review of data as they are gathered and comparison to data that have been interpreted to support or reject earlier conclusions.

Theoretical sampling:
Selecting additional members for the sample, often based on loosened inclusion criteria, to ensure divergent opinions are heard; a requirement for grounded theory development.

Characteristics of Qualitative Analysis

Qualitative analysis may not follow a standard, but it does have some steps that are common to all approaches. All qualitative researchers must take the following actions:

- Prepare the data for analysis.
- Conduct the analysis by developing an in-depth understanding of the data.
- Represent the data in reduced form.
- Interpret the larger meaning of the data (Creswell, 2013).

These may look like sequential steps, but the distinctions among them are often virtually undetectable because the researcher moves back and forth among the processes of data collection, analysis, and drawing conclusions. Unlike quantitative studies, when analysis is postponed until all data have been collected, qualitative analysis begins nearly as soon as data collection has begun. As data are collected, they are reviewed and re-reviewed, and analytic memos are written. Newly collected data are compared to existing data to confirm or refute conclusions and to decide when saturation has been reached. This **constant comparison** of new findings to existing results is a key characteristic of qualitative analysis. It is sometimes called "intensive engagement with the data" to reflect the depth at which the analyst considers the meaning of the information collected (Creswell & Clark, 2011). This approach enables the researcher to pursue interesting ideas or to sort through confusing input while informants are still available and data collection is still in progress. The researcher is then free to follow where the informants lead instead of taking a predetermined path leading to a single conclusion.

Using a constant-comparison process allows the analysis to guide subsequent data collection, with the researcher amending or adding interview questions or changing observational methods based on the findings. The researcher may even recruit new informants or change selection criteria to illuminate issues raised during analysis. This highly flexible process, which is essential for the grounded theory approach, is called **theoretical sampling**. Theoretical sampling involves the selection of a second sample of informants to whom less restrictive criteria are applied, with the goal of encouraging diverse viewpoints to emerge (Creswell & Clark, 2011). These secondary sites or cases are purposely selected to compare with the sample that has already been studied. Although this may sound like a sampling issue, theoretical sampling is, in effect, a source of triangulation—that is, it is one of the means by which qualitative analysts confirm their results.

It is characteristic of qualitative inquiry that data collection and analysis—even sampling and measurement strategies—may be indistinguishable during the research process. Data collection and data analysis are symbiotic in that the researcher must go back and forth between the two to identify the point at which results are trustworthy and data saturation occurs.

Styles of Qualitative Analysis

Qualitative researchers use multiple methods of analysis. Some influential qualitative methodologists have suggested general directions for the approach to overall analysis.

Generally, three major analytic styles are distinguished that fall on a continuum between structure and lack of structure:

- Template analysis style
- Editing analysis style
- Immersion/crystallization style

At one extreme is a style that provides a highly systematic and standardized approach to analysis; at the other end is a more intuitive, subjective, and interpretive style. Neither style is right or wrong for a particular study. Instead, the selection of the best approach and process depends on the research question, the study design, and the sensibilities of the researcher (Bazeley, 2013; Miles, Huberman, & Saldana, 2013).

The most highly structured style is **template analysis**, which requires developing a template that provides an analysis guide for sorting narrative data. This style is appropriate when a study has a clear theoretical perspective, because it requires using codes that are devised *a priori*. These codes may be developed theoretically, or they may be based on established literature. The advantage of template analysis is its simplicity—it is a focused and structured approach to analysis. Template analysis is more time efficient than the other analytic styles, and it is a commonly adopted approach in content analysis. The use of codebooks, inter-rater reliability assessment, and data definitions are characteristic of this approach, which is widely used in nursing research.

The **editing analysis** style is geared toward interpretation of text to find meaningful segments. Researchers using grounded theory, phenomenology, or hermeneutic traditions tend to employ this approach (Bazeley, 2013; Miles et al., 2013). Editing analysis is commonly encountered in nursing research and is used to discover the meaning of experiences, relationships, and interactions.

The least structured approach is **immersion/crystallization analysis**. It is appropriate when a researcher desires total immersion in and reflection on text, especially during case research and ethnography. Stemming from the notion that the researcher is the true analytic tool, this analytic approach requires that the investigator be immersed in the data and rely heavily on intuition to arrive at conclusions (Creswell & Clark, 2011; De Chesnay, 2015). Insights do not necessarily come after the data have been collected but might arise during data collection as well, so this analytic technique also employs constant comparison. As the analysis is being carried out and the conclusions are "crystallizing," the researcher can better decide how to proceed in further data gathering. Immersion/crystallization analysis is not a style that appears in the nursing research literature as much as template analysis and editing analysis, but it is still useful in healthcare research. Its primary downsides are its time-consuming nature and its requirement that the researcher constantly hold his or her biases at bay.

These three qualitative analysis styles may be employed in a variety of ways. Each has specific characteristics that apply to a particular type of research question and analysis procedure, but all qualitative analysts will not use the same single process. The primary considerations described in this chapter are generally applicable to qualitative analysis, but a single study may include all of these steps or only a few of them.

Template analysis:
A style of analysis that includes developing a template to sort narrative data.

Editing analysis:
A style of analysis geared toward interpretation of text to find meaningful segments.

Immersion/crystallization analysis:
A style of analysis that uses total immersion in and reflection on the text, usually in personal case reports.

Parsimonious:
Reduced to the fewest components; a parsimonious model is the simplest one that will demonstrate a concept.

Recontextualizing:
A qualitative data analysis and cognitive process undertaken by the researcher to search for meaning that may lead to a theory.

The Qualitative Analysis Process

Qualitative data analysis is an active and interactive process. The researcher looks at the data deliberately and in depth to become thoroughly familiar with them. It is not unusual for the researcher to examine and re-examine the data many times in the search for meaning. Thus this investigative process requires integrating multiple ways of knowing to get at the heart of the data. Fitting the data together is similar to putting the pieces of a puzzle together. The researcher becomes embedded in the data, like a detective at a crime scene, looking for clues that might lead to an intuitive conclusion about the data. As the researcher progresses through the process of conjecture and verification, corrections and modifications are made, leading to the development of patterns and themes.

Qualitative analysis may be viewed as a cognitive process that evolves through the following phases:

1. *Comprehending* occurs early in the process of analysis. The researcher attempts to make sense of the data that have been collected and get a sense of their overall tone.
2. *Synthesizing* leads the researcher to sift through the data using inductive reasoning to put the pieces of the puzzle together.
3. *Theorizing* brings the researcher to the point of what he or she believes has truly emerged from the data. This phase continues until the best and most **parsimonious** explanation has evolved. A parsimonious explanation is one that is the most focused while providing the best overview of the final conclusions.
4. **Recontextualizing** is a process that involves applying the theory that was derived from the analysis to different settings or groups. This extended exploration can result in the increased generalizability of the newly developed theory. The premise is that if a theory can be recontextualized, it can be generalized (Thorne, Stephens, & Truant, 2016).

Even though these phases are presented here in a linear fashion, they are rarely accomplished in that way. Instead, these phases typically intertwine with one another and may occur sequentially or simultaneously.

Management and Organization of Data

To make sense of the narrative data, the researcher must establish a method of managing and organizing the information early in the research process. The analysis process then can proceed in a logical—if not exactly linear—fashion. Organization and preparation of the data include transcription of audio recordings, optical scanning of artifacts and other documents, addition of field notes to transcripts, and other preparatory activities.

It is imperative to organize data effectively, so that they can be thoroughly evaluated and their confidentiality can be preserved. Data that are not well controlled are at risk for misuse and unauthorized access. Given this risk, data management is a primary consideration for the qualitative researcher.

Each piece of information that has been collected should be cataloged in some fashion. For each piece of data, the source, date of collection, and type of data should be noted. Because qualitative inquiry often generates multiple types of data, the same study may include electronic transcripts, hard-copy notes, photography, and audio recordings. Finding a method to track and maintain all of these data can pose quite a challenge. The data management process should be determined early in the study so data can be cataloged, reviewed, and analyzed as they are collected.

GRAY MATTER

Developing themes and codes in qualitative research proceeds through five steps:
- Reduce the raw data.
- Identify themes with subsamples.
- Compare themes across subsamples.
- Create a coding scheme.
- Determine the reliability of the coding scheme.

Schematic:
A system of organizing data into preset categories to allow for examination and further analysis.

Codes:
Labels, descriptions, or definitions assigned to data to allow them to be categorized and analyzed in qualitative research.

Review the Data for Initial Impressions

Once the data have been sorted and cataloged, the researcher undertakes the first of many reviews of the data. The data will be examined in their entirety many times, but the first read-through is helpful for establishing an overall impression of the data. It is recommended that the first reading be just that—a reading, rather than a review or note-taking session. Performing this initial review without preconceptions can give the researcher a sense of the data and some time to reflect on their meaning. The initial review should leave the researcher with general ideas about the tone of the data, impressions of the depth and clarity with which informants presented their ideas, and thoughts about where the research should go next.

Identify a Classification System

After a general impression has been gained from the read-through of the data, the researcher must develop a classification system. The researcher may establish a schematic to increase the manageability of the data. A schematic is an outline of the categories of meaning that may be expected from the data. In the template approach, this schematic is predetermined. In other approaches, it will likely be a work in progress. **Table 15.1** depicts a schematic for a qualitative analysis.

The development of a schematic as a classification system requires either substantial theoretical and literature background or an intense examination of the data. The development of general categories for data requires that the analyst elicit underlying consistencies, concepts, and clusters of concepts. This intense examination raises many questions: What is this informant saying? What is going on? What does it mean? What is this similar to? What is it different from?

Develop Codes and a Codebook

After completing an intense examination of the data and developing an overall schematic, the researcher develops more-specific categories of meaning based on what has been gathered. These categories of meaning are called codes. Codes support a more detailed analysis

Table 15.1 An Example of a Coding Schematic: Nurses' Reactions to a Perinatal Death

Theme	Codes
Getting through the shift	Flight mode: focusing on the nursing care Going through the motions Holding it together until later
Symptoms of pain and loss	Responses to loss: shaken to the core Feeling the loss: physical symptoms Feelings of self-doubt Emotional toll of the loss
Frustrations with care	Disagreements about provision of care among healthcare providers Dealing with language barriers
Showing genuine caring	A means to make the situation more bearable Protective feelings for the mother Handling the deceased infant with care and respect Creation of special bonds with patients Prayer while caring for the patient and afterward
Never forget: holding onto grief	Memories that will not go away Remembering the intense emotions involved Changed forever by the experience

Modified from Puia, D., Lewis, L., & Beck, C. (2013). Experiences of obstetric nurses who are present for a perinatal loss. *Journal of Obstetric, Gynecologic, & Neonatal Nursing, 42*, 321–331. Reprinted by permission of Elsevier.

process for the data. They are "chunks of meaning," or pieces of data that demonstrate patterns or themes in the responses.

An infinite range of possible codes exists for qualitative data. Nevertheless, the qualitative analyst can reflect on the following general categories of meaning to guide the code-development process:

- *Setting and context codes:* Identify elements of the setting or the environment that form patterns.
- *Perspective codes:* Relate the unique viewpoints of informants to the topic under study.
- *Subjects' ways of thinking:* Describe how informants frame their thoughts and actions about the topic.
- *Process codes:* Outline the ways things get accomplished.
- *Activity codes:* Describe things informants or others do.
- *Strategy codes:* Relate the strategies informants use to accomplish goals.
- *Relationship codes:* Identify the ways individuals interact and relate to one another.
- *Social structure codes:* Describe the ways individuals interact in groups.

This list is not all-encompassing, but it does give the analyst a lens through which to examine potential patterns and themes in the data.

Table 15.2 A Codebook Excerpt		

Staffing Research: Characteristics of Patients/Families That Affect Workload

Transcript Number:

Coder:

Date Coded:

Theme (Record Phrases Here)	Key Words	Definition: Code Phrases into This Category if They Reflect ...
1.0 Presence	Reassuring Listening Spending time Touching Comforting Offering companionship	A need for a physical presence and actual proximity of the nurse, unrelated to procedures or tasks
2.0 Integrating information	Teaching Acting as liaison Translating Interpreting Explaining Knowing what to expect Educating	An action related to improving knowledge and understanding about either the disease process or ways to achieve health
3.0 Family dynamics	Dysfunctional Poor or limited relationships Alcohol or drug abuse Mental health issues Physical abuse	Family dynamics related to interpersonal interactions and physical or mental problems that affect these interactions
4.0 Physical condition of the patient	New or worsening diagnosis Comorbidity/complexity Pain/anxiety/nausea Life-threatening conditions Chronic conditions	Interpersonal, emotional, and physical conditions that are a result of a presenting or emerging medical problem

Codebook:
A guide for the qualitative analysis that outlines individual codes with definitions, criteria for inclusion, and examples.

Unit of analysis:
The definition of the major entity that will be considered a "subject" for analysis.

Table 15.2 provides an example of a **codebook** for a qualitative study of nursing workload related to caring behaviors. This codebook was developed for the categorization of phrases from transcripts of focus groups of nurses responding to questions about patient and family characteristics that increase workload on a patient care unit of a hospital.

Code the Data

After a codebook has been developed, the analyst then codes the existing data by classifying each unit of analysis into a coded category. This step requires that the researcher determine the unit of analysis within each piece of data. The **unit of analysis** is the most basic segment, or element, of the raw data or information that can be assessed in a meaningful way regarding the phenomenon (Munhall, 2010). A unit of analysis might comprise a word, a phrase, an artifact, a photograph, or a descriptive paragraph. The researcher reviews the data again, this time identifying and labeling each unit of analysis. **Table 15.3** provides an excerpt from a transcript in which the units of analysis—in this case, phrases—have been identified and labeled. This transcript is taken from the study of nursing workload described earlier.

The units of analysis are then reread and categorized into the appropriate code. An example of a coded excerpt appears in **Table 15.4**. Each phrase number is assigned to a specific code in the codebook. By reviewing the transcript, the reader can see how

Table 15.3 An Excerpt from a Transcript
Houser: What are the things that patients depend on you for that you would call caring, not doing?
Nurse: I think one of the big things I see over and over again is that patients and their families rely on us as nurses to be some sort of interpreter between physicians and them. [1] I mean, a lot of us have stood in the room when the doctor leaves and the patient will look at you and say, "Huh? What did he say?" And you know you kind of bring it down to their level [2] and whatnot. So I think one of the things they truly rely on us for other than starting the IV or giving the shot is to be that intermediary, the communicator [3].
Houser: Nurses have called that translating. Or being an interpreter. Is that what you are meaning?
Nurse: Yeah. Yeah. In a sense.
Nurse: Sometimes just sitting in the room.
Nurse: Uh-huh. If you sit, usually if you sit and listen [4], as opposed to standing and listening, that makes a different impression. The time might not be any different. But because you sat, the impression is that you listen, whereas if you stand, sometimes the impression doesn't always come across as that.
Houser: What several of you have said is it requires a presence. This is not something that can be done over the intercom or can be delegated. Are there other things?
Nurse: Specifically taking care of their pain [5] in a timely fashion. Even if you are real busy, pain is real important to people; hunger [6] is only about the next thing.
Nurse: That is really hard to do when you are busy.
Houser: Can you describe some characteristics of patients who seem to need more in the way of caring?
Nurse: Well, I think the patient who grieves in general, and it doesn't necessarily have to be about death. It could be about their own death. Maybe they have just gotten the death sentence. Maybe they lost a body part. [7] I myself and most of the ICU nurses will sit down with that patient [8] and try to draw them out, as far as helping their grief. And often you see their vital signs just get better—just by talking with them and showing them there is another human being who wants to share that pain and grief [9] with them.
Nurse: The families, a lot of families, they have fear, too. And some families bring in baggage [10]. They haven't seen grandma or mom in six months and they got a call from the neighbor, who said, "You know, I think you better go see her." And then they realize maybe they should have seen mom sooner than six months ago. And so they are dealing with the guilt [11].

Table 15.4 A Coded Excerpt

Staffing Research: Characteristics of Patients/Families That Affect Workload

Transcript Number:

Coder:

Date Coded:

Theme (Record Phrases Here)	Key Words	Definition: Code Phrases into This Category If They Reflect ...
1.0 Presence: phrases coded: 4 8	Reassuring Listening Spending time Touching Comforting Offering companionship	A need for a physical presence and actual proximity of the nurse, unrelated to procedures or tasks
2.0 Integrating information: phrases coded: 1 2 3 9	Teaching Acting as liaison Translating Interpreting Explaining Knowing what to expect Educating	An action related to improving knowledge and understanding about either the disease process or ways to achieve health
3.0 Family dynamics: phrases coded: 10 11	Dysfunctional Poor or limited relationships Alcohol or drug abuse Mental health issues Physical abuse	Family dynamics related to interpersonal interactions and physical or mental problems that affect these interactions
4.0 Physical condition of the patient: phrases coded: 5 6 7	New or worsening diagnosis Comorbidity/complexity Pain/anxiety/nausea Life-threatening conditions Chronic conditions	Interpersonal, emotional, and physical conditions that are a result of a presenting or emerging medical problem

phrases are coded into categories of meaning in the codebook. Each identified unit of analysis is assigned to a specific code or placed in a "leftover" category. These leftovers may be used to develop individual codes, or they may be isolated responses that are later ignored. Qualitative analysis is rarely about single instances of occurrences, but rather looks for overall patterns and themes in the data. Codes that have a large number of entries are likely candidates for emerging themes; codes with very few entries should be scrutinized to assess whether they represent common meanings or isolated anecdotes. During the coding process, it is not unusual to require modifications to the code labels, definitions, or key words as new data are constantly compared and analyzed in relation to existing data.

Themes:
Implicit, recurring, and unifying ideas derived from the raw data in qualitative research.

Evaluate the Codes to Identify Overall Themes

The coding process is used both to generate descriptions and to begin interpretation of themes and patterns in the data. Using codes for description results in a detailed rendering of information common to the people, places, or events in the research setting. Descriptive codes are particularly useful in case studies and ethnography.

Identifying themes requires in-depth scrutiny of the codes and the data. As a result of this scrutiny, themes emerge that encompass several codes. A qualitative study may have a substantial number of codes—it is not uncommon for researchers to report anywhere from 10 to 60 codes for an analysis—but only a small number of themes should emerge. Often an analyst will arrive at one central theme, with a small number of subthemes, based on several dozen codes.

Themes are, as the word implies, overall patterns that are recognized in the data through categorization and analysis of individual units of meaning. These common threads appear frequently in the analysis, and they should be fairly self-evident by the end of the laborious analysis process. Themes are not single anecdotes, but rather recurring meanings that appear woven throughout all the data that are collected. It is through identification of these overall themes that qualitative analysis makes its greatest contribution to evidence for nursing practice.

Table 15.5 illustrates how a group of codes may be organized into themes. The themes in this case were the result of a study investigating environmental elements that affect workload on a patient care unit. Conclusions based on recurrent themes are specific enough to be applicable to practice, yet common enough to transfer to other settings and people.

The processes described so far in this chapter are completed as part of one type of general approach to content analysis. This analytic process may be modified, adapted, or otherwise changed when a specific tradition has been employed as a research method. Each of the traditions includes some unique characteristics that must be considered in the

Table 15.5 The Organization of Codes into Themes

Overall	Theme Individual Codes
Leadership	Behaviors support staff work Nurses serve as role models Attitudes that inspire others Skills reduce demand on staff
Expertise of staff	Skill and knowledge in clinical specialty Demonstrates good judgment Committed to quality patient care Patient-centered attitude
Staff stability	Vacant positions Rate of turnover Acquisition of new employees
Resources	Access to financial and material resources for patient care Equipment in working order Enough people, time to get job done

analysis procedures and may be the basis for their customization. **Table 15.6** compares the unique characteristics of three traditions (phenomenology, grounded theory, and ethnography) that require substantial adaptation of the analysis procedure.

Software for Qualitative Analysis

As noted previously, the analysis process involves coding segments of data into meaningful categories and developing overarching themes. This coding process is based on units of analysis that may consist of entire paragraphs of information, so it can become laborious from a practical standpoint. Although this process is often done manually, it may also be computerized.

Computer software for qualitative analysis is less widely available than quantitative analysis software. Often, researchers have no choice except to resort to manual data management; indeed, they follow this path nearly 65% of the time, according to one study (Vaughn & Turnere, 2016). Although it can be a cumbersome, time-consuming undertaking, many qualitative researchers prefer manual analysis because they believe it enables them to remain immersed in the data (Denzin & Lincoln, 2011).

Use of computer-based qualitative analysis continues to inspire controversy among qualitative researchers. Some perceive that a process otherwise viewed as holistic, interpretive, and humanistic becomes mechanical when it is automated. Others voice concerns

Table 15.6 Comparison of Qualitative Analysis Traditions

Tradition	Common Approaches to Analysis	Research Outcome
Phenomenology	Reflection on the data Explication of themes Discernment of patterns that form the essence of the experience	Full, rich description of the essence of a human experience
Grounded theory	*Open coding:* Generating categories of meaning *Axial coding:* Positioning each category in a theoretical model that demonstrates the overall relationships *Selective coding:* Creating a story from the interconnectedness of the categories *Theoretical sampling:* Adding informants as the theory unfolds to illuminate/refute specific conclusions	Integrated, parsimonious theory with concepts that have analytic imagery
Ethnography	Triangulation of multiple sources of information Use of thick description	Well-described cultural scene

that the efficiencies of automation will tempt qualitative researchers to use larger samples and sacrifice depth in favor of breadth (King, 2010; Mavrikis & Geraniou, 2011).

Others believe that using a computer for qualitative analysis makes the process go much more quickly and easily without causing the researcher to lose touch with the data. Computerized analysis may make coding less burdensome, freeing the researcher to find creative ways of looking at the data. By offering assistance in processing, storing, retrieving, cataloging, and sorting through data, software for qualitative analysis leaves the researcher with more time for review and reflection on meaning. Such software allows the transcribed data to be entered and coded based on a dictionary of codes that has been developed by the researcher in an identical manner to one that is manually based (Morris & Ecclesfield, 2011).

Qualitative analysis software provides some very real advantages. Multiple copies of data can be made, so the researcher is not tied to a paper system. Blocks of data can be sorted and moved to other codes, and the relative ease of assigning data to codes may enable the researcher to try several coding schemas before settling on a single one. The capacity to categorize the same data into multiple codes may also help the researcher see patterns that might not emerge when all units of analysis have one exclusive code assigned to them. During the software-based process, automation allows the researcher to maintain the original data in their intact form so that the data can be reread in their context rather than as individual units of analysis. Most computerized systems also have a search capacity, such that they can identify specific words or phrases that support the coding process. Using these systems can enhance the reliability of a qualitative study by applying standard rules that are built into the programs (Bazeley, 2013; Cruz & Higginbottom, 2013; Leech & Onwuegbuzie, 2011; Miles et al., 2013). Table 15.7 lists some of the most widely used qualitative software analysis products, along with their related features.

Table 15.7 Software for Computerized Qualitative Analysis

	Media Accepted	Capability	Analytic Memos
Atlas.ti	Text, graphics, audio, Web, and video	Strings of words, categories, phrases, and individual words	Can be attached to documents, codes, and other memos; can be written for all object types
HyperResearch	Text, graphics, audio, and video	Text searches for phrases or words	One memo per coded segment
MAXqda	Text, .pdf images, audio, and video	Text searches for phrases, words, or memos	Can be attached to text passages or codes
The Ethnograph	Text	Single-code search, linked-code search, identifiers as code searches	Can be attached to a project, data file, or line of text
QSR NVivo10	Text, surveys, social media posts, video, photos, websites	String, category, and text searches	Memos can be linked to documents, passages, or codes

The use of qualitative analysis software is likely to remain the subject of controversy for some time due to the interpretive nature of qualitative inquiry. It is clear, however, that such software can help the researcher complete data analysis more efficiently, while leaving the interpretation of the analysis results to the researcher. Software can sort, document, and copy data with ease, but it cannot yet perform reflection, analysis, and interpretation. Those steps require the human component—that is, a skilled researcher who can reduce a large amount of data to a manageable, meaningful form.

Reliability and Validity: The Qualitative Version

Quantitative researchers are concerned with reliability and validity because the generalization of cause-and-effect findings to populations requires a certain level of evidence based on statistical significance. Applying quantitative standards for reliability and validity to qualitative studies often results in frustration for researchers and a shortage of studies used as evidence for nurses (Turpin, Asano, & Finlayson, 2015). The qualitative researcher should not focus on quantitatively defined indicators of reliability and validity—but that does not mean that application of rigorous standards is not appropriate for evaluating findings from qualitative studies.

Guba and Lincoln (1989) established the classic standards for qualitative research, which call for an overriding emphasis on trustworthiness, or the "true value" of the data that have been collected. These authors recommend that researchers use four criteria to establish the trustworthiness of qualitative conclusions:

- Credibility
- Dependability
- Confirmability
- Transferability

These criteria may seem familiar, because they also apply to design decisions. The discussion here focuses primarily on how trustworthiness is instilled during the analysis process. The qualitative researcher has several means of ensuring that the ability to meet each criterion is evident in a final study.

Credibility of Results

Qualitative researchers are concerned with the credibility of their study results. How confident is the researcher that his or her interpretations represent truth? Several techniques can be used to ensure that credibility exists.

First, a prolonged engagement with the participants in the study supports in-depth analysis. Time is also needed to test interpretations and conclusions for misinformation or misinterpretation. The amount of time spent on these activities should be documented as part of the analytic report.

Second, triangulation is useful to enhance the credibility of the researcher's conclusions. Triangulation occurs when the analyst uses a variety of sources and data to confirm his or her interpretations and conclusions (Denzin & Lincoln, 2011; Thomas & Magilvy, 2011). The researcher should report both the type and the source of triangulated results.

Peer debriefing:
An external check of the credibility of results in which objective peers with expertise in the qualitative method of analysis review and explore various aspects of the data.

Cohen's kappa:
A measure of inter-rater or inter-coder reliability between two raters or coders. The test yields the percentage of agreement and the probability of error.

Inquiry audit:
A review of data and relevant documents, procedures, and results by an external reviewer.

Decision trail:
A detailed description of the researcher's decision rules for data categorization and inferences made in the analysis.

Third, external checks performed on the analysis may establish credibility. One type of check is **peer debriefing.** Peer debriefing involves reviewing methods, procedures, and conclusions with objective peers who have expertise in the study methods or content. In addition to performing peer debriefing, the researcher may ask study participants to validate the preliminary findings and interpretations. Member checking is not used by all qualitative researchers, but it is a solid method for checking the credibility of any themes or categories that the researcher may have identified from data analysis.

Dependability of the Analysis

If the data are not dependable, then the credibility of the qualitative analysis will suffer. In contrast, the dependability of the analysis is supported when multiple raters are able to achieve similar results when applying the codebook to identified units of analysis. Confirming inter-rater reliability or inter-coder reliability is a step taken by qualitative researchers to ensure the dependability of the data analysis. Measures of inter-rater reliability quantify the amount of agreement between two coders who use the same codebook to categorize units of analysis.

Two methods are available to assess qualitative agreements. Simple agreement is the tallying of the percentage of time that both coders agreed on a categorization. **Cohen's kappa** takes this analysis one step further and generates a p value for the probability that random error was responsible for the agreement. Agreement of at least 80% is considered acceptable for qualitative coding, with an associated p value less than 5% that the agreement was due to chance (Fain, 2013).

Considerable controversy surrounds the use of this quantitative method to assess agreement among qualitative raters—or even the need to do so. On a practical level, qualitative studies that have subjected an interpretive process to an objective evaluation are often more widely accepted as evidence by the scientific community. In addition, documenting reliability of a codebook can help later if replication of the study is attempted. A codebook that has been substantiated through measures of inter-rater reliability can confidently be considered a reliable set of codes for future use as a template (Creswell & Clark, 2011).

A less quantitative technique that lends itself to assessing dependability is the **inquiry audit.** In this process, an outside reviewer examines the data and any other relevant documents. An inquiry audit involves asking one or more external research peers to view the data separately and conduct two independent inquiries, during which interpretations and conclusions can be compared (Creswell, 2013).

Confirmability of the Analysis

Confirmability is present when the findings of two or more independent researchers achieve congruence. An inquiry audit can also support confirmability as well as dependability of the analysis. A more widely used method to ensure confirmability, however, is the audit trail. This carefully documented record enables an independent auditor to follow how the researcher arrived at his or her conclusions. To further enhance auditability, the researcher should maintain a **decision trail;** it details the researcher's decision rules for data categorization and the inferences made in the analysis (Fain, 2013).

Transferability of the Findings

When findings from the data can be transferred to other settings or groups, transferability has been achieved. For a study to reach this level, it is imperative that the researcher provide enough information to allow judgments about the context of the data. This information is referred to as thick description—a label that refers to the richness and complete description of the research setting, transactions, and processes observed during the inquiry (Denzin & Lincoln, 2011). Such a deep level of detail enables the reader to draw conclusions about whether the findings can be transferred to a particular set of patients in a specific setting.

Reporting Qualitative Results

A qualitative report, which is often written using the first person voice, is interesting and engaging to read because of the informal writing style and the liberal use of quotations from informants. The report must still provide information about the topic under study, however, and most qualitative researchers reflect on the "fittingness" of the results as well. Fittingness refers to how well the study findings fit the data and are explicitly grounded in the lived experience being investigated. It also reflects both the typical and atypical elements of that experience. References to theoretical and literature support are often used in this context. In addition, direct quotes from the informants may support this aspect of confirmability (Fain, 2013).

One popular way to illustrate and support themes is to use "low-inference descriptors"—that is, examples of participants' verbatim accounts. Integrating quotations from informants within the written report of the findings demonstrates that this portion of the report is grounded in the data. Liberal use of quotations ensures the reader that the author has not "cherry-picked" quotations that support his or her point of view, thereby supporting the study's credibility. When reporting supporting quotations, the researcher should find quotes that represent the feelings and thoughts of all the informants best—not just dramatic or particularly vivid examples that represent a single person's viewpoint (Creswell, 2013).

Conclusions in qualitative reports are generally reported in a similar fashion:

- The sample and setting are described using codes and thick description.
- The main themes and subthemes are identified.
- Each theme and subtheme is described in detail.
- Quotations from informants are used to illustrate the themes and subthemes.
- The overall implications for nursing practice are described.

The last section is where questions are raised as to how these results can apply to practice, education, and research. Which implications do the results have for nursing theory? Which additional aspects of the topic under study need exploration? Did the results generate a hypothesis that might subsequently be tested with a quantitative design? The qualitative report ends with suggestions for future research and should provide sufficient detail that transferability can be assessed.

Reading the Qualitative Analysis Section of a Report

Qualitative analysis is often more difficult and time consuming to accomplish than quantitative analysis, but its report is usually engaging and interesting to read, and it provides intuitive insights into human behavior. Few consistent standards apply to the qualitative analysis process; there are no rules about which test to use or how to interpret an outcome. As a consequence, the qualitative evaluation process is also more difficult and time consuming because it is more challenging to determine whether the author "got it right."

When performing such an evaluation, it is helpful if the research process is transparent so that the reader can trace the decision processes the author used to carry out the study (Bazeley, 2013; Miles et al., 2013). The reader of qualitative research depends on the reporting of the study author to establish the link between data and results. In such a report, there are no numerical tables to review or statistical values to scrutinize—but neither is there an objective way to determine whether the data were interpreted correctly. The qualitative reader, then, is challenged to determine whether a study meets his or her standards for credibility, dependability, confirmability, and transferability. Critique is also difficult because space limitations mean that the researcher can provide only excerpts from the data; the reader must take on faith that the researcher used good judgment when coding the narrative data, eliciting themes, and integrating the findings into a meaningful whole.

The author of a qualitative research report should explicitly identify the approach to data analysis and the specific methods used to accomplish it. The reader should be able to see clear links among the research question, the tradition used to answer it, the data collection procedures, and the analytic process. These should all be consistent and appropriate for the purposes of the study.

When critiquing qualitative analysis, the main objective is to determine whether the researcher used the appropriate process to validate inferences and conclusions. Evidence of bracketing serves to minimize the effects of preconceptions and biases. Purposive sampling and inclusion criteria—and perhaps the presence of theoretical sampling—support the credibility of the study. Documentation of triangulation and measures of inter-rater reliability are helpful in supporting the dependability of the conclusions. Peer debriefing, member checking, and an inquiry audit also increase confidence in the results, and an audit trail supports confirmability. The authors should explicitly describe these procedures and any others used to support confidence in the results.

WHERE TO LOOK FOR QUALITATIVE RESULTS

- The report of qualitative data analysis is typically the third or fourth major heading in a qualitative research report. It is usually easily identified by the title "Results" or "Findings."

- The author should describe the process that was used to analyze the data in the methods section, although it is occasionally reported simultaneously with the results. A reasonably informed reader should be able to reconstruct the analysis process given the author's description.

- If the author used a predetermined schematic, it should be provided in a table or figure. The process for arriving at the schematic should be described in the methods section.
- The report should begin by highlighting the major themes identified and subsequently describe the more detailed codes that make up each theme.
- Some authors use a figure or a table to report all of the themes and associated codes; nevertheless, charts, graphs, and numerical summaries are not typically found in this type of study.
- Each theme should be accompanied with a definition of that theme and a list of associated codes. Direct quotes from informants should be presented to illustrate and support each reported theme. Examples of verbatim responses are expected for each code, and liberal use of quotes is one method of ensuring trustworthiness.
- The methods used to establish the credibility, dependability, and confirmability of the results should be described thoroughly, although this description is not found in a standard location in the report. Approaches to establishing reliability can be described in the methods, in the results, or even in the conclusions. Multiple methods are often used to ensure the overall trustworthiness of each element.

CHECKLIST FOR EVALUATING QUALITATIVE RESULTS

- ❏ The report of the sample provides enough details to judge the adequacy and characteristics of the sample.
- ❏ The procedure used to analyze the data is described in sufficient detail.
- ❏ The reader can trace the decision processes that the author used to carry out the study (for example, via an audit trail or a decision trail).
- ❏ The analytic method used is appropriate for the qualitative tradition/design.
- ❏ The authors report methods for ensuring the following:
  - Credibility of the findings
  - Dependability of the methods
  - Confirmability of the conclusions
- ❏ Sufficient descriptions and reports of the sample are provided to ensure appropriate transferability.

Using Qualitative Analysis in Nursing Practice

The results of qualitative studies can be applied in nursing practice in a variety of ways. These data provide rich insights into the experiences of patients, their families, and other caregivers. Using the results of qualitative studies in practice requires that the nurse be able to critically appraise the transferability of the data. The nurse must review the descriptions of the setting and the informants to determine whether they are similar enough for the results of the study to be confidently applied to another group of individuals.

The nurse reader should focus on the themes elicited in the study to determine the research's applicability to evidence-based practice. These themes often provide guidance in the development of counseling procedures, teaching plans, discharge preparation, and other means of helping patients manage their health. Results of case research can help nurses understand how individuals may experience threats to their health, uncommon conditions, or exacerbations of their disease states. Phenomenology facilitates an understanding of how patients experience events and situations, enabling the nurse to design better supports for them. Ethnography can assist the nurse in designing culturally sensitive care. Grounded theory, in particular, helps the nurse understand and analyze situations, so as to predict changes in them and to influence outcomes.

Regardless of the type of qualitative study undertaken, the results should be scrutinized for trustworthiness to determine which findings can be used in evidence-based practice. The analysis should be subjected to the same critical review. In other words, the study should satisfy general assumptions about the evidence and withstand scrutiny of the methodological quality of the analysis.

Henderson and Rheault (2004) support the use of qualitative results in evidence-based practice, but they also recommend that a stricter standard be applied to qualitative analyses that will be used as evidence for practice. They propose the following criteria for determining whether to include qualitative results in a practice guideline:

- The methods of analysis should be described in detail.
- Two or more researchers should independently judge the data.
- Triangulation of data sources, methods, or investigators should be evident.
- A code–recode procedure should be described.
- Peer examination or external audit should be reported.

In addition, these authors recommend rating qualitative results in much the same way that results of experiments are rated using levels and grades. Based on the four elements of trustworthiness (credibility, dependability, confirmability, and transferability), levels of qualitative evidence can be linked to recommendations. **Table 15.8** identifies the levels of qualitative evidence and associated strength of recommendations that are suggested to integrate qualitative analyses into practice.

Leeman and Sandelowski (2012) offer additional guidance for incorporating qualitative research into evidence-based practice. They suggest that qualitative inquiry has a critical role in providing solid evidence that will enhance quality care to help ensure compliance with treatment plans, explain unintended consequences, and support positive patient outcomes. Following the critical appraisal of qualitative studies, research found to be credible can be used as practice-based evidence in six specific areas:

- *Practice-based interventions and implementation strategies:* Revealing untested but promising interventions
- *Causal mechanisms:* Exploration of underlying mechanisms affecting patient outcomes
- *Approaches to adaptation:* Understanding how nurses adapt strategies to diverse practice settings
- *"How to" guidance:* Revealing the steps required to implement an intervention, including barriers and facilitators
- *Unanticipated effects:* Unexpected consequences of an intervention at both patient and system levels
- *Contextual factors:* Provider willingness, capacity, and need for a new intervention

Table 15.8 Decision Rules for Incorporating Qualitative Research into Evidence-Based Nursing Practice

Decision	Considerations
The study satisfies general requirements for inclusion in an integrative review.	The journal in which the research appears is peer reviewed. The problem addressed in the study meets the inclusion criteria for the review.
The study meets screening criteria as a qualitative study.	The study involves observation of social problems in a naturalistic setting. The researchers interpret the data to arrive at conclusions. Observations are linked to theory. Researchers adhere to ethical guidelines for research involving human subjects.
The level of evidence is evaluated based on standards for trustworthiness.	Level 1: Meets the standards for credibility, transferability, dependability, and confirmability. Level 2: Meets three of the four standards. Level 3: Meets two of the four standards. Level 4: Meets one of the four standards. Level 5: Does not meet any of the standards.
The strength of recommendations is based on the quality of the evidence.	Grade A: Recommended; supported by one or more Level 1 studies. Grade B: Optional; supported by at least one Level 2 study. Grade C: Optional; supported by multiple Level 3 or 4 studies.

Adapted with permission from Henderson, R., & Rheault, W. (2004). Appraising and incorporating qualitative research in evidence-based practice. *Journal of Physical Therapy Education, 18*(3), 35–40.

Creating Qualitative Analyses

There are few rules for qualitative analyses; however, following some general guidelines can help the novice researcher conduct a trustworthy analysis that results in meaningful themes:

- *Establish the goal of the analysis.* The design of the study will provide guidance as to the overall goal of the analysis. The goal of analysis may be to determine content, find meaning, describe a culture, or develop a theory. Beginning the analytic process with a general goal provides the analyst with direction and structure as the analysis proceeds.
- *Organize the data.* There will almost certainly be an enormous amount of data to manage, so developing an organizational system early in the qualitative analysis process helps keep this process manageable. Determine a way to identify each piece of data by source, timing, and type as it is collected, and store all data in a secure location.

Margin notes:
Reflective notes
manually inserted into
qualitative transcripts
that describe ideas
about meaning that
occur to the analyst
during reading.

Dictionary:
Specified definitions
of codes included
in the qualitative
analysis codebook.

- *Begin analysis early*. Data should be evaluated and analyzed as they are collected. This constant-comparison method enables the researcher to make changes in the data collection plan while informants are still available.
- *Read individual pieces of data in their entirety for tone*. The first read-through of a data source should be undertaken purely to get a sense of the tone of the overall response, not for analysis.
- *Reread each piece of data for meaning*. Subsequent readings begin to reveal meaning. As the data are examined, analytic-oriented notes should be written in the margins of transcripts, and relevant quotations and examples should be identified. At this stage, the analyst will begin identifying units of analysis such as words, phrases, or entire documents for later analytic coding.
- *Develop codes*. Potential categories for codes were introduced earlier in this chapter. During this phase of analysis, units of meaning are categorized into codes.

Data may be coded in an infinite number of ways, but Creswell (2013) provides some structural guidance for this process. His approach includes the following steps:

1. Select a document from the data.
2. Reread the document to get a sense of the whole. Ask questions, such as "What is this about?" The concern at this point is not substance, but rather underlying meaning. Write thoughts in the margins. These **margin notes** should describe the ideas about meaning that come to mind while reading the data.
3. Make a list of all the ideas that have been written in the margins. Cluster together the ideas that have similarities. Organize these topics into columns such as "major topics," "unique topics," or "leftovers."
4. Take the list and revisit the data. Note which segments of the data represent each of these categories. Evaluate this preliminary organizing schematic to see if the codes capture most of the data segments. Review multiple pieces of data to determine whether the code categories are sufficient or whether additional categories emerge.
5. Find the most descriptive label for each topic and turn it into a category. Write a definition for it and identify representative words in the informants' language.
6. Group topics that are redundant, overlapping, or reflective of similar concepts. Look for ways to reduce the total list of categories.
7. Label the final categories of meaning, and develop a codebook that outlines each code, its definition, and any criteria for placing data into the category. The result of this process leads to the development of a **dictionary** to guide the further analysis of the remaining data.[1]

Once all data have been coded, the analyst scrutinizes the data for overall themes. These themes are identified and reported, with supporting quotations from informants being supplied as well. Qualitative analysis is complete when no new codes or themes emerge from data analysis.

---

[1]Modified from Creswell, J. W. (2013). *Qualitative inquiry and research design: Choosing among five approaches*. Thousand Oaks, CA: Sage. Reproduced with permission of SAGE Publications Inc.

Summary of Key Concepts

- The sheer volume of data that is characteristic of qualitative inquiry creates challenges related to both managing data and drawing sensible conclusions.
- The goal is to reduce the data to meaningful units that can be described, interpreted, and reported in an understandable way.
- Qualitative analysis is challenging because no standard rules exist for interpreting the data that are generated, and concise conclusions must be drawn while retaining the rich description that is a qualitative characteristic.
- Although not standard, some steps apply to most qualitative analysis:
  1. Prepare the data for analysis.
  2. Conduct the analysis by developing an in-depth understanding of the data.
  3. Represent the data in reduced form.
  4. Interpret the larger meaning of the data.
- As data are collected, they are reviewed and re-reviewed, and analytic memos are written. Using this kind of constant-comparison process allows the analysis to guide subsequent data collection, with the researcher amending or adding interview questions or changing observational methods based on the results.
- The three general styles of qualitative analysis are template analysis, editing analysis, and immersion/crystallization analysis.
- To make sense of the narrative data, a method of managing and organizing the information must be established early in the research process.
- After gaining a general impression from a first read-through of the data, the researcher develops a classification system.
- Upon the conclusion of an intense examination of the data and the development of an overall classification schematic, the researcher develops more specific categories of meaning called codes.
- Units of analysis, such as a phrase, word, or document, are categorized into specific codes that reflect overall meaning.
- The coding process is used both to generate descriptions and to begin interpretation of themes and patterns in the data.
- The most widely used qualitative analysis procedure is simple content analysis. This method may be adapted to the specific research tradition used, such as ethnography, phenomenology, or grounded theory.
- The use of automated systems for coding continues to inspire controversy but is also becoming more common. Computerized systems for coding can enhance reliability of the data, although researchers must be careful not to substitute breadth for depth of analysis.
- Standards have been established to determine the trustworthiness of qualitative data analysis—namely, credibility, dependability, confirmability, and transferability.
- Qualitative results are reported as themes, supported by their descriptive codes and verbatim reports from informants. Quotes should be used that represent patterns, not individual anecdotes.

CRITICAL APPRAISAL EXERCISE

Retrieve the following full-text article from the Cumulative Index to Nursing and Allied Health Literature or similar search database:

Zamanzadeh, V., Jasemi, M., Valizadeh, L., Keogh, B., & Taleghani, F. (2015). Effective factors in providing holistic care: A qualitative study. *Indian Journal of Palliative Care, 21*(2), 214–224.

Review the article, focusing on the sections that report the analytic procedures and results. Consider the following appraisal questions in your critical review of this research article:

1. What is the specific design used for this research study? Was the design explicit in the article? Would you describe it in the same way?
2. What was the sample for this study? How were the subjects selected for recruitment?
3. Describe the data collection strategies. Were they appropriate for the study objectives?
4. Describe the procedure used for analysis. In what ways did this approach support the credibility and trustworthiness of the results?
5. Was the coding scheme emergent or predetermined?
6. What was appropriate about the reporting format? How could it have been strengthened?
7. Appraise the strength of this research as evidence for practice. In what ways could these findings be applied to nursing care?

References

Bazeley, P. (2013). *Qualitative data analysis: Practical strategies.* Thousand Oaks, CA: Sage.

Creswell, J. W. (2013). *Qualitative inquiry and research design: Choosing among five approaches.* Thousand Oaks, CA: Sage.

Creswell, J. W., & Clark, V. L. (2011). *Designing and conducting mixed methods research.* Thousand Oaks, CA: Sage.

Cruz, E. V., & Higginbottom, G. (2013). The use of focused ethnography in nursing research. *Nurse Researcher, 20*(4), 36–43.

De Chesnay, M. (2015). *Nursing research using ethnography: Qualitative designs and methods in nursing.* New York, NY: Springer.

Denzin, N. K., & Lincoln, Y. S. (2011). *Qualitative research.* Thousand Oaks, CA: Sage.

Fain, J. (2013). *Reading, understanding, and applying nursing research* (4th ed.). Philadelphia, PA: F. A. Davis.

Guba, E., & Lincoln, Y. (1989). *Fourth generation evaluation.* Newbury Park, CA: Sage.

Henderson, R., & Rheault, W. Q. (2004). Appraising and incorporating qualitative research into evidence-based practice. *Journal of Physical Therapy Education, 17*(3), 35–40.

Jackson, D., Hutchinson, M., Luck, L., & Wilkes, L. (2013). Mosaic of verbal abuse experienced by nurses in their everyday work. *Journal of Advanced Nursing, 69*(9), 2066–2075.

King, A. (2010). "Membership matters": Applying membership categorisation analysis (MCA) to qualitative data using computer-assisted qualitative data analysis (CAQDAS) software. *International Journal of Social Research Methodology, 13*(1), 1–16.

Leech, N. L., & Onwuegbuzie, A. J. (2011). Beyond constant comparison qualitative data analysis: Using NVivo. *Social Psychology Quarterly, 26*(1), 70–84.

Leeman, J., & Sandelowski, M. (2012). Practice-based evidence and qualitative inquiry. *Journal of Nursing Scholarship, 44*(2), 171–179.

Mavrikis, M., & Geraniou, E. (2011). Using qualitative data analysis software to analyse students' computer-mediated interactions: The case of MiGen and Transana. *International Journal of Social Research Methodology, 14*(3), 245–252.

Miles, M. B., Huberman, A. M., & Saldana, J. (2013). *Qualitative data analysis: A methods sourcebook* (3rd ed.). Thousand Oaks, CA: Sage.

Morris, D., & Ecclesfield, N. (2011). A new computer-aided technique for qualitative document analysis. *International Journal of Research and Method in Education, 34*(3), 241–245.

Munhall, P. (2010). *Nursing research: A qualitative perspective* (5th ed.). Sudbury, MA: Jones and Bartlett.

Thomas, E., & Magilvy, J. K. (2011). Qualitative rigor or research validity in qualitative research. *Pediatric Nursing, 16*, 151–155.

Thorne, S., Stephens, J., & Truant, T. (2016). Building qualitative study design using nursing's disciplinary epistemology. *Journal of Advanced Nursing, 72*(2), 451–460.

Turpin, M. J., Asano, M., & Finlayson, M. (2015). Combining qualitative and quantitative data collection and analysis methods in understanding multiple sclerosis fatigue management. *International Journal of Qualitative Methods, 14*(2), 53–68.

Vaughn, P., & Turnere, C. (2016). Decoding via coding: Analyzing qualitative text data through coding and survey methodologies. *Journal of Library Administration, 56*, 41–51.

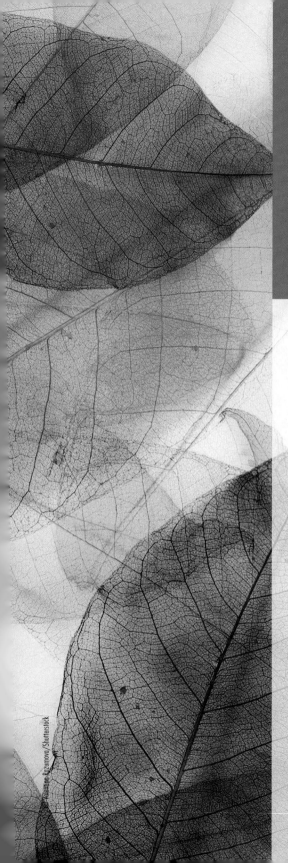

Part VII

Research Translation

16 Translating Research into Practice

Chapter 16

Translating Research into Practice

CHAPTER OBJECTIVES

The study of this chapter will help the learner to

- Verbalize the relationship between nursing research and nursing practice.
- Describe areas where research can be used to resolve issues in practice.
- Communicate research findings to the broader professional community.
- Describe the submission steps for a manuscript, podium, or poster presentation.
- Discuss methods to aggregate research as evidence for nursing practice.
- Explain strategies for implementing a research program in a health organization.
- Compare six models for knowledge translation.

KEY TERMS

Integrative review	Practice guidelines	Systematic review
Meta-analysis	Qualitative meta-synthesis	

Introduction

The best research starts with the words "I wonder." Curiosity motivates the process. Designs help researchers answer the following questions: "What is going on now?" "Which nursing interventions are effective?" "How do people feel about this?" Statistics answer the logical next question: "Are you sure about that?" After all of these questions have been asked and answered, the most important question is left for last: "Can we use this knowledge to improve someone's life?" Research without application is a tremendous amount of work for nothing. Even the most theoretical research is used to build models that will, eventually, benefit patients or the nurses who care for them. Our shared profession does not benefit from contributions to knowledge that are never put to use. Translating research into practice, then, is the final and most important step in the research process; it is vital for the progress of evidence-based practice (EBP) (Drolet & Lorenzi, 2011).

Other chapters have described methods of critiquing and conducting research. This chapter turns to the relationship of research to nursing practice. Even well-designed and

© Valentina Razumova/Shutterstock

executed research studies do not help patients in and of themselves. Instead, research as evidence is helpful only when it is translated into nursing practice. Wallace, Byrne, and Clarke (2012) argue that "the gap between what we know and what we do undermines the benefits realized from advances in healthcare science" (p. 339). As the accessibility of research and evidence for practice has increased, so has the need to ensure that knowledge translation occurs. Nurses are being asked both to provide the evidence for patient care and to translate existing research knowledge into practice. This paradigm shift is one that is affecting all healthcare professions. The heightened demand for benefit from research has driven such initiatives as the National Institutes of Health's (NIH) Roadmap and the Clinical Translational Science Awards, as well as increased requests for NIH and Agency for Healthcare Research and Quality (AHRQ) grants to support studies of translational efforts (Woods & Magyary, 2010).

Many driving forces conspired to create the current climate. Whenever change is instituted, plans for reducing resistance to that change and methods of facilitating strengths and capitalizing on opportunities must be considered. New skill sets—deeply rooted in systematically generated evidence—are needed by nurses at all levels of experience and in almost all clinical settings.

VOICES FROM THE FIELD

As facilitator of a grant-funded home health project, I was responsible for leading a collaborative group of home care leaders charged with creating a sustainable, stable nursing workforce for the agencies. Gathered around the table were stakeholders from practice and academia. They represented organizations that were competing for the same scarce resources, while challenged to recruit enough qualified home care nurses to meet their patients' care needs. The harsh reality of the situation was that some of the home care agencies were already experiencing diversion of patients to other agencies because of an inadequate supply of competent nursing staff. The urgency for a quick solution was evident. These leaders were faced with reducing unnecessary hospital readmissions, ensuring their patients had access to care, and meeting increasing demands for documentation—and doing it all within a challenging economy and a dramatically changing industry. Asking home care executives to slow down and collaborate with their competitors to find a solution was extremely challenging. One CEO said, "My organization is bleeding and you are asking me to take off the only Band-Aid I have to wait until you collect data. Are you serious?"

I met with our external evaluator, an established nurse researcher, and presented our challenges. I was certain that if we could collect the right evidence and translate it into language the executives understood, we could demonstrate a return on investment worthy of their time and resources. The researcher suggested a novel approach to analyze turnover data—survival analysis. This tool is usually reserved for medical studies, but if you thought of retention as "surviving" the first few years of employment, it made sense. This approach allowed our group to examine turnover in a statistically sound way, and helped identify risk points for losing new nurses. I could see the value of these data; they produced actionable information that could immediately be translated into strategies for reducing turnover. I was further intrigued by the researcher's suggestion that we calculate the actual cost of recruiting, hiring, and orienting a new home care nurse as evidence of the true cost of instability of the workforce. This effort helped the executives appreciate the costs of not using the evidence to reduce turnover, and it gave us a basis for determining the return on investment of support systems developed during the grant period.

A quote from Benjamin Franklin has been a memorable touchstone for me: "Tell me and I forget. Teach me and I remember. Involve me and I learn." I knew the only way to have a long-term impact in this chaotic environment was to involve the stakeholders in every step of the research. It was also apparent that we needed a mix of evidence; both quantitative measures and qualitative themes would help us understand the challenges we faced in trying to stabilize this workforce. We conducted an extensive search of the literature, collected surveys from both practice and academic members of the collaborative, conducted focus groups to find recurrent themes about workforce challenges, and interviewed individual partners. The agencies provided us with historical workforce data related to their voluntary terminations. Using a formula we found in the literature, we examined hiring and orientation processes of these agencies and calculated both direct and indirect costs. Based on these data, our researcher was able to calculate the actual cost of an unstable workforce and predict the amount of time before a home care nurse could be considered productive enough to recapture hiring and orientation costs. Using this evidence, we calculated the true cost of workforce instability for each partner agency, and we were able to show them how much money they could save if they reduced turnover. This information was not just helpful at the project level: The survival analysis provided each agency with individualized evidence of the risk points for losing new employees. The findings were dramatic—one agency was losing half of its new employees within six months. The study results made an impact and got the attention of the leaders of the agencies. The real-time individualized data created a significant spark for change, and motivated the agencies to examine their recruitment and orientation processes.

We followed up with periodic presentations of the research evidence as it was generated. This stimulated dialogue among the collaborative partners that helped them understand the implications of the data for their agency. The home care leaders began making recruitment and hiring changes based on the evidence. They adapted their orientation programs, created coordinated coaching and mentoring programs, and implemented cohort support groups for new hires. They enhanced these efforts at times just before the identified risk points for loss. Their goal was to provide support to new hires, enhance their confidence, and, they hoped, hang on to their nurses. The strategies identified as a result of this evidence are beginning to stop the bleeding and have created a sustainable impact.

With the help of the nurse researcher, we were able to involve our partners throughout the entire evidence-gathering process to help them learn, motivate action, and generate meaningful, sustainable outcomes. Collecting data together and reviewing those data's meaning through dialogue was powerful in motivating immediate change. Using evidence in this way engaged researchers, academics, and practitioners in the collaboration, and helped explain the results in a language that was understandable, relevant, and timely for our partners. In this case, there was a direct relationship between the use of evidence and a change in practice. In the end, the grant created a significant collective impact that will ultimately ensure that patients are cared for by a competent, stable workforce.

Deborah Center, MSN, RN, CNS

The Nurse's Role in Knowledge Translation

Translational research entails the transformation of scientific findings into interventions that are widespread and improve patient care (Layde et al., 2012). This complex process requires both research activities and implementation efforts. The pathway of translational research was originally envisioned as unidirectional, moving from research laboratory to practice. Callard, Rose, and Wykes (2011) argue, however, that translational research should be visualized as a loop, rather than as a linear process. Indeed, there is growing awareness that practitioners must provide feedback to researchers if their work is to ultimately benefit patients. Researchers need to understand much more about how the interventions they test actually benefit patients. It is far from guaranteed that research findings will reach those persons whom they were intended to help; involving both practitioners and researchers in translational processes ensures that everyone will benefit.

Nurses are in a unique position to foster the translation of research into practice. Woods and Magyary (2010) identified two critical skills for knowledge translation: team science and transdisciplinary efforts. In the past, traditional models of research dissemination involved researchers working in isolation, focusing on a single problem grounded in a single discipline, and sharing information only when the research was complete. By comparison, contemporary models of research have been transformed into teams of investigators representing diverse disciplines that are better able to investigate multidimensional patient problems. True transdisciplinary work requires understanding the contributions made by the relevant disciplines, integrating their individual perspectives, and focusing on a shared problem. Nurses are often central figures in organizing and leading these transdisciplinary research teams and, therefore, are capable facilitators of knowledge translation.

Contemporary research translation requires a variety of methods for gathering data that are relevant for clinicians. Ensuring that interventions will be acceptable to patients necessitates a focus on more than quantitative analysis. Attention to the acceptability and desirability of evidence-based treatments is also needed. The nursing profession has long relied on mixed methods of inquiry, so mixing research paradigms is not a foreign concept to members of this discipline. Indeed, integrative reviews—or the systematic evaluation of both quantitative and qualitative studies in determining practice guidelines—were embraced early on by the nursing profession.

A key element of research translation, though, relies on the human component. A growing body of evidence suggests that a therapeutic alliance between caregiver and patient may be the most important predictor of intervention success. Partnership building and effective communication with patients are proving to be some of the most significant predictors of successful treatment outcomes (Woods & Magyary, 2010). Nurses are in a unique position to ensure that emphasis is placed on how relationships contribute to the effects of treatments when translating evidence-based clinical guidelines, protocols, and standard order sets. This role may be particularly important in culturally diverse populations.

Identifying Problems for Knowledge Translation

Problems that are suitable for knowledge translation may be identified in a multitude of ways. Direct patient care, patient and colleague questions, conferences, journals, hospital and other healthcare delivery agency data, professional organizations, government agency research priorities, and quality reports can all generate inquiries. In daily nursing practice, nurses face problems that are easily translated into questions that can be answered with research evidence.

Patient questions and outcomes can also prompt the identification of EBP problems. Focus groups of patients, which are often convened for marketing purposes, can be a means of identifying these issues. Follow-up calls with patients after discharge can elicit areas ripe for research to prevent readmission. Conferences and journals can be wonderful sources of both information and research questions. Studies can be replicated and presented at conferences; such presentations provide an opportunity to interact with researchers in an informal way. Professional organizations and government agencies, such as those involved in the *Healthy People 2020* initiative, often have research priorities that are also good sources of EBP problems.

Another excellent source of translational research questions is the patient care report. Length of stay for various diagnoses, nosocomial problems, and patient safety issues are only a few issues that become apparent in the unit report.

Knowledge translation cannot occur if studies have not been communicated to a broad audience and combined with like evidence to create strong practices. The first step is to find an appropriate target for communicating research findings, and to use posters, podium presentations, or publication to disseminate recommendations. The second step is to aggregate these individual studies into compelling practice guidelines.

Communicating Research Findings

Part of the purpose of research—applied or otherwise—is to make a contribution to the body of empirical knowledge that serves as the foundation of a profession. There are many ways to communicate research so that it can be incorporated into practice. Local, regional, and national conferences often solicit both poster and podium presentations, and journals are always receptive to solid research studies on relevant clinical topics. Contrary to what many clinicians may think, journals are often anxious to publish reports by staff-level practitioners, because those closest to clinical processes are often in the best position to determine how to improve them.

Inexperienced researchers may worry that their work is not sophisticated or important enough for publication or presentation. In reality, good work is good work, no matter who performs it. The process of getting a research study reviewed is a systematic one that can be completed by any researcher, seasoned or novice. For the new researcher, a common approach to communicating research results is to first submit research for peer review as a poster in a regional or national conference. The researcher can then submit research for podium presentations and, finally, for publication in a peer-reviewed journal. Regardless of the venue chosen for peer review, the basic steps followed are the same.

Finding the Right Audience

The first step in communicating the findings of a research study is to select the right audience for the work. The target audience should be carefully considered before writing the abstract or preparing the manuscript. The best venue for reporting results is one that has a clearly defined focus that fits with the goal of the research. Some research studies have a clearly defined audience—a study on reducing infections would obviously be appropriate for conferences and journals that focus on infection control—but others may have less obvious audiences. In the latter case, the researcher may have to dig a little deeper to find the appropriate venue for presenting the study results. Some journals publish lists of priorities or solicitations for articles on their webpages or in the journal itself. Conferences generally identify an overall theme, and include a list of conference objectives or goal statements that cover the types of information that are of interest. The more closely the study topic is matched with a topic of interest for the journal or conference, the more likely the submission is to be successful.

The best audience is one that can put the research results into practice. Many clinical conferences or periodicals, for example, provide access to the clinicians who are in the best position to apply research results on a day-to-day basis.

Preparation of an Abstract

Conferences have very specific requirements for submissions from would-be presenters, including those related to spacing, margins, and method of submission of the initial document. The form for submission generally requires an abstract of the work, which conference organizers use to make decisions about acceptance for a poster or podium presentation. An abstract is a summary of the most important aspects of the research. An abstract also appears in the beginning of a publication and as a summary in searchable databases, so it should be constructed carefully.

The researcher should pay particular attention to limits on the number of words and to the deadlines for the submission. The personnel who screen submissions for reviewers often discard abstracts that violate the fundamental instructions; thus an abstract may not reach reviewers if it is too long or in the wrong format. Submissions after the deadline are generally not reviewed at all, so abstracts absolutely must reach the conference organizers prior to the deadline.

The abstract of the research study is the only description that most conference reviewers will see, and it may be the first description that a journal editor sees, so it should be clear, compelling, and concise. The abstract should report the most important elements of the research in a way that generates interest and even excitement about the project. Think of the abstract as an advertisement for the research, focusing on the strongest points and most interesting findings.

The submission guidelines will include a limit for the number of words or even characters permitted in the abstract. Some guidelines limit the abstract to as few as 100 words, whereas others allow up to 500 words. Because exceeding the word length generally results in the submission being screened out, meeting this requirement is a critical consideration.

If no specific guidelines are provided for the submission, use the generally accepted standards for what is included; they appear in **Table 16.1**. It helps to put each required element as a heading in bold font so that the reviewer can find the various sections easily and determine that all are present without having to read the submission multiple times.

The most successful authors write the abstract, and then edit it multiple times until the necessary word length is achieved. At all times, it is critical to focus on the results and their implications for practice. The abstract should provide the most important information that communicates the study's strengths and usefulness.

The peer review process can take from two weeks to several months to unfold. When an abstract is accepted, the real work of preparing the presentation begins.

Table 16.1 Anatomy of an Abstract	
Element	**Specific Guidelines**
Introduction	• Begin simply, usually with no more than a sentence or two. • Explain why this research is important. • Include provocative sentences or an interesting lead-in that will "grab" the readers so they will want to read the whole abstract. • Call this section "Introduction," "Summary," or "Background."
Objective	• Report the primary purpose of the study; this can be one or two sentences that describe the aim of the study in detail. • If the research question is a restatement of the purpose statement, do not include both. • If the purpose is achieved with an unconventional research question, then include both. • Call this section "Objective," "Purpose," or "Aims."
Methods	• Describe the design of the study, the methods used to achieve the purpose, and the procedures applied to control internal validity. • Include the sampling strategy and the analytic plan. • Identify the independent and dependent variables, which may also be called "predictors" and "outcomes," respectively. • Present enough detail so the reader understands the fundamental process for the research, but do not overload the readers with details. • Include only minimal statistics; these usually include at least the sample size and the calculated power. • Explicitly identify the actual statistical tests that were run.
Results	• Summarize the most important results (whether they were statistically significant or not). • Keep in mind that a lack of effect may be as important as the presence of an effect. • Report some statistical results here, but limit them to test statistics and associated p values. • Do not use this section to comment on the meaning of the results—simply report them.
Conclusions	• Focus on the most important implications of the findings and the usefulness for practice. • Address application issues here.

The Compelling Poster Presentation

A poster presentation at a conference is a research report presented as a visual display so that it can be read and viewed by large groups of professionals in an informal setting. The author stands near the poster at specified times to discuss the details of the research and answer questions. A poster presentation gives the author an opportunity to interact with conference participants and discuss the research. Poster presentations are a good place for a novice researcher to start the communication process because they are less intimidating than a podium presentation and require less preparation than a formal manuscript. Nevertheless, abstracts for poster presentations are peer reviewed and accepted based on merit, so they require the researcher to begin the scholarly review process that is the hallmark of professional research.

Once an abstract has been accepted as a poster presentation, the process of poster development begins. The elements of the poster must be chosen, developed, and translated into physical form. Allow adequate time for this process; it requires the help of specialists in both research and media development, and time is required for others to make their contributions.

Each conference will have specific requirements for the size of the poster, the length of time it can be displayed, and the amount of time the author is expected to be present. A researcher should take advantage of all the space available for the poster and plan to be present whenever allowed to maximize exposure and communication of the findings.

The purpose of a poster is to translate ideas and images into graphic form, and a good poster will show viewers what was done instead of telling them (Hedges, 2010). It is helpful to develop a mock-up of the poster using graph paper and sticky notes to get an idea of which layout will be most effective as well as how much space is needed for each element.

The poster should serve as a stand-alone description of the research. The researcher should determine the information that is critical to understanding the study and its clinical implications; good poster development begins with this content and expands on it as space allows. The usual components of a poster are as follows:

- *Introduction.* The introduction attracts attention to the poster, summarizes the identified need for the research, and describes the significance of the study. Statistics reporting the prevalence of the clinical problem and the clinical implications are helpful for meeting these criteria.
- *Research purpose and question.* The purpose statement and research question help focus the study and identify the exact aim of the work.
- *Methods and design.* This section should include a concise description of the design, procedures, measures, and analytic tests used in the study.
- *Results.* Results should be presented primarily in visual form using tables or graphs, with limited text.
- *Conclusions.* Although brief, the conclusions are the heart of the poster. This section should highlight the most important findings and implications for clinicians.
- *Acknowledgments.* It is appropriate to include recognition of staff who helped with the research or the poster and the sponsors of the project. Also note sources of funding that supported the project.
- *References.* A brief references list, focusing on the most important citations, can be included at the end of the poster.

FIGURE 16.1 represents the typical layout of a poster, with associated text font sizes and content. Of course, there are infinite ways to lay out a poster so that it is readable and draws the viewer in to find out more. A poster can be an effective way to interact with those conference attendees who are interested in the research and to present the study in an informal setting. Podium presentations, by comparison, provide the opportunity to reach a large audience in a relatively short period of time, while providing more information than is possible in a poster presentation.

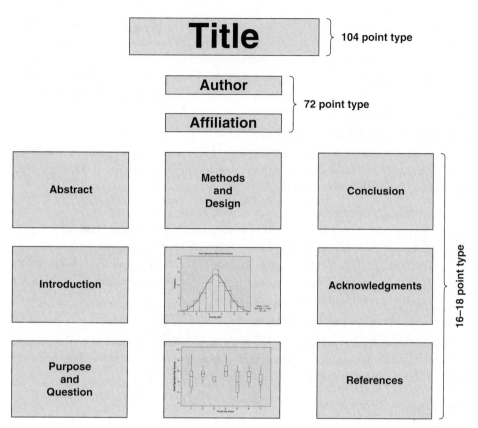

FIGURE 16.1 Anatomy of a Poster Presentation

An Effective Research Presentation

The communication skills that are needed to present research effectively are no different from those needed for any type of group presentation: effective preparation, practice, and focused content development. To prepare for a podium presentation, the researcher needs to know the type of talk that is expected, the composition of the audience, the amount of time allotted, and the objectives for the presentation.

Which Type of Presentation Is Expected?

Types of research presentations can vary from informal roundtable discussions to highly formalized keynote speeches. The kind of presentation will drive the content, as different types of presentations have different objectives. Presentations at general clinical conferences will be focused on practice implications, for example, whereas presentations for research conferences may focus on methods and procedures. The goals of the conference can help guide the particular focus of the presentation.

Who Will Be the Audience for the Presentation?

The composition of the audience will drive the development of the presentation. Whether the audience is composed of generalists or specialists will dictate the level of detail provided. How many participants are present and where they come from is also important—an international audience needs a different presentation style than a domestic one. It is also helpful to know how the audience members may apply the information, and whether they will focus on the usefulness of the information rather than theoretical considerations. An in-depth knowledge of the audience will help the researcher customize the presentation to a particular set of needs, resulting in a better response on the part of the attendees and a greater chance of research utilization.

What Are the Presentation Objectives?

Research results should be presented logically. Most research presentations are brief, so a researcher has to focus on those points that are the most important. The following outline is a suggested format for a podium presentation:

- An introduction to the problem or clinical issue
- The purpose or primary aim of the research and the research question
- Design of the study, including a description of the methods and procedures
- The findings from the study, including the type of analysis and the major results
- A discussion of the results, including the major limitations, as well as the most important findings for clinical practice
- Implications for future research and for clinical practice

The relationship between each stage of the research should be clear to the listener. The conclusion should summarize the overall importance of the study, the main concepts discussed, and the major implications for practice.

Planning for Publication

Poster and podium presentations reach an audience that goes beyond a single university or organization. Even so, the number of people who can learn about and use the research findings is limited to those who are physically present. Publication in a professional journal, by comparison, ensures that the research reaches the largest target audience. This kind of publication is an attainable goal even for novice researchers.

The first step is to find an appropriate journal for the research report. The journal should be selected before the manuscript is written so that it can be tailored appropriately to the readers. Reviewing several articles from journals that are being considered can be very helpful in this regard. Journal websites provide authors with directions for submitting manuscripts and for monitoring the peer review process. These instructions are generally straightforward and labeled "directions for authors" or "authors' guidelines." They provide valuable information for preparing an acceptable manuscript. If specifics are not provided by the journal, the author can follow the guidelines in Table 16.2, which describes the most common elements of a research manuscript.

The review process generally takes from 4 to 12 weeks. A request for revision should not be viewed as a disappointment—most authors are asked to revise their submissions prior to full acceptance for publication. Some requests for revision may be substantial, but should not be viewed as a rejection. The successful author uses the suggestions for revision as a learning tool and considers them as a step toward publication rather than a rejection. Even the most seasoned authors will make revisions to ensure an article meets

Table 16.2 Anatomy of a Manuscript		
Element	**Contents**	**Considerations**
Abstract	Summary of purpose and research question Overview of methods and procedures Major results Implications of the results General conclusions drawn	Generally write after the manuscript is complete. Should be 300 or fewer words. Report the most important parts of the study. Can stand alone as a description.
Introduction	Detailed statement of the problem Relevance to clinical practice Brief review of the most relevant literature Theoretical framework for the study Specific purpose of the study, research question, and hypotheses (if appropriate)	Provide the context for the research question. State the problem and purpose in the first few paragraphs. Limit the literature review to the most relevant literature.
Methods and Procedures	Specific study design and rationale for selection Sampling strategy, including selection criteria and method Description of sample, including sample size Measurement methods with documentation of reliability, validity, and procedures Procedures for implementation of the treatment and placebo Data collection and analysis procedures	If a well-known measurement or treatment is used, give a less-detailed description of it. Use diagrams and photographs to clarify the procedures used for intervention and measurement. Provide description and references only for unique statistical tests.
Results	Textual description of the statistical tests Tables and figures that summarize the results Decisions for each hypothesis	Do not duplicate tables and figures in the text; the information presented in each place should be unique. Use this section for reporting only; discussion of the findings comes later.
Discussion	Interpretation of statistical results Discussion of the clinical relevance of the findings Contributions of the results to practice Comparison of results with previous works of others Discussion of study limitations and strengths Suggested areas for further study	Do not use commentary to reiterate results, but rather expand on them and relate the findings to practical uses.
References	List of all references cited in the manuscript	

the expectations of the journal's peer reviewers and editors. Such feedback can be used to continuously improve both writing and research.

A note is in order here about converting an academic paper into a publishable manuscript. Although considerable condensing of material is required, the author needs to maintain the key substance and meaning of the work. Specifically, the literature review will be substantially shorter for an article, with a focus on only the most relevant citations. To keep the literature review reasonable, do not include any statements that reflect common knowledge in the field or that contribute nothing unique to the study. The writing style should emphasize clarity of expression and use an active voice and simple language. Organize the information logically and take care to remain objective.

Finding and Aggregating Evidence

When research is publicly available, similar studies can be brought together to provide strong evidence for practice. The help of experts in electronic retrieval of documents should be sought to make best use of nurses' time and abilities. Time and training must be provided for nurses to learn how to critique an article and how to evaluate whether findings are useful (Krom, Batten, & Bautista, 2010). Nurse managers may potentially support a differentiated practice model, in which baccalaureate-prepared nurses use their educational preparation to critique and evaluate research, whereas master's and doctorally prepared nurses help initiate projects and translate knowledge into practice (McCloskey, 2008). Holders of a doctor of nursing practice degree are the ideal candidates to act as liaisons between practice and research, and they can be placed in charge of creating knowledge translation projects.

Experts at creating synthesized reviews should be made available to assist and mentor nurses. Organizations interested in encouraging nurses to perform literature searches should have access to databases and a mechanism for obtaining requested literature. A collaborating librarian is most helpful in these circumstances and can assist nurses in finding more obscure materials.

The strongest evidence for nursing practice is provided when multiple studies report the same results. However, multiple studies must still be evaluated for quality and the results aggregated in a way that reveals recommendations for practice. Several processes are available for evaluating, aggregating, and summarizing multiple studies as evidence.

GRAY MATTER

Six primary methods are available for aggregating the results of research studies for translation into practice:

- Scoping review
- Systematic review
- Integrative review
- Meta-analysis
- Meta-synthesis
- Practice guidelines

The Scoping Review

Scoping review is a relatively new method for aggregating evidence into guidelines for practice. Developed as a precursor to the full systematic review, a scoping review is intended to present a broad overview of the evidence pertaining to a topic, irrespective of study quality, and is useful when examining emerging areas for which little evidence is available (Tricco et al., 2016). Scoping reviews are used to identify knowledge gaps, set research agendas, and identify implications for the practice guidelines that should follow a systematic review.

Although related, scoping reviews differ from systematic reviews in the way studies are included or excluded. Both inclusion criteria and quality standards are less stringent than in a formal systematic review, and a broad range of research designs is included. The aims of such reviews are to inform practice (not to guide it) and to provide direction for programs, policy, and future research priorities.

The number of scoping reviews reported in the literature has escalated steadily since this method was introduced in 2012. A scoping review can be helpful as an initial high-level step in evaluating evidence. These reviews are appropriate for guiding policy or informing a research agenda, but should not be used as stand-alone evidence for practice change.

The scoping review is based on a six-stage framework:

1. Identify the research question.
2. Search for relevant studies.
3. Select studies.
4. Chart the data, collate data, and summarize results.
5. Report results.
6. Consult with stakeholders to validate study findings (Colquhoun et al., 2014).

Scoping reviews remain controversial, however, likely because they are implemented inconsistently and the methods used to guide them are not standardized. Variability is evident in scoping studies in terms of definitions, methodology, reporting, and recommendations. The results of scoping reviews should be used with some skepticism and then only for practice implications. These types of reviews lack the rigor that a systematic review provides—rigor that gives the nurse confidence to use the findings in practice.

CASE IN POINT Scoping Review

The way that nursing is taught is changing rapidly due to the demands of the contemporary nurse learner. Peer-assisted learning is being implemented to capitalize on the power of peer teaching and to address the burgeoning number of support services needed by nursing students. In other words, it is often more effective for students to learn from other students. Peer-assisted learning is based on social theory as well as cognitive congruence.

Because peer-assisted learning is relatively new as a teaching method, Williams and Reddy (2016) undertook a scoping review to determine whether peer-assisted learning improves performance, and whether this method holds promise as a standard for future learning design. A wide range of articles was included in these authors' search, including 10 mixed-methods randomized trials, one retrospective study, four controlled trials, two crossover trials, three prospective trials, one thesis, and one comparative effectiveness design.

Williams and Reddy's (2016) analysis revealed three major themes related to student performance. The strongest finding was that the peer students providing services showed the most significant improvement in objective outcomes. Nevertheless, a positive effect on the learner's performance was also identified. Second, in both cases, it appeared that peer-assisted learning was more effective for learning skills than for learning theory and abstract concepts. Third, there did not appear to be any identifiable negative impact on performance. The most common application of peer-assisted learning was in medicine and nursing.

Williams and Reddy's (2016) work was a typical scoping review in that it included a broad range of study types due to the novelty of the topic. The peer-assisted learning method has not been used long enough to generate a broad base of quantitative analyses. The quality of the studies was not evaluated rigorously, so the scoping review primarily provided support that this teaching method may hold promise, but should be tested more thoroughly with quantitative methods. As such, it could guide a research agenda for a researcher who may want to design specific studies or pursue a systematic review.

The Systematic Review

One of the cornerstones of EBP is the systematic collection and analysis of all available research on a topic—that is, the systematic review. These reviews are critical for EBP because they summarize the numerous and sometimes contradictory findings in the literature in an unbiased, methodical way.

A systematic review is a highly structured and controlled search of the available literature that minimizes the potential for bias and produces a practice recommendation as an outcome (Bettany-Saltikov, 2010). Systematic reviews can focus on patient concerns, the prevalence of problems, or the effectiveness of diagnostic procedures. However, in recent years, much attention has been paid to the effectiveness of healthcare interventions.

With regard to systematic reviews of healthcare interventions, the Cochrane Library (http://www.cochrane.org) is widely recognized as one of the most useful sources of high-quality reviews. The reviews conducted within the framework of the Cochrane Collaboration are highly valued because of their methodological rigor. These reviews focus heavily on quantitative analysis and experimental designs and, therefore, provide solid evidence for the effectiveness of interventions. Although the Cochrane Library is the most familiar source of systematic reviews, other databases contribute systematic reviews of interventions.

Because the Cochrane Library had its start in medicine, it is sometimes criticized for providing little evidence for nursing care. However, these concerns appear to be unfounded based on the work of Mistiaen, Poot, Hickox, and Wagner (2004). These researchers found ample evidence of systematic reviews for nursing practice, including studies of psychological interventions, technical procedures, nutritional counseling, educational interventions, organizational studies, and studies of the effectiveness of exercise and positioning. All of these reviews were either focused on or had direct relevance to nursing practice.

The strength of the systematic review as a basis for practice recommendations is its unbiased, exhaustive review of the literature, followed by a rigorous methodological

Systematic review: A highly structured and controlled search of the available literature that minimizes the potential for bias and produces a practice recommendation as an outcome.

Table 16.3 Databases of Systematic Reviews

Database	Focus	Website
Best Evidence Topics (BET)	Systematic reviews for topics with few quality clinical trials. BET allows for inclusion of lower-quality evidence by listing the research weaknesses of papers included in the evaluation.	http://bestbets.org/background/best-evidencetopic-format.php
Cochrane Controlled Trials Register (CCTR)	Systematic reviews, randomized controlled trials, and protocols for systematic reviews.	http://www.cochrane.org/
CRD Database of Abstracts of Reviews of Effects (DARE)	Systematic reviews.	http://www.crd.york.ac.uk/crdweb/
CRD Health Technology Assessment (HTA)	Systematic reviews of the application of technology in health care.	http://www.dimdi.de/static/en/db/dbinfo/inahta.htm
NHS Economic Evaluation Database (NHS EED)	Systematic reviews that focus on the economic evaluation of healthcare interventions.	http://www.crd.york.ac.uk/crdweb/AboutNHSEED.asp
TRIP Database	Clinical search tool designed to allow health professionals to rapidly identify the highest-quality clinical evidence for clinical practice.	http://www.tripdatabase.com/

evaluation and the use of objective rules to link findings to recommendations. Each step of a systematic review is subject to rules intended to minimize the potential for bias in article selection, evaluation, or elimination from consideration. This eliminates the possibility that a practitioner might solicit and summarize only those articles that support his or her current beliefs about practice, rather than testing them. This neutral, objective, and unbiased review of the literature is the hallmark of a systematic review (Gough, Oliver, & Thomas, 2012).

As the name implies, planning the search strategy for a systematic review involves a sequence of carefully considered questions:

1. *Determine the background for the review.* Why is it important to have a systematic review for this intervention? How was the need identified?
2. *State the main review question.* What is the goal of the review? Is the review to test a specific existing intervention or to come up with "best practices"?
3. *Develop inclusion and exclusion criteria.* Who are the patients of interest? Which age groups, diagnoses, or other conditions are of interest? Which specific patient groups will not be included? Which interventions and outcomes are of interest?

4. *Devise a search strategy.* What are the sources of studies that will be searched (including published, unpublished, and "gray literature" such as conference proceedings)? What are key journals that must be hand-searched?
5. *Develop study selection criteria.* Which search terms will be used? Which types of studies are acceptable (e.g., experimental, descriptive, qualitative)? Which time frame will be considered?
6. *Determine study quality criteria.* Which quality indicators will be used to appraise articles for inclusion? Which quality level is acceptable overall? Which quality problems warrant exclusion from the study?

Once the search and evaluation strategies are devised, they are carried out faithfully as planned. Studies that are excluded at any stage of the review must have an objective rationale for their elimination. The systematic reviewer maintains a record of each abstract and article reviewed, along with documentation of the reason for its elimination if the study was dropped from consideration. This ensures that the reviewer uses objective and defensible reasons for selecting studies for final recommendations and minimizes the potential effects of researcher bias on the outcome. **FIGURE 16.2** depicts the process for making decisions about the inclusion of specific studies in the final recommendations from a systematic review.

The outcome of a systematic review is a recommendation for practice. These reviews are considered the strongest evidence in practice because findings are presented only when multiple studies of strong methodological rigor have supported practices (Bettany-Saltikov, 2010). Many recent changes in practice—from the way the third stage of labor is managed, to the way pain is controlled in adults, to the way blood glucose is stabilized in patients with diabetes—have emerged from systematic reviews. Nurses are in key positions to both use and generate systematic reviews. However, many systematic reviews have been criticized for relying exclusively on randomized trials and quantita-

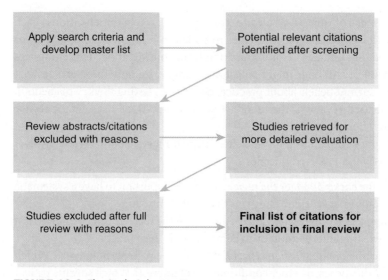

FIGURE 16.2 The Study Selection Process

tive studies. Nursing is a humanistic profession, so attention to the whole person demands that systematic reviews for many nursing practices accommodate more than experiments and incorporate qualitative findings into reviews.

CASE IN POINT Systematic Review

The benefits of exercise for older adults are well documented. Despite these established health benefits, few older adults exercise in a sustainable way. In fact, fewer than 10% of older adults (age 65 or older) meet national standards for aerobic and strengthening activity. In younger people, yoga has been demonstrated to have positive cardiovascular effects. Barrows and Fleury's (2016) systematic review sought to determine if the same benefits could be achieved with older adults.

The researchers selected extensive inclusion and exclusion criteria for articles. A total of 582 articles were retrieved, 142 of which underwent full review. A final sample of 9 articles met both the inclusion and quality criteria. The final review demonstrated that yoga had benefits for cardiovascular health in the older adult population. A variety of indicators were improved when older adults engaged in this activity, including blood pressure, body composition, blood lipids, and blood glucose. These improvements were seen in both healthy older adults and those with chronic health problems. The routine practice of yoga improved a variety of functional and psychosocial outcomes as well, fostering better overall health and quality of life. The participants in these studies indicated that yoga was a sustainable physical activity model for them, so it is expected these cardiovascular benefits could have long-lasting effect.

The systematic review undertaken by Barrows and Fleury (2016) is illustrative of the approach taken by most quantitative reviews. The a priori identified databases, inclusion criteria, and quality assessments were typical of the methods used to reduce the potential for bias in the search. The fact that the initially large number of potential citations was reduced dramatically is not unusual. The inflexible inclusion criteria and rigorous methodological quality required of studies often result in a small number of studies that are actually appropriate for inclusion in the final review.

The Integrative Review

Reviews of evidence in the healthcare literature are some of the most well-established methods of aggregating research into coherent, concise recommendations. **Integrative reviews**, by comparison, are broader reviews that allow for the simultaneous inclusion of experimental and nonexperimental research to more fully understand a phenomenon of concern. Integrative reviews achieve a wide range of review goals: They allow nurses to define concepts comprehensively, review evidence holistically, and analyze methodology from multiple perspectives. The integrative review has the potential to play an extraordinarily important role in the development of evidence-based nursing knowledge.

The integrative review is a methodology that synthesizes quantitative, qualitative, and comparative effectiveness research to provide a comprehensive understanding of the human response to health, illness, and interventions (Weaver & Olson, 2006). Integrative reviews have the potential to contribute to nursing knowledge, inform research, guide practice, and form policy initiatives with a solid foundation on what is known about both science and human behavior. Not surprisingly, combining diverse data sources is complex and challenging. A well-done integrative review adheres to the guidelines for systematic reviews that ensure control of bias in study selection and evaluation. However, integrative reviews require an expansion of two key areas of a systematic review: the criteria used

Integrative review:
A methodology that synthesizes quantitative, qualitative, and comparative effectiveness research to provide a comprehensive understanding of the human condition.

for selecting specific research designs and the standards used to judge the quality of the evidence. Qualitative designs must be considered for applicability to the problem under study and specified as acceptable. Appraisal of the quality of these studies must be based on standards for qualitative trustworthiness—not the standards used for quantitative evaluation. Using quantitative standards to evaluate qualitative research will result in frustration for the reviewer and a dearth of qualitative studies that make the final cut.

One method that has been proposed to evaluate the quality of studies incorporated into integrative reviews is to (1) group studies on the basis of their trustworthiness, using preset criteria, and (2) determine if the research methods moderated the outcome. For example, if studies were less rigorous but supported the findings of randomized trials, then they may be considered trustworthy. Conversely, if studies with less rigorous designs produced results that contradicted those obtained in more highly rated studies, then they may be discarded (Cooper & Koenka, 2011). A key point is that these decisions are made before the analysis begins, so that bias is controlled. Another approach reported by Pentland et al. (2011) is to assess studies for authenticity, methodology, informational quality, and generalizability rather than based on rigid preset quantitative criteria.

The translation of final study findings to recommendations must also be modified in integrative reviews. The link between studies and recommendations must be amended to include grading for both types of studies. If carefully and objectively completed, an integrative review can play a critical role in EBP initiatives, portraying the complexity that is inherent in the human condition.

CASE IN POINT Integrative Review

Health inequity continues to affect the lesbian, gay, bisexual, and transgender (LGBT) population. Biases may arise from both sexual and social stigma. The stigma may take the form of negative attitudes of others, threats to status, and feelings of powerlessness.

The last decade has seen a growing acceptance of LGBT identities and expressions, yet many public groups still struggle with a lack of support. Evidence suggests that LGBT persons have significant health disparities as compared to heterosexuals, and that researchers are only slowly beginning to explore these differences. The purpose of Lim and Hsu's (2016) integrative review was to critically appraise both quantitative and qualitative studies about nursing students' attitudes toward LGBT persons.

Both experimental and nonexperimental designs were searched. A total of 211 articles met the inclusion criteria based on their titles, and 53 remained after the researchers reviewed the abstracts. After inclusion and quality criteria were applied, 12 articles were included in the final review, including 9 qualitative, descriptive, and correlation studies and 3 intervention studies.

Studies conducted before 2000 revealed more negative attitudes toward the LGBT community than studies reported in the 21st century. Nevertheless, nearly half of the nursing student respondents indicated negative attitudes toward these individuals. Some data indicate that negative attitudes toward the LGBT community worsen health disparities, so these findings are of serious concern. The need for professional development of nurses on LGBT health issues is called for to ensure this population has access to quality care.

Lim and Hsu's (2016) integrative review demonstrates the primary distinction of this aggregation approach—the inclusion of both quantitative and qualitative studies in the review. It is unique in that data were available via these studies that essentially allowed for comparisons over time. This comparison resulted in some of the most hopeful findings, even as it revealed that considerable disparities persist.

Meta-Analysis

Meta-analysis is a statistical method of aggregating the results of quantitative studies. When experiments are replicated with similar populations using standard measures, it becomes possible to sum up the aggregate impact of the intervention on outcomes. Meta-analysis involves drawing inferences from a sample of studies; in other words, in a meta-analysis, the study is the "subject" (Card, 2011). When the results of multiple studies are compared, methodological weaknesses become apparent and true effects are revealed. Much as a sampling distribution of means is a curve made up of many group means, so a meta-analysis is a result that comprises the compilation of many effect sizes. This analytic technique is extremely useful in health care for judging the clinical and practical significance of any effects the intervention may have had.

> **Meta-analysis:** A statistical method of aggregating the results of quantitative studies so an overall effect size can be evaluated.

Meta-analyses are complicated to run, and they yield complex output. The challenge of meta-analysis is to find a sufficient number of studies that used similar populations, measures, and statistics. Meta-analysis is particularly challenging because of the diversity of study designs, the potential differences among the sample subjects, and the range of statistics that may be applied. Even so, meta-analyses remain some of the strongest evidence of the clinical significance of interventions. Available software programs can analyze disparate types of data gleaned from multiple studies for commonalities. The numbers that are yielded by a meta-analysis describe typical responses and provide a numerical basis for judging the magnitude of effect across all studies (Berenstein, Hedges, Higgins, & Rothstein, 2009). Interventions that have demonstrated *statistical* significance across several studies may have, in aggregate, relatively little clinical effect. In these cases, meta-analysis reveals that the nurse can conclude with a great deal of certainty that the intervention improves things, but not much. In contrast, when an intervention is very effective, it will demonstrate a strong effect over and over again. In these cases, meta-analysis will reveal the amount of improvement that can be expected, and the nurse can use these findings with confidence.

CASE IN POINT Meta-Analysis

"Fever phobia" is a term that has been used to describe the exaggerated and unrealistic fear of fever expressed by many parents and caregivers. Although more than two decades' worth of evidence shows that fever, in itself, is not dangerous, parents continue to be alarmed by its appearance and often demand unnecessary treatment as a result.

Purssell and Collin (2016) conducted a meta-analysis of publications that demonstrated the prevalence of fever phobia and determined whether this prevalence was associated with child mortality rates and geography. A total of 195 papers were identified via peer review search and another 5 studies from an Internet search.

After screening, 40 papers met the inclusion criteria and provided sufficient data for meta-analysis. The statistics of interest were the proportion of the sample that expressed fear of fever, the number reporting fear of specific outcomes, the proportion that had experienced a youth mortality, and the geographic distribution of participants.

The meta-analysis demonstrated a high prevalence of fever fear; however, significant variation was noted across the studies, with reported prevalence ranging from 8% to 43%. The prevalence was not explained by experience with youth mortality or geography. The most common fears were brain damage, coma, convulsions, death, and dehydration. The authors concluded that fever phobia is common and has not declined significantly over time. They suggest that it is a culturally based phenomenon, rather than an individually learned behavior. Thus, strategies to reduce its prevalence and effects should focus on culturally sensitive interventions, rather than pure education.

The meta-analysis conducted by Purssell and Collin (2016) is typical in that it had inclusion and quality criteria, and used only specific studies that reported an identical prevalence and demographic variable. Use of such strict criteria means that a small sample of studies is to be expected, as was the case in this study. The result, however, is particularly strong evidence in that aggregate clinical significance can be quantified. These authors were able to draw conclusions based on this strong evidence that can better support effective nursing interventions.

Qualitative Meta-Synthesis

Qualitative meta-synthesis is an interpretive process that provides an overall framework for the combination and synthesis of findings from multiple qualitative studies that focus on the same phenomenon of interest (Holly, Salmond, & Saimbert, 2011). This approach appeals to qualitative researchers because it has characteristics of methods that elevate the level of evidence provided by these studies. The inclusion of multiple sites, multiple samples, and replication of qualitative studies enhances trustworthiness and, therefore, the confidence with which one can generalize the results. Meta-synthesis is conducted much as meta-analysis is, but the focus is on recurrent themes rather than aggregate effect sizes. Meta-synthesis represents a family of methodological approaches to developing new knowledge based on rigorous analysis of existing qualitative research findings. Its aim is to find an overall representation of a qualitative phenomenon by treating the qualitative themes, narratives, and descriptions from studies as data for further analysis (Timulak & McElvaney, 2013). As such, these types of studies are the qualitative equivalent of a meta-analysis, providing the nurse with trustworthy evidence about the humanistic aspect of patient care.

Qualitative meta-synthesis: The development of overarching themes about the meaning of human events based on a synthesis of multiple qualitative studies.

CASE IN POINT Meta-Synthesis

The death of a patient is an emotional and demanding time for nurses. This is particularly true for new graduate nurses, who may be unprepared to deliver end-of-life care and who may have never witnessed a death. Zheng, Lee, and Bloomer (2016) set out to summarize new graduate nurses' experiences with patient death by examining the summary findings of qualitative studies. Their meta-synthesis was comprehensive, including searches in 12 databases covering more than two decades of research. While the initial search yielded a total of 686 articles, only 6 met the inclusion and quality criteria that were pre-established by the authors. Data extraction included descriptive data as well as main results or themes.

Synthesis of the themes revealed that new graduate nurses thought caring for dying patients and their family members was an emotionally charged experience. They experienced a range of emotional responses when assisting the patient and family through this time. Negative feelings such as nervousness, helplessness, powerlessness, stress, guilt, frustration, and anger were reported. These feelings were intensified when the nurse believed the dying patient was suffering unnecessarily. Some found the withdrawal of care from dying patients especially difficult. Regardless of the unit—even when working in the trauma or critical care unit—new graduate nurses had difficulty balancing their emotional compassion with carrying out the responsibilities of their role. Particularly difficult was the fact that, despite these emotional challenges, new graduate nurses were often left on their own to perform care for dying patients, making the experience even more intense.

Other themes included facilitating a good death, support for family, inadequacy of training on end-of-life care issues, personal and professional growth, and coping strategies. Overall, though, the new graduate nurses reported they benefited from such challenging encounters, even when they were unprepared for them.

Zheng et al.'s (2016) study was a typical meta-synthesis in that only qualitative studies were selected for inclusion. The themes and codes from all of the studies were synthesized into a single model that was supported in aggregate by the research. This meta-synthesis had a widely seen outcome—namely, the relatively large number of studies was reduced considerably after sampling criteria and quality standards were applied.

Practice Guidelines

All aggregate studies provide strong evidence for nursing practice. Indeed, they are placed at the top of the pyramid of evidence because their replicability and consistency inspire confidence in their results. The practicing nurse, however, will find that **practice guidelines** are among the most practical and understandable ways to read aggregate evidence. Practice guidelines are often developed by a group of clinical experts who are convened by a professional or academic body. The team conducts a rigorous and systematic review of existing research and judges how to best apply the research. Guidelines provide recommendations for practices that are graded as mandatory, optional, or supplemental and may be stated as standards of practice, procedures, or decision algorithms. Practice guidelines can be obtained from many sources, including the U.S. government clearinghouse (http://www.guidelines.gov), which is the most comprehensive source of publicly available evidence-based guidelines.

Clinical practice guidelines must still be appraised for quality before a decision is made in favor of their widespread implementation. Such guidelines may be affected by a host of complicating forces, such as a lack of transparency in developmental processes, limits on the amount of evidence available to support a guideline, conflicts of interest with those who develop treatments, and questions about how to reconcile contradictory evidence. To facilitate the review process, the National Academy of Sciences tasked a group of researchers with developing criteria for evaluating the quality of a clinical practice guideline. Graham et al. (2011) recommended that a guideline be evaluated on the following criteria:

- The scope, purpose, and overall clinical question are explicitly stated.
- Stakeholders (i.e., patients) are involved in the development of the guideline in some way.
- Development of the guideline is rigorous and peer reviewed.
- Recommendations are clear and easily identified; both summary and patient education information are included.
- Implementation considerations—including cost and patient acceptability—are considered in the final guidelines.
- The group funding the practice guideline development has no financial interest in the outcome.

The results of aggregate studies offer the most direct link between research and practice. Even so, EBPs must be open to change as new evidence emerges, and that requires a systematic approach to ensuring efficient, timely research uptake.

Practice guidelines: Research-based recommendations for practices that are graded as mandatory, optional, or supplemental and that may be stated as standards of practice, procedures, or decision algorithms.

Models for Translating Research into Practice

Translating research into evidence requires the ability to find, appraise, and synthesize research results into recommendations. In addition, myriad other support systems must be available to ensure knowledge translation. For example, systems for communicating findings in a comprehensive and accurate way must be available. Ongoing support from nursing leadership is a requirement, including providing support, being accessible, modeling the use of evidence, and providing resources (Sandstrom, Borglin, Nilsson, & Willman, 2011). Systems for monitoring the effects of change must be in place. Using a tested model for a systematic organizational approach to knowledge translation enhances the potential for ongoing success.

Of course, no single model will fit every patient care environment. The model of evidence translation that will prove most useful depends on the type of practice, the setting, and the practitioner's needs. Six models are presented here: the Iowa Model of Evidence-Based Practice, a guide for practicing nurses; the Johns Hopkins Nursing Evidence-Based Model, based on clinical–academic collaboration; a model for integrating evidence into a Magnet hospital environment; a framework for outcomes-focused knowledge translation; the Collaborative Model for Knowledge Translation, which focuses on interaction between researchers and practitioners; and a model for translating evidence into community-based practice.

Iowa Model of Evidence-Based Practice

The Iowa model, which was first described by Titler (2001), is based on a five-step process:

1. *Identify a nursing problem and conduct a search of the literature.* Topics might include clinical care issues, cost-effectiveness, and operational issues, among others.
2. *Determine whether the issue is a priority for the organization.* Considering the resources required to conduct research, this is an important determination. Higher-priority issues will be those that fit organizational, departmental, and unit goals; those that are high volume or high cost; and those that are driven by market forces. The organization's administration will be able to guide nurses regarding which topics are most appropriate.
3. *Form a team to develop, implement, and evaluate the project.* A research committee may already be in place that can provide oversight. The authors of the model suggest that representatives of all stakeholders and disciplines be involved in the team. For example, a pain management project should include pharmacists, physicians, nurses, and psychologists, whereas the team for a project concerning effective bathing should include nursing staff and experts in skin care.
4. *Assemble the relevant literature.* Existing systematic reviews are important to secure. In addition to published literature, the authors suggest looking at bibliographies, abstracts published as part of conference proceedings, master's theses, and doctoral dissertations.
5. *Begin the process of critiquing the literature.* Guidance from advanced practice nurses (APNs) should be sought in this stage as the literature is synthesized. A group approach will help distribute the workload and aid staff nurses in understanding

the scientific basis for implementing changes. At this point, the group decides if there is enough research to guide practice. The following are some of the questions to consider when reviewing the literature:

- How consistent are the findings across studies?
- What are the types and the quality of studies?
- How relevant are the findings to clinical practice?
- Are there enough studies using a population similar to that of the organization in which the findings will be applied?
- How feasible is the prospect of applying the findings in practice?
- What is the risk–benefit ratio?

Doody and Doody (2011) further refined this model by expanding on the grading criteria:

- *Effectiveness*: Does the evidence support interventions that achieve an intended and beneficial outcome?
- *Appropriateness*: Does the evidence provide support for the consumer's experience (i.e., is there adequate concern for psychosocial as well as physical outcomes)?
- *Feasibility*: Does the broader environment within which the care will be delivered have the resources and support necessary to implement the recommendations?

The Iowa model is widely recognizable, easy to understand, and straightforward to implement in a clinical setting. It does require time, support from management, and training in research critique as elements for success. Often, training and mentorship can be provided by individuals who have a research record and the capacity to provide practical advice. Seeking out a collaborative relationship with an academic organization often provides this support.

Johns Hopkins Nursing Evidence-Based Practice Model

Clinical–academic collaborations can form the basis for effective EBP uptake because the relationship is mutually beneficial. Through such partnerships, clinicians get the education and mentorship needed for bedside science projects, and researchers often gain access to the living laboratories that make for the best applied studies.

The Johns Hopkins Nursing Evidence-Based Practice Model was developed through collaboration between hospital nursing staff and nursing faculty and was first described by Newhouse et al. (2005). This model incorporates the impact of internal and external environmental factors on nursing problems. The core of this model (represented in **FIGURE 16.3**) is the use of best available evidence. All sources of evidence are used to consider a nursing issue in the domains of practice, research, and education. A multidisciplinary approach is used to identify problems, search out evidence, and implement a plan. There are three phases to the model:

- *Practice question phase*: A clinically relevant practice question is generated that is endorsed by the organization's administration. The scope of the research question is defined, and a nurse is assigned to lead the project. A multidisciplinary team is recruited, and a team conference is held.

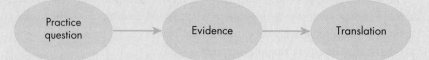

Practice question

Step 1:   Identify an EBP question
Step 2:   Define scope of practice question
Step 3:   Assign responsibility for leadership
Step 4:   Recruit multidisciplinary team
Step 5:   Schedule team conference

Evidence

Step 6:   Conduct internal and external search for evidence
Step 7:   Critique all types of evidence
Step 8:   Summarize evidence
Step 9:   Rate strength of evidence
Step 10: Develop recommendations for change in processes of care or
             systems on the basis of strength of evidence

Translation

Step 11: Determine appropriateness and feasibility of translating
             recommendations into the specific practice setting
Step 12: Create action plan
Step 13: Implement change
Step 14: Evaluate outcomes
Step 15: Report results of preliminary evaluation to decision makers
Step 16: Secure support from decision makers to implement recommended
             change internally
Step 17: Identify next steps
Step 18: Communicate findings

FIGURE 16.3 The Johns Hopkins Model of EBP Implementation

Reproduced from Newhouse, R., Dearholt, S., Poe, S., Pugh, L., & White, K. (2005). Evidence-based practice: A practical approach to implementation. *Journal of Nursing Administration, 35*(1), 37. Reprinted with permission of Lippincott Williams & Wilkins.

- *Evidence phase:* A internal and external search for evidence is conducted. The evidence is critiqued, summarized, and rated for strength (credibility based on the types of studies and their outcomes). The last step in this phase is to develop recommendations for modifying processes of care or systems based on the strength of the evidence.
- *Translation phase:* This final phase may be the most important. An evaluation is conducted to determine the appropriateness and feasibility of translating the recommendations into the clinical setting. An action plan is created, and the change is implemented as a pilot program. The outcome of the change is evaluated, and the results reported to decision makers. A decision is made by administration as to whether to support institution-wide changes in the process, and this decision is communicated to the stakeholders.

Newhouse and Spring (2010) have since outlined the skills and competencies needed for EBP:

- Expertise in performing evidence-based analytic processes
- Ability to formulate practice questions and carry out the evidence appraisal and aggregation process
- Assessment of those who receive evidence-based care as well as one's ability to implement the care
- Communication capacity and ability to collaborate across professional lines
- Proficiency at engaging a variety of professionals in the evidence appraisal and change process

The strength of the Johns Hopkins model is its reliance on a strong academic–clinical collaboration as a foundation for mutual benefit. This type of partnership provides motivation for those involved in educating nurses to work closely with those providing care. Even more motivation comes into play when a healthcare organization decides to pursue Magnet recognition. Specific requirements for the generation and use of evidence are in place for those organizations for which becoming a Magnet designate is a goal.

Such clinical-academic partnerships are not limited to large academic medical centers and urban universities. Highfield, Collier, Collins, and Crowley (2016) applied the model to a small, community-based hospital in partnership with a state university. They formally identified a nurse research facilitator role that served to increase the amount of research and EBPs implemented by staff nurses. The partnership included career development, education, and leadership of research teams. Through this collaboration, the academic partner gained an understanding of appropriate practice-based problems and access to subjects for research; the staff nurses (the clinical partner) gained valuable research consultation and mentoring to sustain EBPs.

Knowledge Translation as Part of Magnet Recognition

Magnet hospitals, in particular, are required to have operational and clinically influential EBPs in place. Turkel et al. (2005) created a model for integrating EBP as part of the Magnet recognition process that is considered an exemplar by the appraisers who award the Magnet designation (Messmer & Turkel, 2010) (see **FIGURE 16.4**). This model consists of five steps:

1. *Establish a foundation.* Critical to step 1 is the support of leadership. The chief nurse executive (CNE) must create a supportive environment to change the nursing and healthcare culture in favor of EBP. The CNE's responsibility is to obtain resources for EBP, including electronic databases, a consulting librarian, technology, release time for nursing staff, and/or funding for an APN consultant. RNs and APNs should work together to come up with areas of concern, create EBP protocols, educate peers, facilitate journal clubs, and conduct research projects. The CNE may form a nursing research committee to guide projects. Including participation in EBP projects as part of the annual performance review or as part of clinical leader advancement will motivate staff nurses to become involved in the work.

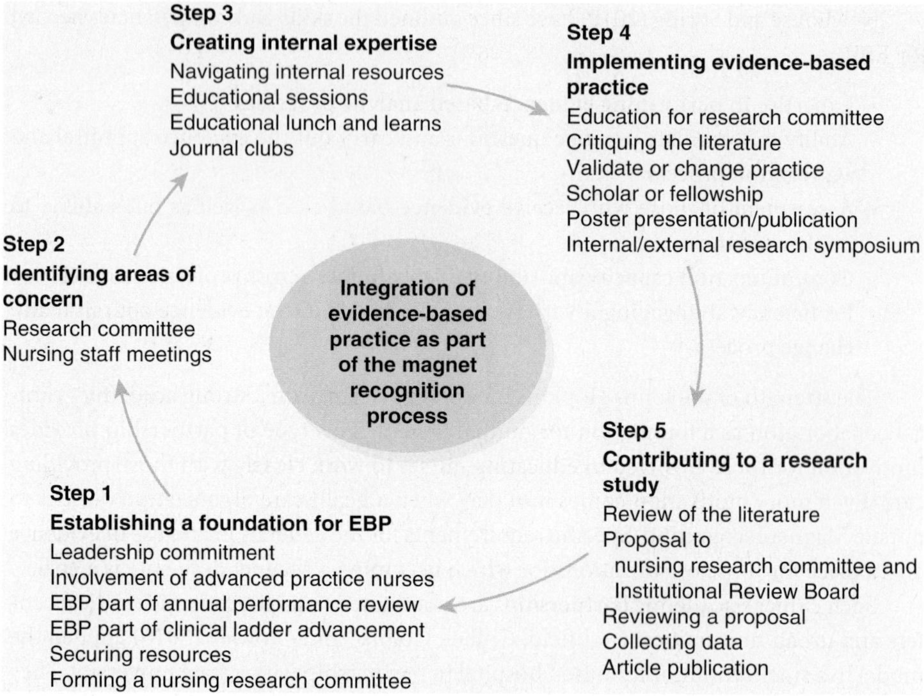

Step 3
Creating internal expertise
Navigating internal resources
Educational sessions
Educational lunch and learns
Journal clubs

Step 4
Implementing evidence-based practice
Education for research committee
Critiquing the literature
Validate or change practice
Scholar or fellowship
Poster presentation/publication
Internal/external research symposium

Step 2
Identifying areas of concern
Research committee
Nursing staff meetings

Integration of evidence-based practice as part of the magnet recognition process

Step 5
Contributing to a research study
Review of the literature
Proposal to
   nursing research committee and
   Institutional Review Board
Reviewing a proposal
Collecting data
Article publication

Step 1
Establishing a foundation for EBP
Leadership commitment
Involvement of advanced practice nurses
EBP part of annual performance review
EBP part of clinical ladder advancement
Securing resources
Forming a nursing research committee

FIGURE 16.4 A Model of EBP Integration in a Magnet Facility

Reproduced from Turkel, M., Reidinger, G., Ferket, K. & Reno, K. (2005). An essential component of the Magnet journey: Fostering an environment for evidence-based practice and nursing research. *Nursing Administration Quarterly, 29*(3), 254–262. Reprinted by permission of Lippincott Williams & Wilkins.

2. *Identify areas of concern.* Ideally, the research committee will provide a forum for interested nurses to discuss areas of interest and begin to learn about EBP. Topics need to be staff-nurse driven to ensure excitement, buy-in, and acceptance of the outcome. Nursing staff meetings can be a good starting point.

3. *Create internal expertise.* This is the time to begin reading and discussing the literature. The discussion focuses on the relevance of the article to practice.

4. *Implement EBP.* The nursing research committee will need education to help its members come up with a process for reviewing articles, synthesizing reviews, and determining whether the results validate current practice or require a change in practice. The committee should disseminate its findings through both internal communications and externally, through a poster presentation and/or a publication. Dissemination of the results is important to increase awareness of the developing EBP nursing knowledge base. Consideration should be given to establishing an annual internal research symposium where units can display their work. Likewise, nurses can attend external research symposia to present their findings.

5. *Contribute to a research study.* With an evolving foundation of EBP knowledge, it is not a difficult task to advance to this final step. Previously critiqued articles from journal clubs can serve as the basis for the literature review. The internal or external nurse expert can review the staff nurses' work and assist with development

of a research proposal to be submitted to the research committee and institutional review board. Nurses on the committee can review the proposal with the expert, furthering the members' development of expertise. Nurses can assist with research in the organization by collecting data.

Magnet organizations are obligated to contribute new knowledge to the profession of nursing. This means applying existing evidence, creating practice guidelines, designing research, and making other contributions to nursing science (Messmer & Turkel, 2010). All of the other elements of Magnet recognition related to quality patient care—that is, achieving excellent outcomes for patients, demonstrating the highest level of professional nursing practice, and contributing to the profession—are dependent upon the appraisal, use, and generation of evidence.

Some models delve deeper into the implementation of knowledge translation and actually collect outcomes to inform this process. By monitoring and acting on outcomes achieved with evidence-based care, nurses are able to continuously adapt their care to the changing needs of patients. The next two models described add to the basic knowledge translation process by incorporating this outcomes feedback loop into the formal knowledge translation model.

Outcomes-Focused Knowledge Translation at the Bedside

The outcomes-focused knowledge translation model aims to influence nursing-sensitive outcomes such as patient functional status, patient symptoms, therapeutic self-care, pressure ulcers, and fall outcomes. This simplified model includes four elements: sources of evidence, patient preferences, context of care, and facilitation. These four elements contribute to the uptake of evidence at the point of care by the nurse, which results in first the nursing intervention and then the (desired) patient outcomes. Outcomes link back to the initial four elements as feedback to inform the system. This model, depicted in **FIGURE 16.5**, is easy to interpret and understand and is a good model for use by staff nurses.

Collaborative Model for Knowledge Translation

The Collaborative Model for Knowledge Translation was created to reflect a shift in communication from unidirectional research utilization toward an interactive model of knowledge transfer (Baumbusch et al., 2008). Research champions (staff nurses) establish and maintain connections between researchers and nurses, help researchers navigate the complexities of the healthcare system, negotiate entry into various clinical areas, and provide ongoing feedback on how research is perceived and applied in a practice setting. This model has two dimensions: process and content.

The *process* dimension is the dynamic part of the model and is made up of the collaborative relationship between researchers and nurses. This relationship is characterized by accountability, reciprocity, and respect. The process reflects an ongoing dialogue focused on emerging findings and their effect on patient care. This dynamic interchange allows practitioners to use findings in a rapidly evolving healthcare system and helps researchers to refine research questions in the context of real-world care.

The *content* dimension of this model translates knowledge from a program of research into practice. This feedback element allows outcomes information to be shared with nurses in a way that can be immediately synthesized into practice.

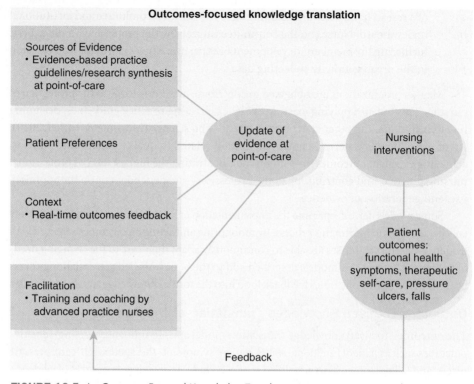

Outcomes-focused knowledge translation

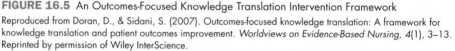

FIGURE 16.5 An Outcomes-Focused Knowledge Translation Intervention Framework

Reproduced from Doran, D., & Sidani, S. (2007). Outcomes-focused knowledge translation: A framework for knowledge translation and patient outcomes improvement. *Worldviews on Evidence-Based Nursing, 4*(1), 3–13. Reprinted by permission of Wiley InterScience.

Community-Based Research Translation Model

Most of the models described here are applied most effectively in an organizational setting. Community health settings, however, have long been subject to a tension between expert-driven public health interventions and evidence-based ones. Layde et al. (2012) developed a model focused on translating research into evidence that can be used in community-based settings and that incorporates the best of both worlds (**FIGURE 16.6**).

The community-based research translation model proceeds in two phases. In the first phase, the focus is on expert analysis of the critical health issues facing a population. This analysis is performed by convening stakeholders, analyzing community health data, reviewing available resources, and taking an inventory of evidence-based interventions. The result is identification of a specific health issue to be addressed.

In the second phase, the EBP is developed. During this phase, nurses analyze the causes of morbidity and mortality, appraise and select evidence-based interventions, adapt the interventions to the community, and develop measures that will reflect outcomes. Implementation of the strategy and monitoring of results lead to a continuous process of evaluating and refining interventions.

Translation of research into practice can sound daunting, but unless the results of studies are put to use, research has achieved little. These models provide clinicians with a way of thinking about knowledge translation and EBP and help them to choose a process that effectively ensures that research ultimately benefits patient care.

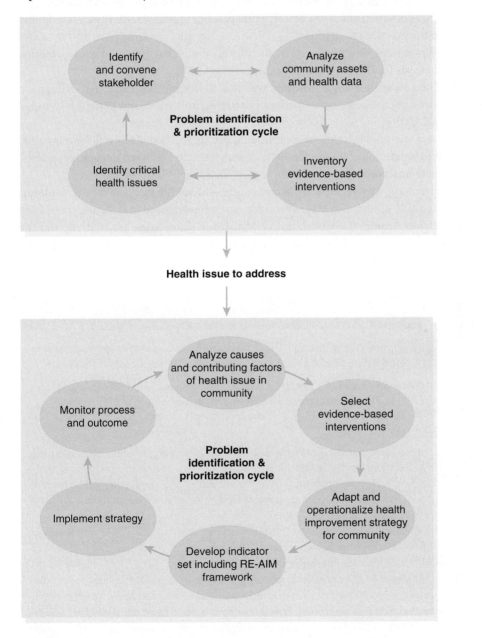

FIGURE 16.6 A Model for Translating Research into Community Health Settings

Reproduced from Layde, P., Christiansen, A., Peterson, D., Guse, C., Maurana, C., & Branderburg, T. (2012) A model to translate evidence-based interventions into community practice. Used with permission from *American Journal of Public Health, 102*(4), 621. Reprinted with permission of The American Public Health Association.

Summary of Key Concepts

- It is important to promote nursing research to improve the health of individuals and groups in society.
- The accountability for transferring research to the bedside lies with nurses.
- The translation of nursing research into practice provides authority and credibility to the practice of nursing.
- Nurses must be empowered by the organizations that employ them to examine the basis for their own practice.
- The reward for organizations will be quality patient care, cost-efficiency, cost-effectiveness, better patient outcomes, and increased patient and nurse satisfaction.
- Many methods exist for the identification and aggregation of research for translation into practice, including scoping reviews, systematic reviews, integrative reviews, meta-analyses, and meta-syntheses.
- Systematic models for knowledge transfer—including the Iowa model, the Johns Hopkins model, the Magnet model, outcomes-focused knowledge translation at the bedside, the Collaborative Model for Knowledge Translation, and the community-based health knowledge translation model can guide the implementation of EBPs.

CRITICAL **APPRAISAL EXERCISE**

Retrieve the following full-text article from the Cumulative Index to Nursing and Allied Health Literature or similar search database:

Strickland, S., Rubin, B., Haas, C., Volsko, T., Drescher, G., & O'Malley, C. (2015). AARC Clinical Practice Guideline: Effectiveness of pharmacologic airway clearance therapies in hospitalized patients. *Respiratory Care, 60*(7), 1071–1077.

Consider both the design of the evidence and its strength when discussing the following. Be sure to provide specific examples for your answers:

1. Identify the clinical problem that is the subject of the guideline. What are the reasons this is an important question to study? What are the implications of care that is not evidence-based in this population?
2. The authors discuss the impact of using treatments that are not evidence-based on three kinds of harm. What are they? Explain each, and give any example of how this harm might be prevented.
3. In this example of translational research, the authors suggest that healthcare costs can be constrained without incurring adverse health outcomes. Several examples are provided. Pick two and discuss how these improvements could affect cost and quality.
4. The authors state that "absence of evidence is not the same as absence of effectiveness." Does this practice guideline dispel completely the effectiveness of inhaled agents?
5. How can the practicing nurse put these findings into practice?

References

Barrows, J., & Fleury, J. (2016). Systematic review of yoga interventions to promote cardiovascular health in older adults. *Western Journal of Nursing Research, 38*(6), 753–781.

Baumbusch, J., Reimer Kirkham, S., Basu Khan, K., McDonald, H., Semeniuk, P., Tan, E., & Anderson, J. (2008). Pursuing common agendas: A collaborative model for knowledge translation between research and practice in clinical settings. *Research in Nursing and Health, 31*, 130–140.

Berenstein, M., Hedges, L., Higgins, J., & Rothstein, H. (2009). *Introduction to meta-analysis: Statistics in practice.* West Sussex, UK: Wiley InterScience.

Bettany-Saltikov, J. (2010). Learning how to undertake a systematic review: Part 1. *Nursing Standard, 24*, 47–55.

Callard, F., Rose, D., & Wykes, T. (2011). Close to the bench as well as at the bedside: Involving service users in all phases of translational research. *Health Expectations, 15,* 389–400.

Card, N. (2011). *Applied meta-analysis for social science research.* New York, NY: Guilford Press.

Colquhoun, H., Levac, D., O'Brien, K., Straus, S., Tricco, A., Perrier, L., ... Moher, D. (2014). Scoping reviews: Time for clarity in definition, methods, and reporting. *Journal of Clinical Epidemiology, 67,* 1291–1294.

Cooper, H., & Koenka, A. (2011). The overview of reviews: Unique challenges and opportunities when research syntheses are the principal elements of new interactive scholarship. *American Psychologist, 67*(6), 446–462.

Doody, C., & Doody, O. (2011). Introducing evidence into nursing practice using the Iowa model. *British Journal of Nursing, 20*(11), 661–664.

Drolet, B., & Lorenzi, N. (2011). Translational research: Understanding the continuum from bench to bedside. *Translational Research, 157,* 1–5.

Gough, D., Oliver, S., & Thomas, J. (2012). *An introduction to systematic reviews.* Thousand Oaks, CA: Sage.

Graham, R., Mancher, M., Wolman, D., Greenfield, S., & Steinberg, E. (Eds.). (2011). Trustworthy clinical practice guidelines: Challenges and potential. In *Clinical guidelines we can trust* (pp. 53–74). Washington, DC: National Academies Press.

Hedges, C. (2010). Research corner. Poster presentation: A primer for critical care nurses. *AACN Advanced Critical Care, 21,* 318–321.

Highfield, M., Collier, A., Collins, M., & Crowley, M. (2016). Partnering to promote evidence-based practice in a community hospital. *Journal for Nurses in Professional Development, 32*(3), 130–136.

Holly, C., Salmond, S., & Saimbert, M. (2011). *Comprehensive systematic review for advanced nursing practice.* Philadelphia, PA: Springer.

Krom, Z., Batten, J., & Bautista, C. (2010). A unique collaborative nursing evidence-based practice initiative using the Iowa model. *Clinical Nurse Specialist, 24*(2), 54–59.

Layde, P., Christiansen, A., Peterson, D., Guse, C., Maurana, C., & Brandenburg, T. (2012). A model to translate evidence-based interventions into community practice. *American Journal of Public Health, 102*(4), 617–624.

Lim, F., & Hsu, R. (2016). Nursing students' attitudes toward lesbian, gay, bisexual, and transgender persons: An integrative review. *Nursing Education Perspectives, 37*(3), 144–154.

McCloskey, D. (2008). Nurses' perceptions of research utilization in a corporate health care system. *Journal of Nursing Scholarship, 40,* 39–45.

Messmer, P., & Turkel, M. (2010). Magnetism and the nursing workforce. *Annual Review of Nursing Research, 28*(1), 233–252.

Mistiaen, P., Poot, E., Hickox, S., & Wagner, C. (2004). The evidence for nursing interventions in the Cochrane Database of Systematic Reviews. *Nurse Researcher, 12*(2), 71–82.

Newhouse, R., Dearholt, S., Poe, S., Pugh, L., & White, K. (2005). Evidence-based practice: A practical approach to implementation. *Journal of Nursing Administration, 35*(1), 35–40.

Newhouse, R., & Spring, B. (2010). Interdisciplinary evidence-based practice: Moving from silos to synergy. *Nursing Outlook, 58,* 309–317.

Pentland, D., Forsyth, K., Maciver, D., Walsh, M., Murray, R., Irvine, L., & Sikora, S. (2011). Key characteristics of knowledge transfer and exchange in healthcare integrative literature review. *Journal of Advanced Nursing, 67*(7), 1408–1425.

Purssell, E., & Collin, J. (2016). Fever phobia: The impact of time and mortality: A systematic review and meta-analysis. *International Journal of Nursing Studies, 56,* 81–89.

Sandstrom, B., Borglin, G., Nilsson, R., & Willman, A. (2011). Promoting the implementation of evidence-based practice: A literature review focusing on the role of nursing leadership. *Worldviews on Evidence-Based Practice, 8*(4), 212–223.

Timulak, L., & McElvaney, R. (2013). Qualitative meta-analysis of insight events in psychotherapy. *Counseling Psychology Quarterly, 26*(2), 131–150.

Titler, M. (2001). The Iowa model of evidence-based practice to promote quality care. *Critical Care Nursing Clinics of North America, 13*(4), 497–509.

Tricco, A., Lillie, E., Zarin, W., O'Brien, K., Colquhoun, H., Kastner, M., ... Straus, S. (2016). A scoping review on the conduct and reporting of scoping reviews. *BMC Medical Research Methodology, 16*(15), 15–26.

Turkel, M., Reidinger, G., Ferket, K., & Reno, K. (2005). An essential component of the Magnet journey: Fostering an environment for evidence-based practice and nursing research. *Nursing Administration Quarterly, 29*(3), 254–262.

Wallace, J., Byrne, C., & Clarke, M. (2012). Making evidence more wanted: A systematic review of facilitators to enhance the uptake of evidence from systematic reviews and meta-analyses. *International Journal of Evidence-Based Healthcare, 10,* 338–346.

Weaver, K., & Olson, J. (2006). Understanding paradigms used for nursing research. *Journal of Advanced Nursing, 53,* 459–469.

Williams, B., & Reddy, P. (2016). Does peer-assisted learning improve academic performance? A scoping review. *Nurse Education Today, 42,* 23–29.

Woods, N., & Magyary, D. (2010). Translational research: Why nursing's interdisciplinary collaboration is essential. *Research and Theory for Nursing Practice: An International Journal, 24,* 9–24.

Zheng, R., Lee, S., & Bloomer, M. (2016). How new graduate nurses experience patient death: A systematic review and qualitative meta-synthesis. *International Journal of Nursing Studies, 53,* 320–330.

Glossary

A priori Conceived or formulated before an investigation.

Altmetrics The creation and study of new metrics based on the Social Web for analyzing and informing scholarship.

Applicability and transferability The feasibility of applying qualitative research findings to other samples and other settings.

Applied research Research conducted to gain knowledge that has a practical application and contributes in some way to a modification of practice.

Attrition A threat to internal validity resulting from loss of subjects during a study.

Audit trail Detailed documentation of sources of information, data, and design decisions related to a qualitative research study.

Bar chart A graphic presentation for nominal or ordinal data that represents the categories on the horizontal axis and frequency on the vertical axis.

Basic research Theoretical, pure, fundamental, or bench research done to advance knowledge in a given subject area.

Beneficence A basic principle of ethics that states that persons should have their decisions respected, be protected from harm, and have steps taken to ensure their well-being.

Bibliometrics The study of publication patterns.

Bivariate analysis Analysis of two variables at a time, as in correlation studies.

Blinded A type of review in which the peer reviewer is unaware of the author's identity, so personal influence is avoided.

Boolean operators The words AND, OR, and NOT, which are used to join or exclude search terms.

Box plot A graphic presentation that marks the median of the values in the middle of the box and the 25th and 75th percentiles as the lower and upper edges of the box, respectively. It indicates the relative position of the data for each group and the spread of the data for comparison.

Bracketing A method of limiting the effects of researcher bias and setting them aside by demonstrating awareness of potential suppositions of the researcher.

Calibration The use of procedures to minimize measurement error associated with physical instruments by objectively verifying that the instrument is measuring a characteristic accurately.

Case-control study An intact-group design that involves observation of subjects who exhibit a characteristic matched with subjects who do not. Differences between the subjects allow study of relationships between risk and disease without subjecting healthy individuals to illness.

Case research methods The meticulous descriptive exploration of a single unit of study such as a person, family group, community, or other entity.

Case study The meticulous descriptive exploration of a single unit of study such as a person, family group, community, or other entity.

Causal-comparative study An intact-group design that involves categorization of subjects into groups. An outcome of interest is measured and differences are attributed to the differences in classification of subjects.

Cited reference search A search that finds articles that are cited by another article.

Closed questions Questions that have a fixed number of alternative responses. Respondents are forced to select answers or ratings on a scale provided by the researcher.

Codebook A guide for the qualitative analysis that outlines individual codes with definitions, criteria for inclusion, and examples.

Codes Labels, descriptions, or definitions assigned to data to allow them to be categorized and analyzed in qualitative research.

Coefficient of variation (CV) A calculation that produces a number that depicts the standard deviation relative to the mean $[CV = 100(SD/\bar{x})]$.

Cohen's kappa A measure of inter-rater or inter-coder reliability between two raters or coders. The test yields the percentage of agreement and the probability of error.

Comparison group A subgroup of the sample of a quasi-experimental design from which the intervention is withheld. Subjects are similar to and compared with the experimental group, but they are not randomly assigned.

Concepts Abstract ideas or topics of interest that must be narrowed to researchable questions to be investigated.

Conceptual definition Clearly stated meaning of an abstract idea or concept used by a researcher in a study.

Confidence interval A range of values that includes, with a specified level of confidence, the actual population parameter.

Confirmatory studies Research in which a relationship between variables has been posed and the study is designed to examine this hypothesis.

Consent effect A threat to internal validity that occurs because the subjects who consent to the study may differ from those who do not in some way that affects the outcome of the study.

Constant comparison A method of analysis in qualitative research that involves a review of data as they are gathered and comparison to data that have been interpreted to support or reject earlier conclusions.

Constructivist research Research that attempts to discover the meaning and interpretations of events, phenomena, or experiences by studying cases intensively in their natural settings and by subjecting data to analytic interpretation.

Control group A subgroup of the sample of an experimental study from which the intervention is withheld.

Convenience sampling A nonprobability method of selecting a sample that includes subjects who are available conveniently to the researcher.

Correlation analysis A measure that depicts the strength and nature of the relationship between two variables.

Correlation research Research designed to quantify the strength and the direction of the relationship of two variables in a single subject or the relationship between a single variable in two samples.

Correlation study A design that involves the analysis of two variables to describe the strength and direction of the relationship between them.

Cross-sectional design Study conducted by examining a single phenomenon across multiple populations at a single point in time with no intent for follow-up in the design.

Cross-sectional methods Studies conducted by looking at a single phenomenon across multiple populations at a single point in time, with no intention for follow-up in the design.

Data source triangulation A type of triangulation in which multiple data sources are used in a study.

Decision trail A detailed description of the researcher's decision rules for data categorization and inferences made in the analysis.

Deductive A process of reasoning from the general to the specific.

Dependent variable An outcome of interest that occurs after the introduction of an independent variable; the "effect" of "cause and effect."

Derived variable A new variable produced when data from other variables are combined using a simple formula.

Descriptive data Numbers in a data set that are collected to represent research variables.

Descriptive studies Research designed to describe in detail some process, event, or outcome. Such a design is used when very little is known about the research question.

Descriptive variables Characteristics that describe the sample and provide a composite picture of the subjects of the study; they are not manipulated or controlled by the researcher.

Dictionary Specified definitions of codes included in the qualitative analysis codebook.

Directional hypothesis A one-sided statement of the research question that is interested in only one direction of change.

Ecological validity A type of external validity where the findings can be generalized and applied to other settings.

Editing analysis A style of analysis geared toward interpretation of text to find meaningful segments.

Effect size The size of the differences between experimental and control groups compared to variability; an indication of the clinical importance of a finding.

Empirical literature Published works that demonstrate how theories apply to individual behavior or observed events.

Epidemiology The investigation of the distribution and determinants of disease within populations or cohorts.

Error of multiple comparisons The increased error associated with conducting multiple comparisons in the same analysis; the 5% allowable error for each test is multiplied by the number of comparisons, resulting in an inflated error rate.

Ethics A type of philosophy that studies right and wrong.

Ethnography A study of the features and interactions of a given culture.

Evidence-based practice The use of the best scientific evidence, integrated with clinical experience and incorporating patient values and preferences in the practice of professional nursing care.

Evidence-based practice guideline A guide for nursing practice that is the outcome of an unbiased, exhaustive review of the research literature, combined with clinical expert opinion and evaluation of patient preferences. It is generally developed by a team of experts.

Evidence pyramid A pyramid diagram illustrating evidence-based information that depicts the potential quality of information, the amount available, and the amount of searching required to find evidence.

Ex post facto research An intact-group design that relies on observation of the relationships between naturally occurring differences in the intervention and outcome.

Exclusion criteria Characteristics that eliminate a potential subject from the study to avoid extraneous effects.

Exempt review A review of study proposals that pose no risk to subjects; the full institutional review board is not required to participate.

Expedited review A review of study proposals that pose minimal risk to subjects; one or two institutional review board members participate.

Experimental designs Highly structured studies of cause and effect applied to determine the effectiveness of an intervention.

Experimental research Highly structured studies of cause and effect, usually applied to determine the effectiveness of an intervention. Subjects are selected and randomly assigned to groups to represent the population of interest.

Experimenter effect A threat to external validity due to the interaction with the researcher conducting the study or applying the intervention.

Exploratory studies Research to explore and describe a phenomenon of interest and generate new knowledge.

External validity The ability to generalize the findings from a research study to other populations, places, and situations.

Extraneous variables Factors that exert an effect on the outcome but that are not part of the planned experiment and may confuse the interpretation of the results.

Extreme case sampling Sampling of unusual or special participants who exhibit the phenomenon of interest in its extremes.

Factors Independent variables in an analysis of variance (ANOVA) that are measured as categories.

Field notes Detailed descriptions of the context, environment, and nonverbal communications observed during data collection and inserted by the researcher into the transcripts to enrich the data interpretation process.

Frequency A count of the instances that an event occurs in a data set.

Full disclosure Reporting as much information about the research as is known at the time without threatening the validity of the study. This practice allows the subject to make an informed decision as to whether to participate.

Full review A review of study proposals that pose more than minimal risk to subjects, that do not qualify for exempt status, and in which the full institutional review board committee participates.

Grounded theory Research aimed at discovering and developing a theory based on systematically collected data about a phenomenon. The intent is to discover a pattern of reactions, interactions, and relationships among people and their concerns.

Guttman scale A scale with a set of items on a continuum or statements ranging from one extreme to another. Responses are progressive and cumulative.

h-Index An indicator of a researcher's lifetime impact in his or her field.

Habituation A process that occurs when an observer has extended contact with the subjects of a study. The subjects revert to natural behaviors and come to disregard the observer's presence.

Health Insurance Portability and Accountability Act (HIPAA) Legislation passed by Congress in 1996, which protects the privacy of personal health information.

Histogram A type of frequency distribution in which variables with different values are plotted as a graph on x-axes and y-axes, and the shape can be visualized.

Historical threats A threat to internal validity because of events or circumstances that occur during data collection.

Hypothesis A restatement of the research question in a form that can be analyzed statistically for significance.

Immersion/crystallization analysis A style of analysis that uses total immersion in and reflection on the text, usually in personal case reports.

Inclusion criteria Guidelines for choosing subjects with a set of characteristics that include major factors important to the research question.

Independence A condition that occurs when the selection of one subject has no influence on selection of other subjects; each member of the population has exactly the same chance of being in the sample.

Independent variable A factor that is artificially introduced into a study explicitly to measure an expected effect; the "cause" of "cause and effect."

Inductive A process of reasoning from specific observations to broader generalizations.

Inferential analysis Statistical tests to determine if results found in a sample are representative of a larger population.

Information literacy The competencies necessary to access, retrieve, and analyze research evidence for application to nursing practice.

Informed consent A process of information exchange in which participants are provided with understandable information needed to make a participation decision, full disclosure of the risks and benefits, and the assurance that withdrawal is possible at any time without consequences. This process begins with recruitment and ends with a signed agreement document.

Inquiry audit A review of data and relevant documents, procedures, and results by an external reviewer.

Institutional review board (IRB) The board required in research institutions that reviews and oversees all research involving human subjects and ensures studies meet all federal regulation criteria, including ethical standards.

Instrumentation A threat to internal validity that occurs because the instrument or data collection procedure has changed in some way.

Integrative review A methodology that synthesizes quantitative, qualitative, and comparative effectiveness research to provide a comprehensive understanding of the human condition.

Internal reliability The extent to which an instrument is consistent within itself as measured with the alpha coefficient statistic.

Internal validity The confidence that an experimental treatment or condition made a difference and that rival explanations were systematically ruled out through study design and control.

Inter-rater reliability The extent to which an instrument is consistent across raters, as measured with a percentage agreement or a kappa statistic.

Investigator triangulation A type of triangulation in which more than one person is used to collect, analyze, or interpret a set of data.

Journal club A formally organized group that meets periodically to share and critique contemporary research in nursing, with a goal of both learning about the research process and finding evidence for practice.

Journal impact factor A way to measure the visibility of research by calculating a ratio of current citations of the journal to all citations in the same time period.

Justice A basic principle of ethics that incorporates a participant's right to fair treatment and fairness in distribution of benefit and burden.

Levels The categories that make up factors in an analysis of variance (ANOVA.)

Levels of evidence A scale that provides the user with a quick way to assess the quality of the study design and, therefore, the strength of the study conclusions.

Likert scale A scale that uses attitude statements ranked on a five- or seven-point scale. The degree of agreement or disagreement is given a numerical value and a total can be calculated.

Line graph A graphical presentation that plots means for a variable over a period of time.

Theoretical literature Published conceptual models, frameworks, and theories that provide a basis for the researcher's belief system and for ways of thinking about the problem studied.

Longitudinal studies Studies conducted by following subjects over a period of time, with data collection occurring at prescribed intervals.

Magnet status A designation for organizations that have characteristics that make them attractive to nurses as workplaces.

Magnitude of effect The size of the differences between experimental and control groups; it supports clinical significance of the findings.

Margin notes Reflective notes manually inserted into qualitative transcripts that describe ideas about meaning that occur to the analyst during reading.

Maturation A threat to internal validity because the changes that occur in subjects do not happen as a result of the intervention, but rather because time has passed.

Mean The average; a measure of central tendency.

Measurement Determination of the quantity of a characteristic that is present; it involves assigning of numbers or some other classification.

Measurement error The difference between the actual attribute (true score) and the amount of attribute that was represented by the measure (observed score).

Median A measure of central tendency that is the exact midpoint of the numbers of the data set.

Member checking A method of ensuring validity by having participants review and comment on the accuracy of transcripts, interpretations, or conclusions.

Meta-analysis A statistical method of aggregating the results of quantitative studies so an overall effect size can be evaluated.

Method triangulation A type of triangulation in which multiple data collection methods are used, such as interviews, observation, and document review.

Mixed methods A research approach that combines quantitative and qualitative elements; it involves the description of the measurable state of a phenomenon and the individual's subjective response to it.

Mode A measure of central tendency that is the most frequently occurring value in the data set.

Multiple-treatment effect An inability to isolate the effects of a treatment because multiple treatments are being used at the same time.

Multivariate analysis The simultaneous analysis of multiple variables.

National Institute of Nursing Research (NINR) A federal agency responsible for the support of nursing research by establishing a national research agenda, funding grants and research awards, and providing training.

Nondirectional hypothesis A two-sided statement of the research question that is interested in change in any direction.

Nonequivalent comparison group before/after design The strongest type of quasi-experimental design in which subject responses in two or more groups are measured before and after an intervention.

Nonequivalent comparison group posttest only A type of quasi-experimental design in which data are collected after the intervention is introduced. Lack of baseline data may introduce extraneous variables in the results.

Nonparametric tests Statistical tests that make no assumptions about the distribution of the data.

Nontherapeutic research Studies that are carried out for the purpose of generating knowledge. They are not expected to benefit the research subject but may lead to improved treatment in the future.

Novelty effect A threat to external validity that occurs when subjects react to something because it is novel or new, rather than to the actual treatment or intervention itself.

Null hypothesis A statement of the research question that declares there is no difference between groups as a result of receiving the intervention or not receiving the intervention.

Nursing process A systematic process used by nurses to identify and address patient problems; includes the stages of assessment, planning, intervention, and evaluation.

Nursing research A systematic process of inquiry that uses rigorous guidelines to produce unbiased, trustworthy answers to questions about nursing practice.

Open access Information that is freely available online with few or no copyright restrictions.

Open-ended questions Questions with no predetermined set of responses.

Operational definition An explanation of the procedures that must be performed to accurately represent the concepts.

Outcomes measurement Measurement of the end results of nursing care or other interventions; stated in terms of effects on patients' physiological condition, satisfaction, or psychosocial health.

Paradigm An overall belief system or way of viewing the nature of reality and the basis of knowledge.

Parametric tests Statistical tests that are appropriate for data that are normally distributed (that is, fall in a bell curve).

Parsimonious Reduced to the fewest components; a parsimonious model is the simplest one that will demonstrate a concept.

Participant observation Involvement of the researcher as an active participant in the culture under study to more thoroughly understand the culture without changing it.

Peer debriefing An external check of the credibility of results in which objective peers with expertise in the qualitative method of analysis review and explore various aspects of the data.

Peer review The process of subjecting research to the appraisal of a neutral third party. Common processes of peer review include selecting research for conferences and evaluating research manuscripts for publication.

Phenomenology Investigation of the meaning of an experience among a group whose members have lived through it.

Photovoice A method used in participatory action research in which subjects take pictures to exemplify their lived experiences, and record accompanying reflections.

Point estimate A statistic derived from a sample that is used to represent a population parameter.

Population The entire set of subjects that are of interest to the researcher.

Population validity The capacity to confidently generalize the results of a study from one group of subjects to another population group.

Power An analysis that indicates how large a sample is needed to adequately detect a difference in the outcome variable.

Practice guidelines Research-based recommendations for practices that are graded as mandatory, optional, or supplemental and that may be stated as standards of practice, procedures, or decision algorithms.

Precision The degree of reproducibility or the generation of consistent values every time an instrument is used.

Prediction study Research designed to search for variables measured at one point in time that may forecast an outcome that is measured at a different point in time.

Predictive research Research designed to search for variables measured at one point in time that may forecast an outcome that is measured at a different point in time.

Primary data Data collected directly from the subject for the purpose of the research study. Examples include surveys, questionnaires, observations, and physiological studies.

Primary sources Reports of original research authored by the researcher and published in a scholarly source such as a peer-reviewed research journal or scholarly book.

Principal investigator The individual who is primarily responsible for a research study. The principal investigator is responsible for all elements of the study and is the first author listed on publications or presentations.

Probability or random sampling A sampling process used in quantitative research in which every member of the available population has an equal chance of being selected for the sample.

Problem statements Statements of the disparity between what is known and what needs to be known and addressed by the research.

Prolonged engagement Investment of sufficient time in the data collection process so that the researcher gains an in-depth understanding of the culture, language, or views of the group under study.

Prospective studies Studies planned by the researcher for collection of primary data for the specific study and implemented in the future.

Psychometric instruments Instruments used to collect subjective information directly from subjects.

Purpose statements Declarative and objective statements that indicate the general goal of the study and often describe the direction of the inquiry.

Purposeful sampling A technique used in qualitative research in which the subjects are selected because they possess certain characteristics that will enhance the credibility of the study and because they can reliably inform the research question.

Purposeful selection A technique used in qualitative research in which the subjects are selected because they possess certain characteristics that enhance the credibility of the study.

Qualitative meta-synthesis The development of overarching themes about the meaning of human events based on a synthesis of multiple qualitative studies.

Qualitative research A naturalistic approach to research in which the focus is on understanding the meaning of an experience from the individual's perspective.

Quality improvement The systematic, data-based monitoring and evaluation of organizational processes with the end goal of continuous improvement. The goal of data collection is internal application rather than external generalization.

Quantitative research A traditional approach to research in which variables are identified and measured in a reliable and valid way.

Quasi-experimental designs Studies of cause and effect similar to experimental designs but using convenience samples or existing groups to test interventions.

Quasi-experimental studies Studies of cause and effect similar to experimental design but using convenience samples or existing groups to test interventions.

Random error A nonreproducible error that can arise from a variety of factors in measurement.

Random selection A method of choosing a random sample using mathematical probability to ensure the selection of subjects is completely objective.

Randomized controlled trial An experiment in which subjects are randomly assigned to groups, one of which receives an experimental treatment while another serves as a control group. The experiment has high internal validity so the researcher can draw conclusions regarding the effects of treatments.

Range A measure of variability that is the distance between the two most extreme values in the data set.

Rate A calculated count derived from dividing the frequency of an event in a given time period by all possible occurrences of the event during the same time period.

Recontextualizing A qualitative data analysis and cognitive process undertaken by the researcher to search for meaning that may lead to a theory.

Reflexivity A sensitivity to the ways in which the researcher and the research process have shaped the data; based on introspection and acknowledgment of bias.

Replicability The likelihood that qualitative research outcomes or events will happen again given the same circumstances.

Replication Repeating a specific study in detail on a different sample. When a study has been replicated several times and similar results are found, the evidence can be used with more confidence.

Replication study A study generated from previous research studies in which the research is reproduced to validate findings, increase generalizability, or eliminate or minimize limitations.

Research design The overall approach to or outline of the study that details all the major components of the research.

Research question A question that outlines the primary components to be studied and that guides the design and methodology of the study.

Respect for persons A basic principle of ethics stating that individuals should be treated as autonomous beings who are capable of making their own decisions. Persons who have limited autonomy or who are not capable of making their own decisions should be protected.

Responsiveness A measure that indicates change in the subject's condition when an intervention is effective.

Retrospective studies Studies conducted using data that have already been collected about events that have already happened. Such secondary data were originally collected for a purpose other than the current research.

Reversal designs Single-subject designs that continue to measure the response of the individual as the intervention is withdrawn or withdrawn and reinitiated.

Right of privacy A person's right to have his or her health information kept confidential and released only to authorized individuals and to have his or her body shielded from public view.

Robust tests Statistical tests that are able to yield reliable results even if their underlying assumptions are violated.

Sample A carefully selected subset of the population that reflects the composition of that population.

Sampling error A number that indicates differences in results found in the sample when compared to the population from which the sample was drawn.

Sampling frame The potential participants who meet the definition of the population and are accessible to the researcher.

Saturation The point at which no new information is being generated and the sample size is determined to be adequate.

Scales Type of closed-question format in which respondents put responses in rank order on a continuum.

Scatter plot A graphic presentation that indicates the nature of the relationship between two variables.

Schematic A system of organizing data into preset categories to allow for examination and further analysis.

Scholarly Concerned with or relating to academic study or research.

Search concepts Major ideas or themes in a research question.

Search strategy The identification of search concepts and terms and the way they are combined that will be used to search for resources for the literature review.

Search terms Words or phrases that describe each search concept used to conduct the literature search. They may include variables in the research question, characteristics of the population of interest, or the theoretical framework of the research problem.

Secondary data Data collected for other purposes and used in the research study. Examples include electronic health records, employee or patient satisfaction surveys, organizational business reports, and governmental databases.

Secondary sources Comments and summaries of multiple research studies on one topic such as systematic reviews, meta-analyses, and meta-syntheses, which are based on the secondary author's interpretation of the primary work.

Selection bias Selecting subjects or assigning them to groups in a way that is not impartial. This type of bias may pose a threat to the validity of the study.

Seminal work A classic work of research literature that is more than 5 years old and is marked by its uniqueness and contribution to professional knowledge.

Sensitivity A measure of discriminant validity in the biomedical sciences that indicates an instrument has the capacity to detect disease if it is present.

Single-subject design An investigation using a single case or subject in which baseline data are collected, an intervention is applied, and the responses are tracked over time.

Snowball (referral, respondent-driven) sampling A non-probability sampling method that relies on referrals from the initial subjects to recruit additional subjects. This method is best used for studies involving subjects who possess sensitive characteristics or who are difficult to find.

Specificity A measure of discriminant validity in the biomedical sciences that indicates an instrument has the capacity to determine when the disease is not present.

Spurious relationship A condition in which two variables have an appearance of causality where none exists. This link is found to be invalid when objectively examined.

Standard deviation The most easily interpreted measure of variability of scores around the mean; represents the average amount of variation of data points about the mean.

Standard error The error that arises from the sampling procedure; it is directly affected by variability and indirectly affected by sample size.

Standard normal distribution A bell-shaped distribution in which the mean is set at 0 and a standard deviation at 1.

Standardized score A measure of position that expresses the distance from the mean of a single score in standard terms.

Stratified purposive sampling Sampling of individuals who meet certain inclusion criteria, and who are then stratified according to other criteria (e.g., age, gender, and ethnicity).

Subject headings Fixed "official" keywords used by many databases to describe major concepts and assigned by indexers to bibliographic records.

Subject selection A threat to internal validity due to the introduction of bias through selection or composition of comparison groups.

Suppressor variable A variable that is not measured but is related to each variable in the relationship and may affect the correlation of the data.

Systematic error Any error that is consistently biased; the measure is consistent but not accurate.

Systematic review A highly structured and controlled search of the available literature that minimizes the potential for bias and produces a practice recommendation as an outcome.

Template analysis A style of analysis that includes developing a template to sort narrative data.

Test blueprint An outline for determining content validity that includes the analysis of basic content and the assessment objectives.

Testing A threat to internal validity due to the familiarity of the subjects with the testing, particularly when retesting is used in a study.

Tests of model fit Tests of association used to determine whether a set of relationships exists in the real world in the way the relationships are hypothesized in the researcher's model of reality.

Themes Implicit, recurring, and unifying ideas derived from the raw data in qualitative research.

Theoretical literature Published conceptual models, frameworks, and theories that provide a basis for the researcher's belief system and for ways of thinking about the problem studied.

Theoretical sampling Selecting additional members for the sample, often based on loosened inclusion criteria, to ensure divergent opinions are heard; a requirement for grounded theory development.

Theory triangulation A type of triangulation in which multiple perspectives are obtained from other researchers or published literature.

Therapeutic research Studies in which the subject can be expected to receive a potentially beneficial treatment.

Time-series designs A type of quasi-experimental design in which only one group receives the intervention; an outcome is measured repeatedly over time.

Traditions Particular designs or approaches in qualitative research used to answer specific types of study questions.

Transferability The ability to apply qualitative research findings in other settings or situations.

Treatment effect A threat to internal validity because subjects may perform differently when they are aware they are in a study or as a reaction to being treated.

Triangulation A means of enhancing credibility by cross-checking information and conclusions, using multiple data sources, using multiple research methods or researchers to study the phenomenon, or using multiple theories and perspectives to help interpret the data.

Type I error Often called alpha (α) and referred to as the level of significance, the researcher erroneously draws a conclusion that the intervention had an effect.

Type II error Often called beta (β) and related to the power of a statistical test, the researcher erroneously draws a conclusion that the intervention had no effect.

Unit of analysis The definition of the major entity that will be considered a "subject" for analysis.

Univariate analysis Analysis of a single variable in descriptive statistics or a single dependent variable in inferential analysis.

Validity The ability of an instrument to consistently measure what it is supposed to measure.

Variable Characteristic, event, or response that represents the elements of the research question in a detectable or measurable way.

Variance A measure of variability that gives information about the spread of scores around the mean.

Visual analog scale (VAS) A rating-type scale in which respondents mark a location on the scale corresponding to their perception of a phenomenon on a continuum.

Vulnerable populations Groups of people with diminished autonomy who cannot participate fully in the consent process. Such groups may include children, individuals with cognitive disorders, prisoners, and pregnant women.

Index

Note: Page numbers with *f* and *t* refer to figures and tables, respectively.